To my wife, Lillian Williamson Cahoon, my son John, and my daughter Tula, whose encouragement, suggestions, and help account for many of the accomplishments within the covers of this book for which credit has been given to me.

FORMULATING X-RAY TECHNIQUES eighth edition

John B. Cahoon, R.T., F.A.S.R.T.
Assistant Professor, Duke University Medical Center;
Technical Director, Programs in Radiologic Technology:
Duke University Medical Center,
Durham Veterans Administration Hospital

Duke University Press, Durham, North Carolina   1974

© 1974 by Duke University Press
LCC number 73-81713
ISBN 0-8223-0309-4
Printed in the United States by the
Kingsport Press, Inc., Kingsport, Tennessee
Second Printing, 1975

PREFACE TO THE EIGHTH EDITION

The reception of preceding editions of *Formulating X-Ray Techniques* has been overwhelming and most gratifying. The acceptance of standard radiographic principles and teaching methods has been more rewarding.

Radiographic exposure techniques need revising from time to time. The trends toward standardization in the Radiology Department and diversification of exposure factors to meet the problems at hand have brought about changes in modern radiographic technique. The swing toward the use of higher kilovoltages, new film emulsions, and new processing chemistry has necessitated changes in formulating techniques. Radiographic machine characteristics have created density and contrast differences from room to room in the same department. Specialization of various divisions and subspecialties in radiology have caused various technical changes. Yet, as before, this book is intended to be a compact text on radiographic exposure, radiographic fundamentals and technique conversions, with particular emphasis on the fundamental factors that directly and indirectly affect radiographic exposure technique.

We have deleted many charts which were considered to be superfluous and have added others which we believe to offer a more scientific approach to the fundamentals of radiologic technology. To make room for valuable new material, superseded material, glossary, and tables have been compressed or omitted. Few will regret this exchange. Duplication of some material will be found in various chapters. Such duplication has been found to be helpful in emphasizing to the student and the instructor the importance and application of the material.

New material will be found here concerning density versus contrast, the photographic effect, and charting radiographic exposure. A new chapter (11) on the history of various systems of exposure technique should be of some interest, and a new chapter on Pathology and Injury (9), a new selection on secondary radiation fog, the reciprocity law, kilovoltage-Ma.S. conversion factors, a simplified explanation of the inverse square law, new material on intensifying screens, many new charts on technique and technique conversion, new sections on radiation dosage tables, and new exposure systems have all been added to this eighth edition.

The brevity of this book may shock those who have been encouraged to believe that good radiographic technique may be bought by the page, pound, or hour—or obtained in any way except through experience. I have paid for hundreds of lessons by means of hours of hard work and repeated experiments for thirty-five years. I have been fortunate in being associated at national and state meetings with some of the best men and women in the field, who have taught me not only the foundations of radiologic technology and the basic principles involved but also how to learn. As I have discussed radiologic technology and at times even argued over it with them, I have continued to be the student. Simplicity, concentration, and economy of time and effort have been the distinguishing features of the teaching methods of the fine persons who have added to what I consider my knowledge of the field.

I have often thought of those who might have been great "chiefs" and superb teachers and administrators, as well as radiology associates, had they only been able to master the simple and indispensable elements of the basic principles involved in technique.

Instead of being in my classroom, you are reading my book. That puts me at a disadvantage in my endeavor to teach you the art and science of formulating X-ray techniques and the basic principles involved in radiographic exposure. The most effective instruction obviously calls for a partnership of pupil and instructor that is best achieved by close association, not only in the classroom, but in the radiographic room. Nevertheless, I think that I have come as close as I can to doing my share on these pages. The rest is up to the reader.

ACKNOWLEDGMENTS

I would like to acknowledge my debt to the following persons for invaluable material lent me: the late Arthur W. Fuchs; Clark R. Warren, R.T.; Vinita Merrill; the late James C. Fletcher; Ted Lynch, R.T.; Ralph Tarrant, R.T.; Terry Eastman, R.T.; JoAnn Morgan, R.T.; Charles E. Naron; James Ohnysty, R.T.; Floyd L. Driver, R.T.; William Conklin, R.T.; and the many technologists and friends from all over the country, as well as other countries, who have written and given invaluable advice and suggestions.

I am deeply appreciative and indebted to the following for their many courtesies and for the reproduction rights extended to me for this edition and former editions over the past years: Eastman Kodak Company, E. I. du Pont de Nemours Company, Picker X-Ray Company, General Electric X-Ray Company, Profexray Company, the former Westinghouse X-Ray Company, the Liebel-Flarsheim Company, the 3-M Company, Low X-Ray Company, GAF X-Ray Company, and the Ilford X-Ray Film Company. I am also most appreciative to the representatives of the aforementioned companies who have always given me assistance and valuable advice.

I want to extend my appreciation to Dr. Richard G. Lester, Professor and Chairman, Department of Radiology, Duke University Medical Center, for the many facilities which have made this edition possible.

My appreciation goes to Dr. Dale R. Lindsay, Associate Director of Medical and Allied Health Education, Duke University Medical Center, Chief, Division of Allied Health, Durham V. A. Hospital; Dr. Thomas T. Thompson, Assistant Professor of Radiology, Duke University Medical Center, Chief of Radiology Services, Durham V. A. Hospital, and Medical Director of the Radiologic Technology Programs at the Duke University Medical Center; and Mr. Stanley B. Morse, Director, Durham V. A. Hospital for providing equipment, teaching, and research space in the Allied Health Education Building of the Durham Veterans Administration Hospital.

Preface

My appreciation goes to Mr. Doyle Davis and Mrs. Elma Medley of the Administrative Staff of the Division of Allied Health for their assistance not only to me but to the programs in Radiologic Technology.

My thanks and appreciation to Ann Underwood Van Sise, R.T., for testing the infants' and children's fixed kilovoltage technique while Chief Technologist at the Children's Hospital, Birmingham, Alabama; to Elsie "Bit" Coman, R.T., for her help in typing manuscripts and in early research of former editions; to Leon Winn, R.T., formerly supervising technologist in Pediatrics at the Duke University Medical Center for his help in the original research and development of the fixed kilovoltage for infants and children; to John Cullinan, R.T., F.A.S.R.T.; and to Clark R. Warren, R.T., for their many suggestions and evaluations of the text.

I would like to thank Dr. J. Lamar Callaway, Dr. Edward S. Orgain, Donnie A. Sorrell, Dr. Boyd T. Worde, Dr. William R. Barry, Dr. Fearghus O'Foghludha, Dr. Guy Odom, Dr. John Gehweiler, J. B. Langley, and the staff, students and alumni of the Duke University Medical Center for their valued advice and continued encouragement.

My deep appreciation is extended to my long-time friend, Mary Duke Trent Semans, for her continued support and encouragement: and to the late Dr. Josiah Trent, for his advice and encouragement in standardized radiologic technique, particularly so for bedside chest radiography in post-operative thoracic surgery cases.

I am deeply indebted to the late Dr. Wilbert C. Davison, the first Dean of the Duke University Medical Center, who was to me, and to many others, the modern Osler of medicine and medical education, the man who gave me my real start in the field of Radiologic Technology education.

My appreciation goes to my long-time friend and mentor in orthopaedic radiography, Dr. Lennox D. Baker, former Chairman and Professor of Orthopaedic Surgery, Duke University Medical Center.

My sincere appreciation to my secretary, Mrs. Diane Gerding, and to Mrs. Elinor Hart for typing the manuscript through its many changes.

I would like to thank the members of the Duke University Press and especially John Dowling, Ted Saros, John Menapace, Cathy Perillo, and Ashbel Brice.

My sincere appreciation to Mr. Floyd L. Willard and his staff of the Medical Illustration Service of the Durham Veterans Administration Hospital for their work in photography.

My appreciation is extended lastly to the many radiologic technologists, radiologists, and commercial representatives who have given me invaluable suggestions and consultations which I consider to be the backbone of my training in Radiologic Technology. To you—numerous individuals I am deeply indebted.

John B. Cahoon, R.T., F.A.S.R.T.

Durham, North Carolina
November 1973

TABLE OF CONTENTS

Preface   v

Chapter 1. **RADIOGRAPHIC FILM**   3

    Composition of radiographic film   3
    Duplicating radiographs   6
    Medichrome film   8
    The Polaroid radiographic process   9
    Film storage and handling   12
    Film tests   15

Chapter 2. **CASSETTES AND SCREENS**   18

    Cassettes   18
    Radiographic calibrations   21
    Cassetteless radiography   22
    Intensifying screens   22

Chapter 3. **PROCESSING**   26

    The processing room   26
    Silver recovery   29
    Automatic processing   30
    Film-feeding procedure   31
    Some questions on 90-second processing (automatic)   31
    Miscellaneous artifacts   35
    Film trouble chart; automatic processing troubles   38

Chapter 4. **CONES, DIAPHRAGMS, COLLIMATORS, FILTERS, GRIDS, AND STEREORADIOGRAPHY**   42

    Cones   42
    Collimators   42
    Filters   44
    Wedge and trough aluminum adapter filters   46
    The Potter-Bucky diaphragm   46
    Stereoradiography   49
    Stationary grid   52
    Selection of a grid   53
    Grid absorption   59
    The anode heel effect   59

Chapter 5. **SIMPLIFIED MATHEMATICS IN RADIOGRAPHY**   62

    Fractions   62
    Equations   63

Contents

    Decimals   63
    Percentages   63
    Proportion   65

Chapter 6. **BASIC EXPOSURE EXPERIMENTS**   66

Chapter 7. **PRODUCING A RADIOGRAPH: TECHNICAL CONVERSIONS**   81

    Exposure   81
    The primary exposure factors   81
    The secondary factors   82
    Milliamperage, time, distance, and kilovoltage   84
    Relation of Kv.P.-Ma.S. and density   85
    Relation between kilovoltage and time   87
    Distance   90
    Ma.S.-distance relationship   91
    The reciprocity law   93
    Decimal equivalents of fractional exposures   94
    The photographic effect   98
    Relation between time and distance   99
    Relation between milliamperage, time, and distance   99
    Relation between milliamperage and distance   100
    Relation between milliamperage and time   100
    Maintaining focus-film distance after tube is angled   100
    Correction factors for change in focus-film distance   104
    Cast radiography   104
    Adapting exposure technique from one hospital to another   104

Chapter 8. **ESSENTIALS OF THE RADIOGRAPH AND IMAGE FORMATION**   106

    Density   110
    Contrast   115
    Detail   120
    Distortion   121
    Kilovoltage   124
    Secondary radiation fog   133
    Milliampere seconds   134
    Review: density versus contrast   135
    General summary   139
    Review   141

Chapter 9. **POSITIONS AND PROCEDURES: PATHOLOGY AND INJURY**   143

    Fluid level experiment   151

Chapter 10. **FORMULATING THE TECHNIQUE CHART: VARIABLE KILOVOLTAGE METHOD**   153

    The patient problem   155
    The factor of motion   156
    Tissue absorption   160

FORMULATING X-RAY TECHNIQUES

    The chest   162
    Variable kilovoltage technique—type one   166
    Variable kilovoltage technique chart—type two   172
    Radiographic guide: variable kilovoltage technique   174
    Close subject-focus-film distance technique   180
    Exposure nomograms for Polaroid TLX films   180
    Technique conversion to higher voltage range   183
    Charting radiographic exposure   184

Chapter 11. **THE EVOLUTION OF RADIOGRAPHIC TECHNIQUE**   186

    Modern systems of exposure technique   195
    Higher voltage radiography   198
    Secondary radiation   200
    Common exposure systems   201
    Radiation dosage   203

Chapter 12. **THE FIXED KILOVOLTAGE SYSTEM OF TECHNIQUE**   205

    How the fixed kilovoltages were determined   206
    Exposure guide: fixed kilovoltage technique (adult)   211
    Exposure guide: fixed kilovoltage technique (infants and children)   219
    Special procedures   228
    High kilovoltage technique   231
    Exposure guides for fixed high-kilovoltage technique   234
    High-kilovoltage air-gap technique   239
    Additional exposure guides   240
    Angiocardiography   241

Appendix A. **THE APPLICATION OF RADIOGRAPHIC FUNDAMENTALS**   244

Appendix B. **SENSITOMETRY**   249

Appendix C. **RADIATION DOSE TO THE SKIN: OPTIMUM KILOVOLTAGE TECHNIQUE**   252

Appendix D. **RADIATION DOSE TO THE SKIN: TISSUE MEASUREMENT TECHNIQUE**   256

Appendix E. **X-RAY UNIT TROUBLE SYMPTOMS**   260

GENERAL QUESTIONS   264

ANSWERS FOR GENERAL QUESTIONS   286

STUDY QUESTIONS   289

SOME SAMPLE FINAL EXAMINATION QUESTIONS   345

Bibliography   363

Index   369

FORMULATING X-RAY TECHNIQUES

Chapter 1. **RADIOGRAPHIC FILM**

The radiographic techniques with which this book is concerned are those applied by the radiologic technologist in producing a diagnostic medical radiograph.

Radiography is essentially photography. The only difference between the two is the means employed for exposing the film and producing a latent image[1] which by subsequent processing yields a visible diagnostic image. In ordinary photography visible light is employed, and in radiography invisible light is employed. With photography longer wave lengths, which occur in visible light, are employed; but in producing a radiograph the short wave lengths—x-rays and other forms of radiation—are employed. However, the manner in which radiographic film is exposed is fundamentally the same as in photography.

The ordinary photograph is a *positive,* but the radiograph is a *negative.* In a negative the blackest or darkest areas on the film correspond to the lightest areas in the object being radiographed. Generally speaking the radiograph is always the negative, but an exception is the Polaroid radiograph, for which the original is a positive. To observe the difference, compare Figures 1.9 and 1.10. In the many radiographs reproduced as illustrations in this book, notice how the opaque parts of the body—particularly the bone—show up as lighter shaded areas, whereas there may often be a region surrounding the image of the object that registers as quite black, where little more than air absorption[2] has restricted some passage of the radiant energy.

COMPOSITION OF RADIOGRAPHIC FILM

Radiographic film consists of an emulsion of finely precipitated silver bromide crystals suspended in gelatin that is coated on both sides of a transparent cellulose support called the film base. The film base furnishes support for the emulsion and provides the proper amount of stiffness for handling. The basic ingredients of a radiographic film are (a) the film base and (b) the emulsion.

The emulsion is basically made of gelatin containing silver bromide crystals. The purpose of the silver emulsion is to absorb radiation during radiographic exposure and produce a latent image. The degree of exposure depends on the intensity of the radiation emerging from the object (remnant radiation) that is reaching the radiographic film.

---

1. Latent image: the image produced on photographic or radiographic film by the action of light or radiant energy *before processing.*

2. Air absorption: the amount of absorption by air of x-ray wave lengths before they reach the part being radiographed.

FORMULATING X-RAY TECHNIQUES

Silver emulsion

The silver bromide crystals in the emulsion are made by dissolving silver metal in nitric acid. The product of this chemical reaction is silver nitrate. The silver nitrate is then combined with potassium bromide to form silver bromide crystals.

The silver bromide crystals are mixed with gelatin to form the x-ray film emulsion. When examined under the microscope, the emulsion shows itself to be made up of countless tiny crystals of silver bromide embedded in the gelatin. Upon exposure and development, these crystals are changed into irregular clumps and strands of black metallic silver that, as a whole, compose the radiographic image.

Gelatin

Gelatin is chemically a colloid. When placed in water, it will absorb a volume of water several times its dry bulk and become soft and flexible. Though in water at high temperature gelatin will liquefy and go into solution, it will not dissolve in cold water.

These characteristics make gelatin a useful constituent of the x-ray film emulsion. Incorporated in the emulsion, it swells considerably in a cool solution without dissolving, and thus it allows the processing chemicals to act easily on the silver bromide crystals embedded in the emulsion. The fixing bath (hypo) can then remove the unexposed crystals and can harden and shrink the gelatin containing the metallic silver that is left.

Double coating

Each emulsion layer is about one thousandth of an inch thick. Since x-rays pass readily through x-ray films—and also through x-ray intensifying screens when these are used—both sides of the film base are given an emulsion coating. The effect of exposure to x-rays is thus greater than would be possible with an emulsion coated on only one side.

TYPES OF X-RAY FILM

Medical x-ray films

Two types of x-ray film are used for medical radiography—regular-type film used with or without intensifying screens and direct-exposure (non-screen) film. When regular-type film is used without intensifying screens (with cardboard holders), it is slower in *speed* than direct or non-screen type film. Regular-type film is more sensitive to the fluorescent action of intensifying screens than non-screen film. Non-screen film is more sensitive to *direct* x-ray exposure and should never be used with screens. Non-screen film or regular film in a cardboard holder is usually employed for *small parts only*.

Because of its thicker emulsion, non-screen film cannot at this writing be used with automatic processing and is therefore not used as much as it was in the past.

Mammography film

A special film made for mammography and 90-second automatic processing is now manufactured and designed for radiography of the breasts. It is an extra-fine-grain, high-contrast, direct-exposure film which provides ex-

Radiographic Film

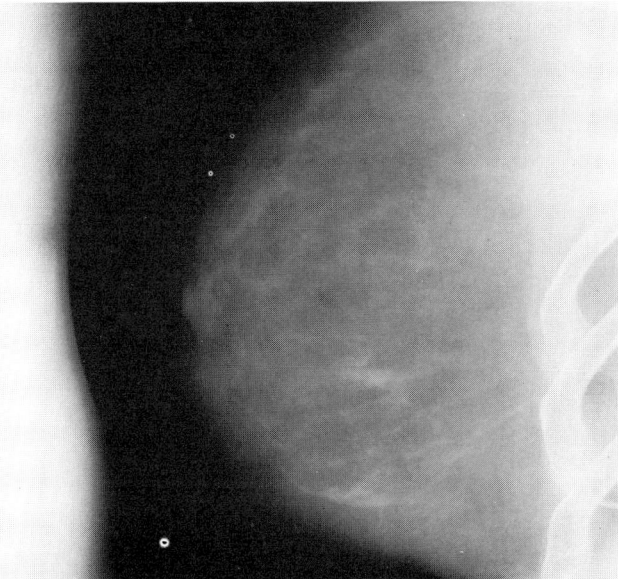

Figure 1.1. Photograph made with Kodak RP/M X-Omat medical x-ray film for mammography. This extra-fine-grain, high-contrast film is designed to show radiographic detail in radiography of the breast, as seen here. [Courtesy, Radiographic Markets Division, Eastman Kodak Company.]

cellent radiographic detail. This film, manufactured by Eastman Kodak Company, has been found valuable also in radiography of the extremities in situations where very fine detail is needed. It can be processed either in longer-cycle automatic processing or manually (Figure 1.1).

Therapy localization film

The Kodak therapy localization film can be processed in a 90-second processor and is designed for therapy localization procedures. It is an extra-fine-grain film intended for direct-exposure techniques and offers excellent radiographic detail over a wide range of exposure to x-ray and gamma radiation. This film can also be processed manually or in a longer-cycle processor.

Dental x-ray films

Dental x-ray films are available in a number of sizes, types, and speeds. The sizes may be classified as periapical, interproximal, and occlusal.

Periapical dental x-ray film is packed in light-tight, moistureproof paper packets. It is useful in examining the roots of teeth. The emulsions are classified as slow, average, and fast as to sensitivity or speed.

Interproximal (bite-wing) film in the form of packets is used for locating cavities between the teeth.

Occlusal film is larger than the periapical film and is employed for examining larger dental areas that cannot be covered with the periapical film.

FORMULATING X-RAY TECHNIQUES

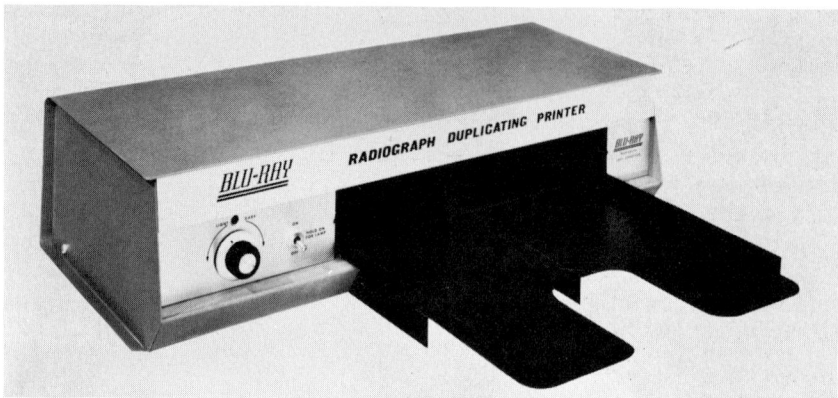

Figure 1.2. The Blu-Ray radiograph duplicating machine.

Dosimeter films

Dosimeter films were developed to measure high-energy radiation dosage. Small dental-size packets containing one or more types of film are used. The different films may be selected to record a wide or narrow radiation-dosage range.

Industrial film

Industrial film is used for high-energy radiography and for special radiographic procedures such as mammography.

DUPLICATING RADIOGRAPHS

Excellent copies of radiographs can be made by employing the Blu-Ray radiograph duplicating machine. The machine is compact and will fit in the darkroom without interfering with loading or unloading cassettes.

To make duplicate radiographs, one need only feed the radiographic duplicating film, which is in contact with the original radiograph, into the Blu-Ray printer. The film is automatically returned in six seconds and is ready

Figure 1.3. Three pairs of radiographs, showing originals and duplicates made by the Blu-Ray machine.

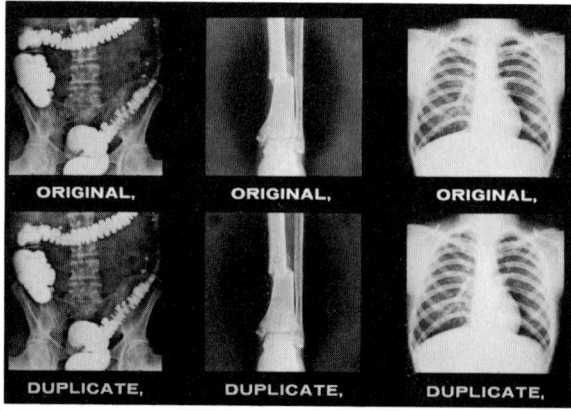

Radiographic Film

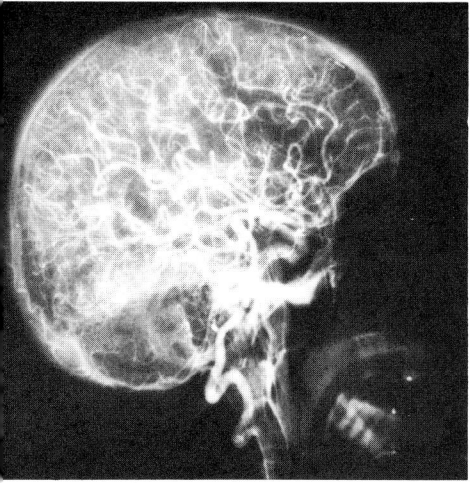 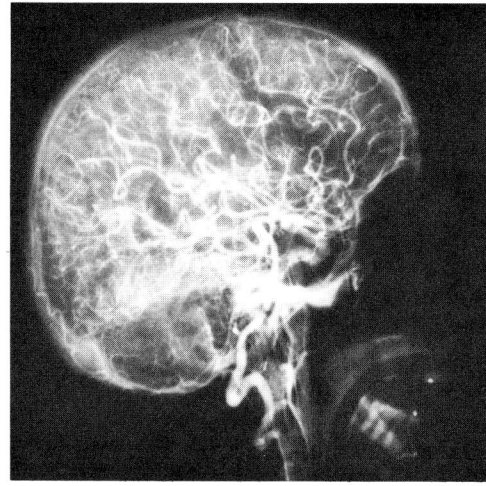

Figure 1.4. Copying with the Kodak RP/D X-Omat radiograph duplicating film. At the left, the original radiograph of the skull; at the right, the copy. [Courtesy, Radiographic Markets Division, Eastman Kodak Company.]

for the processor. Figure 1.2 is a photograph of the Blu-Ray machine. Figure 1.3 shows the original radiograph and the duplicate radiograph made with the Blu-Ray apparatus.

Kodak RP/D X-Omat radiograph duplicating film (Figure 1.4) is designed primarily for reproducing radiographs to accompany patient records, as teaching aids, or in other applications where duplicate radiographs are valuable. This film is also designed to make facsimiles of industrial radiographs. The film can be processed automatically in 90 seconds, in longer-cycle automatic processes, or manually. It may be exposed in a printing frame or in a mechanical contact printer, such as the Blu-Ray radiograph duplicating printer.

Mechanical contact printers, such as the Blu-Ray radiograph duplicating printer, are the most convenient means for exposing duplicating film. These printers are compact and easily portable. Because they are "light type," duplication may be made without interfering with normal processing-room operations.

A conversion kit allowing Blu-Ray printers of an older type to be modified with a BLB fluorescent lamp in order to obtain high-quality duplicate radiographs is available from any dealer in x-ray products.

Subtraction film

For subtraction technique, the Kodak RP/SU X-Omatic subtraction film is a 90-second automatic-processable film designed for preparing the mask for use in the subtraction of radiographic images. It is also suitable for recording on a single film the composite image of a radiograph and subtraction mask. The emulsion, coated on one side of the blue-tinted Estar base, requires about twice the exposure used for the Kodak commercial film 4127 previously recommended for the subtraction technique. The reduced speed simplifies and allows more precise exposure control of the film in a printing frame or in a mechanical contact printer, such as the Blu-Ray radiography duplicating printer. The emulsion characteristics also make this film ideally

FORMULATING X-RAY TECHNIQUES

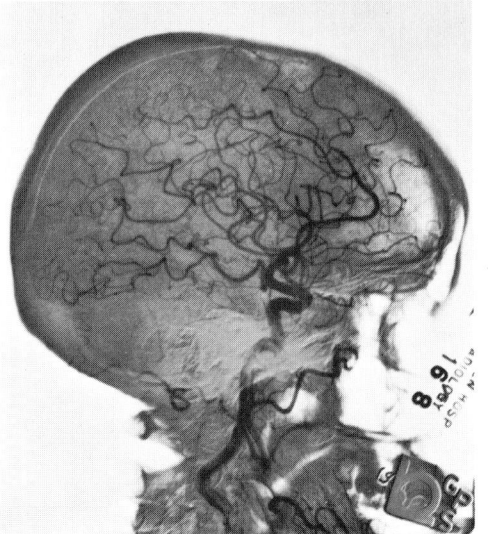 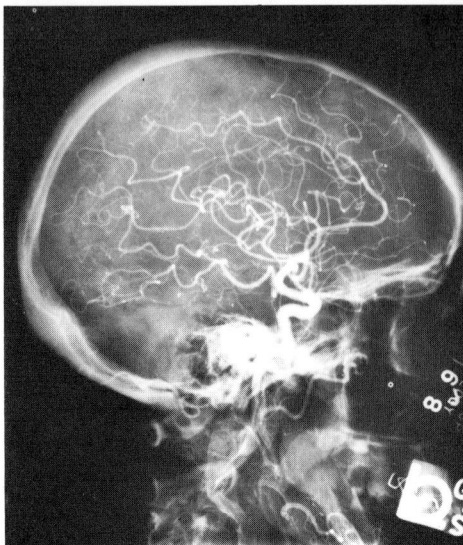

Figure 1.5. Subtraction technique: at the left, the composite image of a radiograph and subtraction mask; at the right, the negative with a high-density mask. Kodak RP/SU X-Omatic subtraction film. [Courtesy, Radiographic Markets Division, Eastman Kodak Company.]

suited for use with LogEtronic equipment. This film may also be processed in longer-cycle automatic processors or manual processing (Figure 1.5). The Du Pont Cronex printer is designed for making subtractions and duplications. The printer will handle all film sizes up to 14" x 17". Three different light sources provide versatility. One is a bright light for registration of the subtraction mask and angiogram. A second is a white light source for exposing the subtraction mask in print. The third is an ultraviolet source for exposing duplicating film. The exposure timer is automatic and permits exposure up to 30 seconds in half-second intervals.

MEDICHROME FILM

Black-and-white radiography has always necessitated a compromise between contrast and exposure range. Medichrome film is a color film (developed by the Agfa-Gevaert Film Company) which makes it possible to vary image contrast, providing a solution to the dilemma of contrast and exposure range. The color radiographic system based on the medichrome film yields a blue image of extremely low graininess. Radiographs can be viewed either on a standard illuminator, with or without the use of color filters, or on a special variable spectrum viewer given a constant brightness level.

The basic medichrome film makes it possible to demonstrate structures of low density within zones of widely varying density, all at the same time. The higher definition of medichrome film (due to its extremely low graininess) aids diagnosis by visualizing minute structures with a low absorption. Vascular or neuroradiological examinations gain substantially from the use of medichrome film; the radiograph will permit study not only of the opacified organ but also, with a comparable exposure, of perivisceral opacities of lesser density.

Radiographic Film

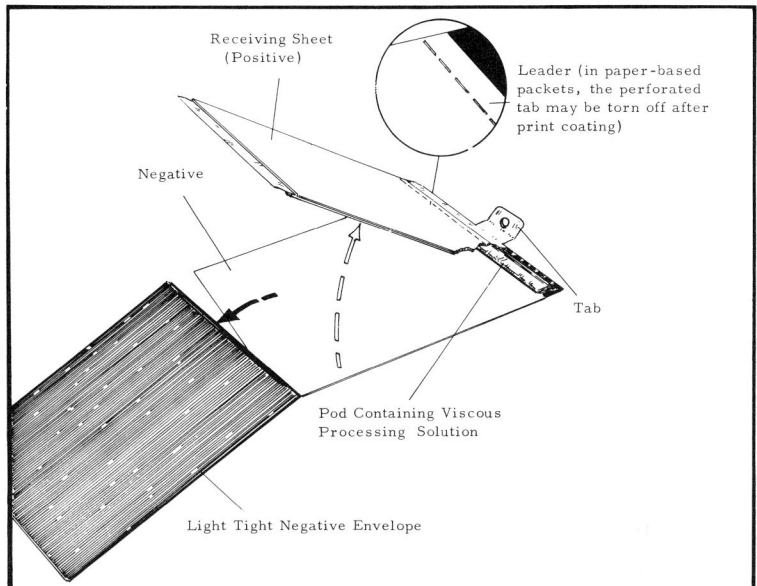

Figure 1.6. The Polaroid radiographic packet.

THE POLAROID RADIOGRAPHIC PROCESS

The Polaroid radiographic packet

The three primary parts of the Polaroid radiographic packet are (a) the negative, which carries the photosensitive emulsion, (b) the pod, a metallic foil envelope which contains the viscous processing solution, and (c) the receiving sheet, which accepts the positive image from the exposed negative. The radiograph obtained may be a paper-based reflection print (Type 3000X and Type 1001) or a film-based (polyester) translucency (Type TLX film).

The remaining parts, shown in Figure 1.6, permit the negative, the receiving sheet, and the viscous processing solution to perform their collective function of producing a finished radiograph.

With Type TLX film, the final result is a translucent positive radiograph, which can be viewed either by transmitted light, such as that from a standard illuminator, or by reflected light, such as that available from room illumination. With Type 3000X and Type 1001, the result is a positive radiographic print which can be viewed by reflected light only.

When Polaroid Type 3000X or Polaroid Type TLX packets are exposed to x-radiation in conjunction with a standard blue-emitting, high-speed fluorescent screen, radiographs of satisfactory density are produced with reductions in radiation exposure ranging from 50 to 84 per cent, depending upon the wet-process film/screen combination used for comparison.

Exposure

Figure 1.7 schematically represents the exposure of a Polaroid radiographic packet. The fluorescent screen emits visible light when excited by x-rays. This visible image is recorded as a latent image on the photosensitive surface of the negative. The exposed Polaroid radiographic packet with its

FORMULATING X-RAY TECHNIQUES

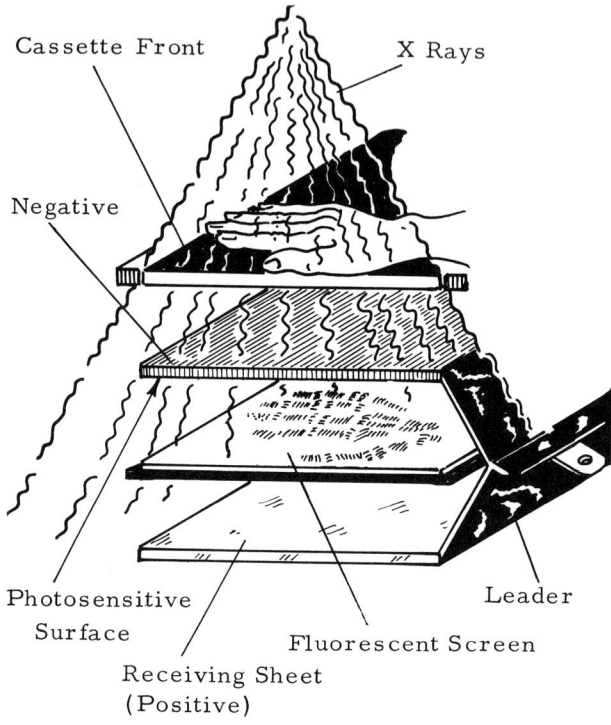

Figure 1.7. The exposure of a Polaroid radiographic packet.

Figure 1.8. The process of diffusion in Polaroid film, shown schematically.

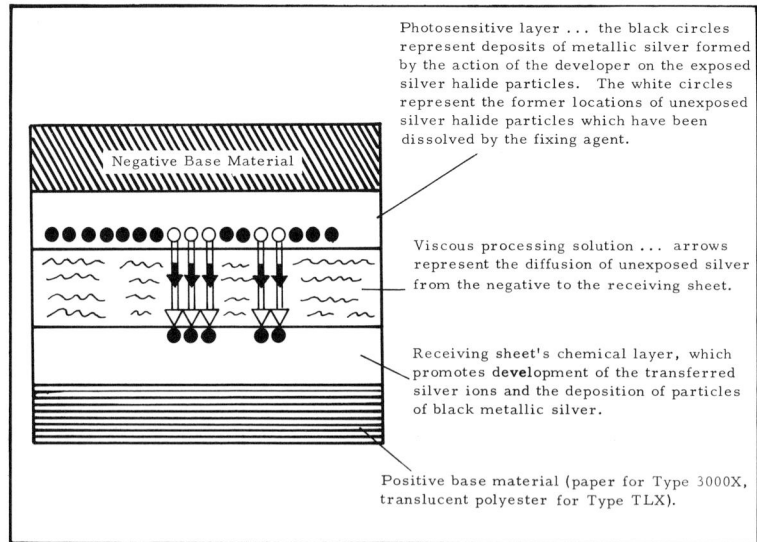

Radiographic Film

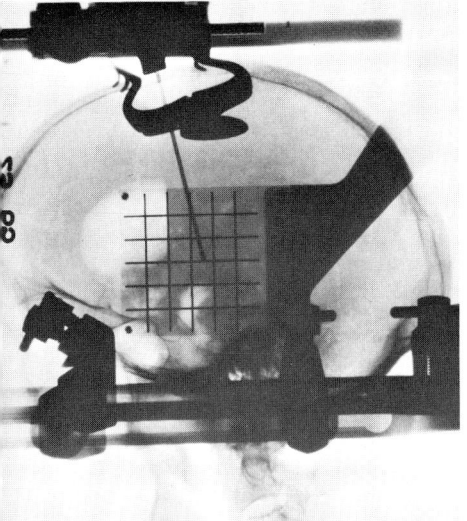

Figure 1.9. Radiograph of lateral skull made with Polaroid TLX film—a positive. The metal clamps show dense black.

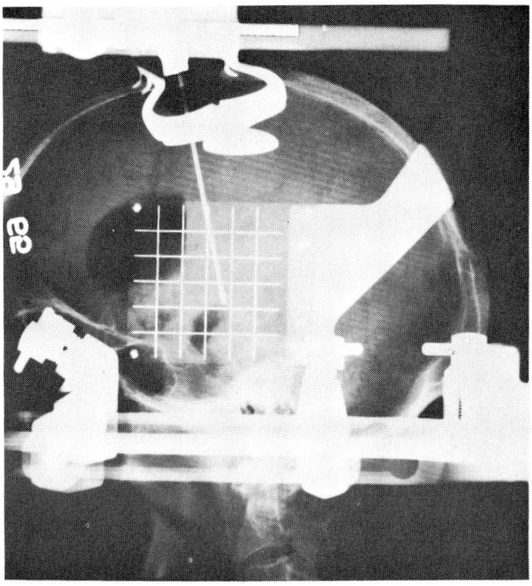

Figure 1.10. Radiograph of the skull of Figure 1.9 made with conventional radiographic film—a negative.

latent image is processed by drawing it through a set of pressure rollers which burst the pod and spread the viscous processing solution between the negative and the receiving sheet. The developing agent in the processing solution reacts with *exposed* silver halide particles and forms a visible, negative image by reducing the silver ions to metallic silver. While this negative image is being formed, another component of the processing solution, a photographic fixing agent, dissolves *unexposed* silver halide particles by forming soluble complexes with their silver ions. These complexes diffuse through the thin layer of viscous processing solution to the receiving sheet, where they contact substances which free the silver ions from their complexes with the fixing agent and make them subject to reduction to metallic silver by the action of the developing agent. The metallic silver so formed is then deposited on the receiving sheet to create the *positive* radiographic image. This entire diffusion transfer reversal process is accomplished in ten seconds with Type 3000X, in sixty seconds with Type 1001, and in forty-five seconds with Type TLX.

Figure 1.8 shows the process schematically. The width of the layers has been exaggerated in this illustration for clarity.

You can perhaps better understand why the final radiograph bears a positive image (compare Figures 1.9 and 1.10) if you remember that it is the silver ions of the *unexposed* silver halide particles that are the source of the metallic silver deposits which form the radiographic image.

Coating

Within one hour after processing, Polaroid radiographic prints should be treated with the print-coating solution that is provided (see instructions accompanying the film). The simple but important treatment quickly neutralizes the small amount of processing solution that remains in the receiv-

FORMULATING X-RAY TECHNIQUES

ing sheet when it is stripped from the negative. Moreover, as soon as the print-coating solution dries, it leaves behind a durable plastic film which protects the surface of the radiograph from scratches, moisture, and atmospheric contaminants which can attack the silver image.

FILM STORAGE AND HANDLING
General

A film is a delicate material and it should not be handled carelessly or roughly. It is sensitive to heat, light, x-rays, radium, chemical fumes, pressure, rolling, bending, etc., and any one of these is capable of adversely affecting the emulsion. Radiographic films can, however, be handled safely in accordance with all the various radiographic needs of the x-ray technologist as long as he knows what he must do to avoid the production of foreign marks, referred to as *artifacts*. From a radiographic standpoint an *artifact* is a mark which is foreign to the x-ray image and which is not necessarily imposed on the film by the action of x-rays.

Radiographic film is packed in metal foil and paper wrapping to protect it from light and moisture, and each sheet is enclosed in a folder of chemically pure interleaving paper. Some film companies supply film with or without interleaving paper.

Heat

Unexposed and unprocessed film should always be kept in a cool, dry place. It should never be stored in basements or near steam pipes or other sources of heat. High temperatures exert injurious effects on the emulsion, causing loss of contrast and the production of fog.

An approximate guide to the storage of film is as follows. If the film is to be used in two months, it can withstand temperatures up to 75° F. without fog. If stored at 60° F., it can be stored for six months, and for one year at 50° F. Ideal storage is 50° to 70° F. and 40 to 60 per cent relative humidity.

Radiation

All radiographic film must be suitably protected from the action of x-rays and all other forms of radiation by the use of lead-lined walls or lead-lined film bins or by keeping the film at a safe distance from radium and x-ray exposure.

Expiration date

Film should be used before the expiration date since film aging causes loss in *speed* and *contrast* and will result in a *mottled* appearance on the finished radiograph. The expiration date will be found on each box of film.

Figure 1.11 shows a lateral lumbar spine thought to be overexposed. Figure 1.12 is a radiograph of the same patient with a reduction of 50 per cent in exposure employing the same cassette. Figure 1.13 is a film taken from the same box of films and processed in the normal manner (without radiographic exposure). This film shows *mottle* from old, outdated film.

Mottle is also caused by "white light" leak in the film bin. The interleaving paper when struck by white light gives the mottle to the film (Figure 1.14). Most film is now supplied without interleaving paper.

Radiographic Film

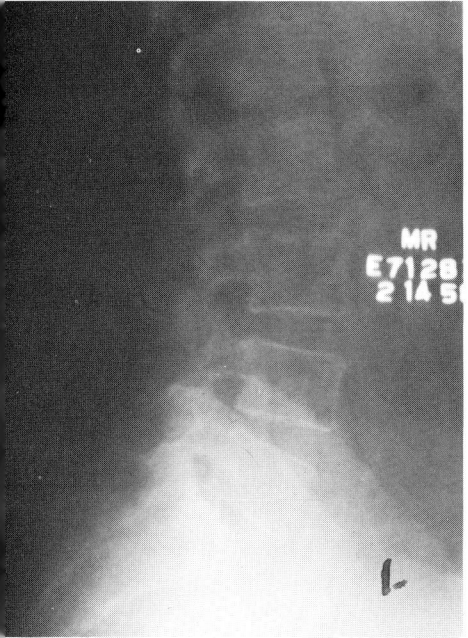

Figure 1.11. Radiograph of lateral lumbar spine, overexposed.

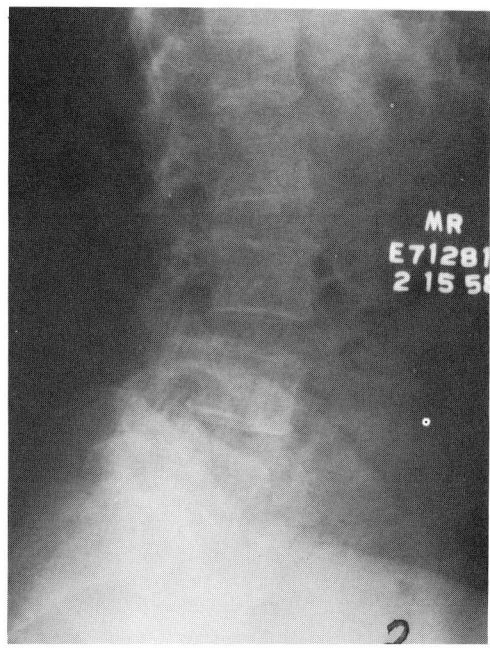

Figure 1.12. Radiograph of the same patient as in Figure 1.11, with 50 per cent reduction in exposure.

Figure 1.13. Non-exposed film from the same box as was used for Figures 1.11 and 1.12.

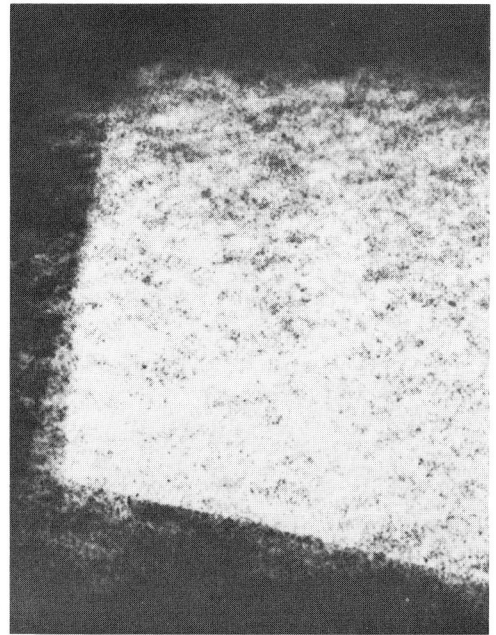

Figure 1.14. Mottle caused by "white light" leak.

FORMULATING X-RAY TECHNIQUES

Handling

When handled, radiographic films should be held as near the edges as possible. The hands should be clean and dry, and hand cream should be avoided. The use of rubber gloves should also be avoided.

Loading and unloading film

Generally, there are two types of containers in which medical x-ray film can be held during exposure—*cassettes* and *cardboard holders.* More recent is the disposable cardboard holder. The choice of holder depends upon the part to be radiographed and the exposure technique. Loading and unloading film is of great importance and requires care. When loading a cassette, place the film *without the paper* in the bottom of the cassette.

Static electricity

When two non-conductors such as interleaving paper and film are separated quickly, a static charge may be established. Electrical charges may be generated when a cassette is open and the two screen surfaces are rapidly separated, or when a film is pulled from the cassette.

The rubbing together of clothing, especially silk, nylon, and rayon, while working in the processing room can build up a static charge.

The three classifications of static markings commonly found on radiographs are *tree static, crown static,* and *smudge static.* Very rapid motions such as removing a film from interleaving paper can build up a charge sufficient to discharge in the form of tree static (Figure 1.15) when the film is touched by the technologist, or when interleaving paper breaks contact with the film. Crown static most often is the result of the rapid withdrawing of a film from a tight or new box of film. Smudge static (Figure 1.16) occurs when

Figure 1.15.   Tree static marks.   **Figure 1.16.**   Smudge static marks.

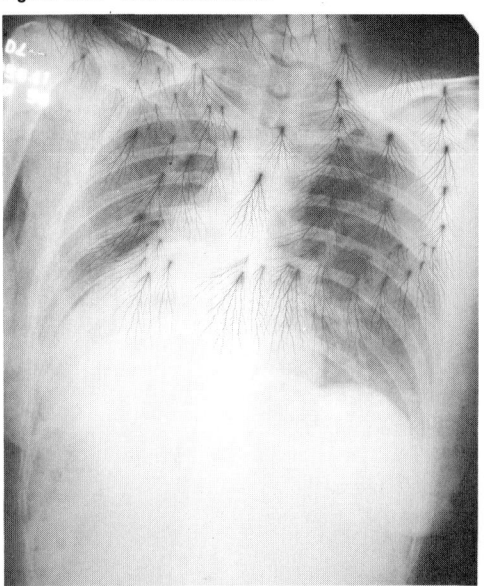
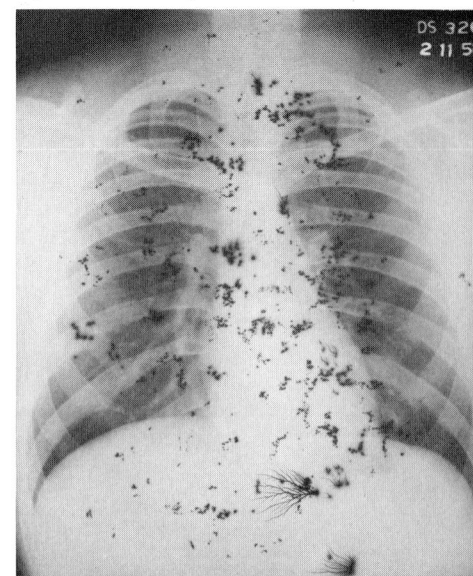

a discharge follows a path induced by dust, lint, or a rough intensifying screen surface.

While grounding the loading bench provides the simplest solution to static problems, moisture in the air around the film area is the greatest aid in the prevention of static. The higher the moisture content of the air, the less chance there will be for static to appear. This is the reason why there is less static with manual processing than with automatic processing.

Film identification data

In studying radiographs, the radiologist must be able to determine readily the side of the body examined, the direction of the central ray, and, if stereoradiography is employed, the direction of the tube shift. The most effective and accurate way to incorporate these data in the radiograph is by means of markers made of lead or other suitable radiopaque materials that can be placed on the cassette or film holder before the exposure is made. Letters, numerals, and holders for this purpose may be obtained from any dealer in x-ray supplies.

It is often necessary to incorporate in the radiograph the name and address or institution of the radiologist, the patient's name, the case number, and the date of the examination. From the standpoint of appearance, efficiency, and medicolegal precautions, the photographic method is excellent for such markings.

FILM TESTS

Every radiologic technologist should learn to make film tests to compare brands of film for contrast and speed values. He should also learn to run chemical tests. Tests should be made, with both a step wedge and body tissues or phantoms, for each brand of film or each brand of chemical to be tested. It is essential to use the same cassette and the same subject matter and to process all the films at the same time. Films should be tested for low and high kilovoltage. All films should be filed for future reference in order to evaluate and compare the contrast and speed characteristics of a film emulsion at a later date with newer film or newer chemistry.

By running a standard test employing the technique used each day in the department, one can easily check the speed and contrast characteristics of a new film by making identical exposures for comparison.

Rather than use patients for film and chemical evaluation, the author prefers to use phantoms and a step wedge. The phantoms shown in Figures 1.17 and 1.18 consist of carefully selected adult human bones, embedded in transparent non-granular plastic. This plastic has the same absorption and secondary-radiation-emitting characteristics as living tissue. One may repeat an experiment, regardless of dosage, as often as necessary with no danger of excess radiation. One may also make critical detailed studies of bone-structure and sharpness comparisons (Figure 1.19).

The tissue-equivalent plastic step wedge, Figure 1.20, is an excellent tool for research and comparative studies. It consists of ten separate blocks which can easily be disassembled and rearranged to obtain different thicknesses. Embedded in the top are several test objects: a 2 x 2 x 2 cm. lead plate for measuring magnification, distortion, and secondary radiation; five

FORMULATING X-RAY TECHNIQUES

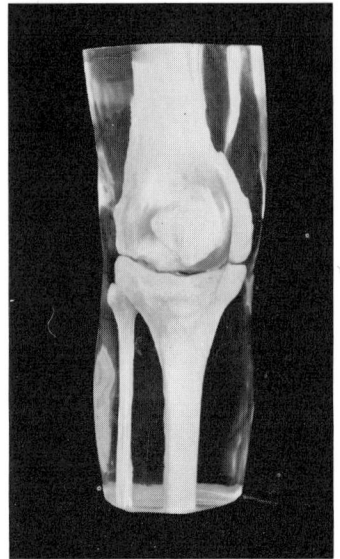

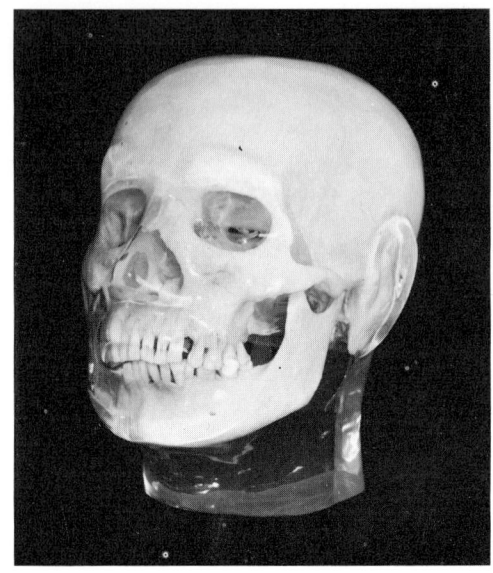

Figure 1.17. Phantom of the knee joint: human bones embedded in a special plastic.

Figure 1.18. Phantom of a human skull, embedded in plastic.

parallel pieces of stainless steel wire to determine sharpness and visibility of detail; a cube of human bone; a gelatin capsule, $\frac{1}{2}$ cm. in diameter, containing bone dust; and an identical capsule containing air.

The steps are wide enough to produce density strips on a radiograph which can be measured with a densitometer. Microdensitometer measurements are possible acrosss the shadow of the stainless steel wire. Densitometer measurements can also be made of shadows cast by other test objects.

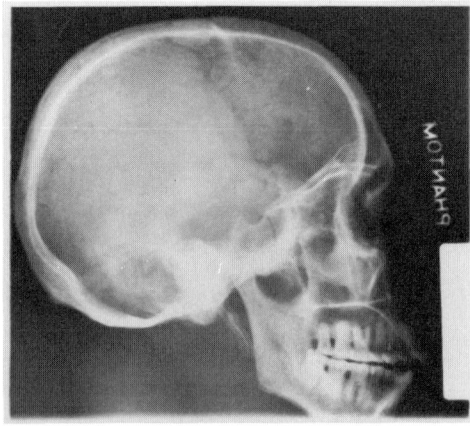

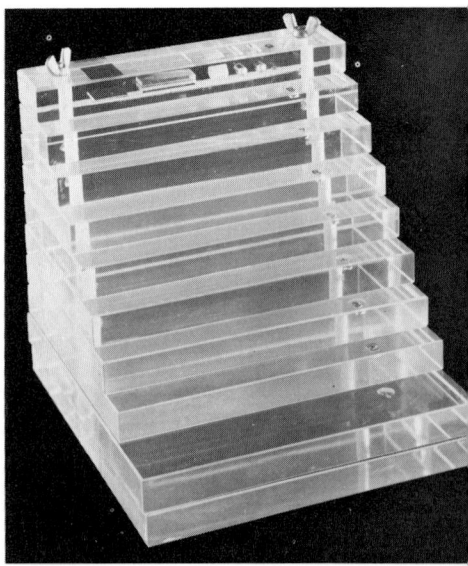

Figure 1.19. Radiograph of a skull phantom.

Figure 1.20. The step wedge made of plastic, described in the text.

Radiographic Film

The wedge is large enough to be placed across two cassetes containing screens and film, permitting screen and film evaluations with a single exposure. These absorption and secondary-radiation-emission characteristics of the wedge have proved remarkably similar to those of human tissues in the voltage range between 50 and 150 Kv.P.

Such a wedge is valuable in teaching and testing. One may demonstrate all the factors which control and affect the quality of the radiograph. It also permits studies of image intensifiers and their allied equipment.

THE LATENT IMAGE

The latent image cannot be seen or detected by any ordinary physical means, but it can be changed into a visible image by chemical processing. Many theories have been advanced as to the nature of the changes in the silver halide molecule that occur in the formation of the latent image. The generally accepted theory regarding the initial effect of x-ray exposure on the film is that a liberation of electrons occurs in the silver halide crystal. Normally, a silver halide crystal is a non-conductor of electricity. Upon exposure to x-rays or light, however, it becomes a weak conductor. From the individual atoms in the crystal, the exposure stimulus releases photoelectrons that flow within the crystal as a tiny electric current. In this movement, some of the electrons are acquired by the silver specks, which thereby assume negative electric charges. The silver halide molecule then undergoes a complicated series of internal changes. The slower-moving silver ions with a positive charge travel to the negatively charged specks, where they are neutralized to form a tiny nucleus of free silver, while the halide portions of the molecule are absorbed elsewhere. Silver ions are attracted and the speck grows larger with free silver until it reaches a size that can initiate chemical reduction of the whole crystal to metallic silver when attacked by the reducing agents in the x-ray developer solution. The exposed silver specks in their aggregate constitute the *latent image.*

Chapter 2. **CASSETTES AND SCREENS**

CASSETTES

A cassette is a thin, light-tight container slightly larger than the film it is intended to hold. The front is made of a radiolucent material such as Bakelite or Magnelite; the back is of steel or light-weight metal. Felt gaskets insure light-proof edges; and the inner, or back, side is lined with a thin layer of lead (except phototimer cassettes) to absorb secondary radiation emitted by the back of the cassette and Bucky tray or table top. A good cassette is light-proof and provides a good contact over the entire area of the film. Unsharpness of the radiographic image is often due to a bent or warped cassette front and/or poor screen contact.

Phototimer cassettes

The cassettes used for conventionally timed radiography have lead-lined backs, to reduce the effect of backscattered radiation on the film. Cassettes used for phototiming must have a radiolucent back to permit the radiation

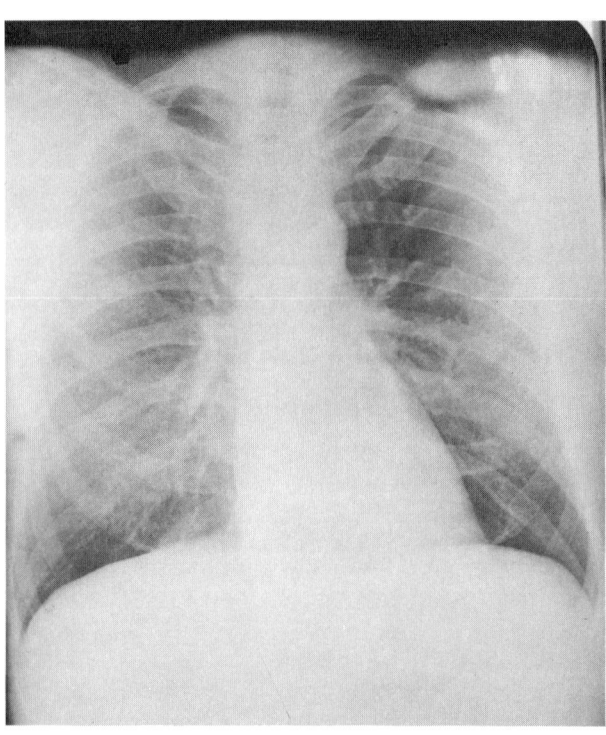

Figure 2.1. Fog caused by light leak.

Cassettes and Screens

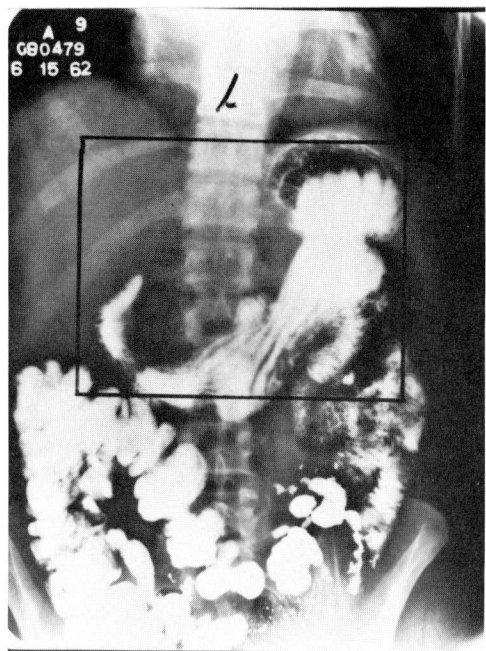

Figure 2.2. Poor definition due to a warped cassette front.

reaching the film to continue on to the photocell, which acts as a timing device, according to a predetermined density scale. Care should be taken for appropriate identification of phototimer cassettes when both types of timing are used.

Worn felt

In many cassettes the lid felt serves a dual purpose. It affords a light-tight seal preventing the enclosed film from being light struck around the edges, which would cause fog. The felt also insures better contact. Figure 2.1 shows fog from light leak.

Poor screen contact

Poor screen contact shows on the finished radiograph as poor definition or detail in certain areas. Figure 2.2 shows a radiograph with poor definition due to a warped cassette front.

Test for cassette or screen contact. Lay a wire screen (about $3/_{16}$ inch mesh) on top of the cassette to be tested. Make an exposure at about 50 Kv.P., $1/_{20}$ second, 50 Ma., 36-inch focus-film distance. Develop the film in the usual manner. If the film shows blurred outlines or is fuzzy, probably the contact is poor between screens and film. It is wise to check the front of the cassette before removing the screens, since it may be warped; or the back of the cassette may be sprung at the hinged area because the cassette has been dropped. Figure 2.3 shows poor contact due to a warped front. Figure 2.4 shows the same cassette after repairs, which resulted in a substantial saving, since the screens did not have to be replaced. It is false economy to

FORMULATING X-RAY TECHNIQUES

Figure 2.3. The result of poor screen contact due to a warped cassette front.

Figure 2.4. The cassette of Figure 2.3 has been repaired, and this is the result.

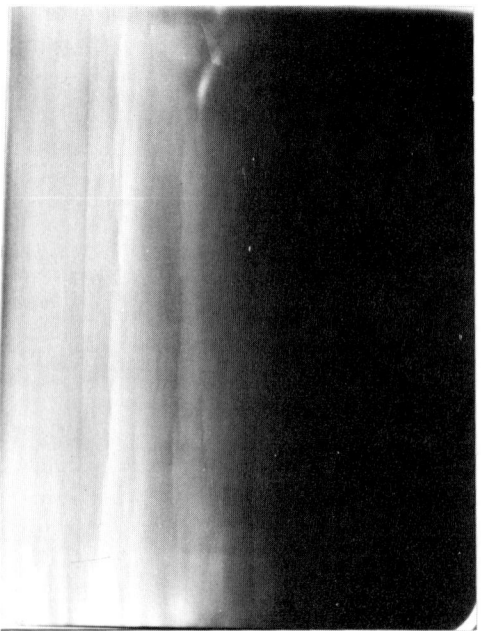

Figure 2.5. Radiograph of a warped grid.

Figure 2.6. Radiograph showing correct exposure but with grid cut-off.

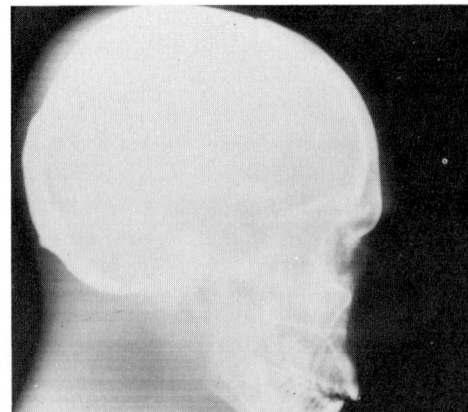

Cassettes and Screens

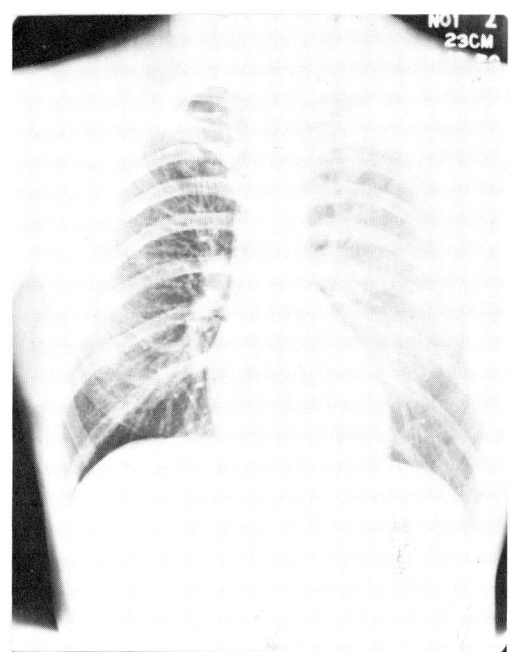

Figure 2.7. Correct exposure, but with grid cut-off on the patient's left side.

mount new screens in faulty cassettes. Other cassette faults which affect film quality include worn felt, loose hinges, dented fronts, or sprung frames. Although cassettes are sturdy and strong enough to withstand normal hard use, they cannot withstand abuse (Figures 2.5, 2.6, 2.7).

RADIOGRAPHIC CALIBRATIONS

The formulation of techniques is extremely difficult, if not impossible, when one is faced with a radiographic machine that has not been calibrated properly. It is ideal, indeed, to formulate techniques on one unit and then transpose the techniques to other units within the same department. Each radiographic unit should be calibrated, and in turn each unit should have equal densities on a film when identical exposures are made.

Inaccuracy of equipment means repeat films, unnecessary exposure to the patient, decreased efficiency to the department, and waste of film.

Each radiographic unit should be calibrated by a service engineer; however, the radiologic technologist should be responsible for the exposure factors, processing, proper cassettes, and film.

The timer should be checked with a spinning top for the exposure of less than 1 second and with a stop watch for exposures longer than 1 second. With a *three-phase unit,* one should use an oscilloscope in place of a spinning top to check the timer for accuracy.

No matter what Ma. station and time-increment values are used, as long as the product is the same, the density level should remain the same.

Example: 100 Ma. at $1/10$ second, 200 Ma. at $1/20$ second, and 300 Ma. at $1/30$ second should all produce the same density.

FORMULATING X-RAY TECHNIQUES

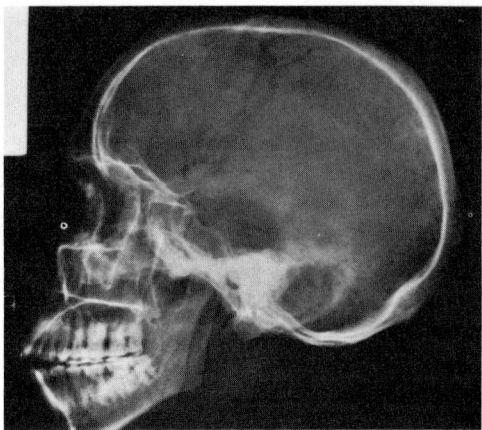

Figure 2.8. This radiograph was made with a properly calibrated machine.

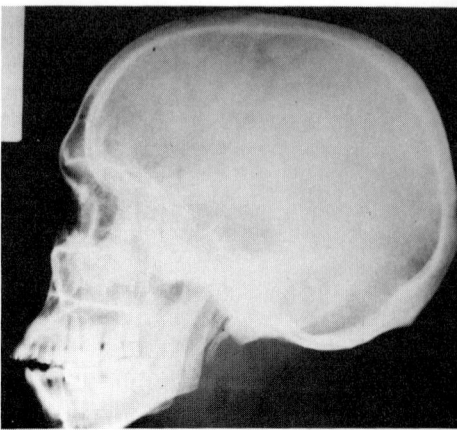

Figure 2.9. This radiograph was made with a machine out of calibration.

Figure 2.8 shows a radiograph made with a machine properly calibrated. Figure 2.9 shows a radiograph with the same exposure, but made with the unit out of calibration.

CASSETTELESS RADIOGRAPHY

Cassetteless radiography is a recent innovation. The Rapido transport and Diplomat processor developed by the Picker X-Ray Company can handle about 70 per cent of the need of the radiology department. This system produces diagnostic images free from artifacts and makes production radiography somewhat easier and quicker, since the finished radiograph is turned out in a one-step operation.

Xeroradiography

The xeroradiographic system represents a new concept in recording radiographic images. The Xerox Corporation manufactures a unit that can be used with one's present radiographic equipment. The system makes high quality images on paper. These units employ developing powder and reusable plates to process dry images in 90 seconds. When employing the 125 Xerox System, film and processing rooms are unnecessary.

Xeroradiographs show excellent resolving power at all levels of contrast. The resolving power of xeroradiography is greater than that of non-screen film techniques, especially for low-contrast applications like mammography.

INTENSIFYING SCREENS

Certain substances have the ability to fluoresce under x-rays; that is, when struck by x-radiation, they emit visible light. These substances are called phosphors; some emit light in the blue and ultraviolet region and others in

Cassettes and Screens

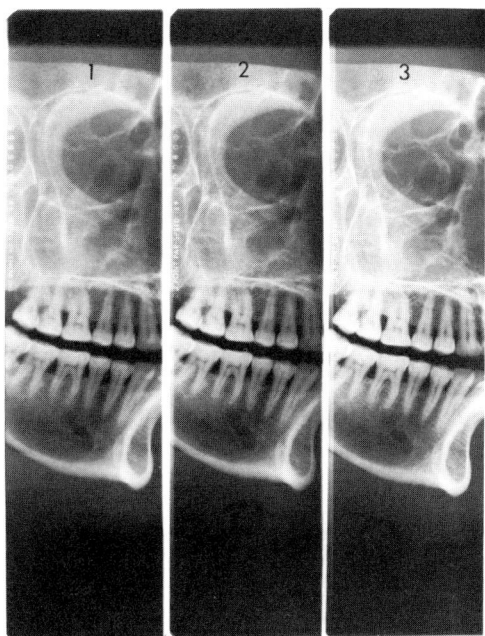

Figure 2.10. Partial radiographs: 1, made with high-speed screen; 2, made with "par-speed" screen; 3, made with detail screen.

the yellow-green region of the spectrum. These characteristics allow the use of different phosphors for different purposes. Three kinds—calcium tungstate, barium lead sulfate, and zinc sulfide—which emit blue light are used in making intensifying screens for conventional radiography. One blue-fluorescent phosphor, zinc sulfide, is used in making a screen for photofluorography (which is now all but obsolete). A green-fluorescing phosphor, zinc cadmium sulfide, is used in making a screen, not only for the outdated photofluorography but for the fluoroscopic screen used for viewing by the radiologist. The intensifying screen is used to help the x-ray film take an image in much shorter time and hence with less exposure than is possible with direct x-rays. It does what its name implies—intensifies the photographic effect of the x-radiation.

The thicker the fluorescent layer of the screen, the greater the intensification. The size of the crystals composing the layer also has a direct influence in this respect: the larger the crystals, the greater the intensity of the light emitted by the screen. Since the thick fluorescent layer allows the light to spread more widely, the *sharpness* of the fluorescent image is decreased accordingly. A choice is usually available in the selection of intensifying screens: fast screens provide high intensification; slow screens produce better image sharpness; medium-speed screens provide a balance between *speed* and *definition*.

An exposure with screens requires only about $1/15$ to $1/40$ of the time required for a direct exposure (one made without screens and using a cardboard holder). Such a reduction in the exposure provides an advantage in general medical radiography.

FORMULATING X-RAY TECHNIQUES

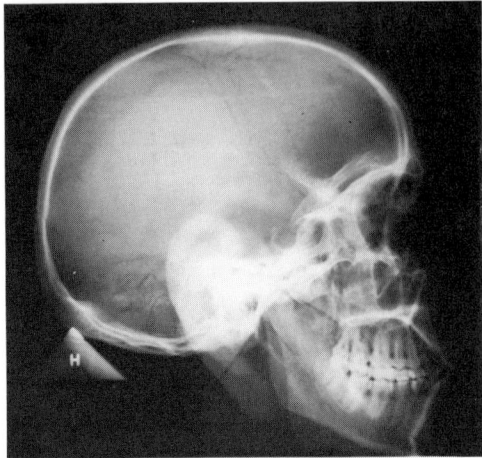 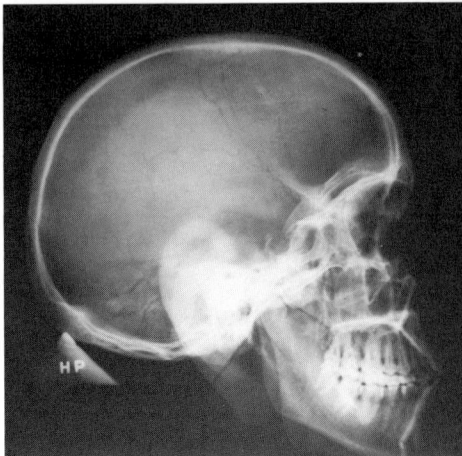

Figure 2-11. Radiograph made with a high-speed intensifying screen.

Figure 2.12. Radiograph made with a high-plus intensifying screen.

Less than 5 per cent of the density on a radiograph is caused by the direct action of x-rays. More than 95 per cent of the film density is due to the light given off by the intensifying screen. The use of screens not only reduces the radiographic exposure time and dosage factor, but adds materially to the contrast of the resultant radiograph.

At the present time there are three general classes of screens, based largely upon application and speed. The most widely used screen is the *medium-speed.* Each manufacturer has his own trade name for screen speed. Generally, the medium-speed screen possesses the best balance between *speed* and *detail* for most radiographic purposes (Figure 2.10). With the increased interest in radiation dosage, the *high-speed* screen has become very popular (Figures 2.11 and 2.12). However, there is a slight loss in detail of the radiographic image. There are many situations in which high-speed screens are very valuable and the slight loss of detail is of very little diagnostic significance. The most common of these are

1. Where reduction of radiation dosage is important;
2. In portable bedside and operating-room radiography where there is a limit on kilovolts and milliamperage;
3. In grid cassettes;
4. In high-kilovoltage radiography;
5. In the radiography of infants and children;
6. In spot-film radiography.

Slow-speed screens render better detail and are used for bone radiography, magnification techniques, and where speed is not at a premium (Figures 2.13 and 2.14).

Multisection screen books for use in body-section radiography represent a special application of intensifying screens: With the multisection screen book, up to seven layers of a body part can be radiographed simultaneously. Each screen pair is balanced in speed to yield the same exposure density on each film.

The DuPont Company manufactures a 14" x 36" Gradient Intensifying

Cassettes and Screens

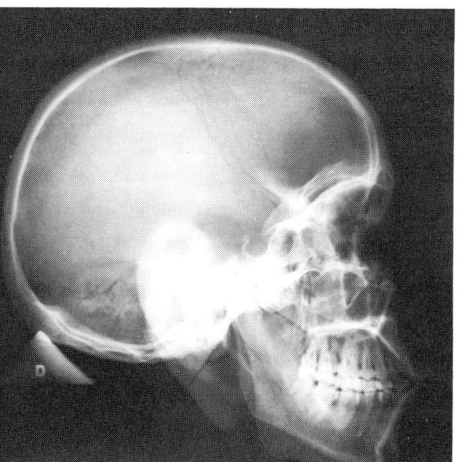

Figure 2-13. Radiograph made with a detail intensifying screen.

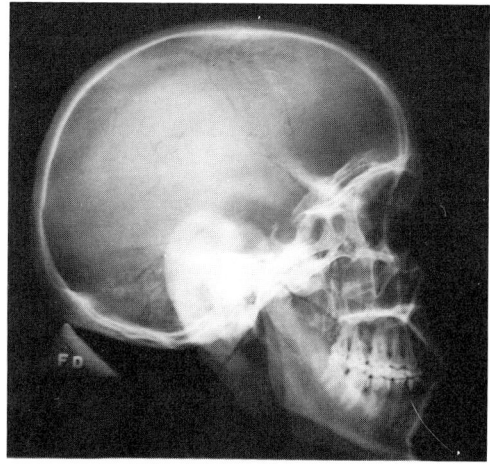

Figure 2.14. Radiograph made with a fast-detail intensifying screen.

Screen which has proved to be advantageous for venograms, femoral arteriograms, leg-length measurements, and radiography of the entire spine. A screen of this type eliminates the need for wedge filters by employing different screen speeds to produce uniform densities of the body parts being radiographed.

The Dupont barium–lead sulfate Hi-Speed screens emit more fluorescence in relation to crystal size than does calcium tungstate. Consequently, it has been possible to produce a fast, high-quality screen of uniformly fine grain.

Stains and abrasions

The most common stains on screens are caused by careless processing-room technique. Developer or hypo smears will stain screens a brownish color and will result in *light areas* on the finished radiograph. Dust and other foreign materials sometimes get into the cassette and will cause damage to screens. Routine periodical cleaning of screens with soap and water or 95-per-cent alcohol is recommended.

Various commercial screen cleaners are available from the x-ray dealer.

Test for lag

Intensifying screens must not continue to fluoresce after the exposure has been terminated; continued fluorescence of screens is called *lag*. Lag will cause a general fogging of the radiographic image, looking like secondary radiation or postexposure fog. Lag is generally due to old, worn-out screens.

To test screens for lag, make a normal exposure of some part with the cassette *empty* of any film; take the cassette to the processing room and place a film in it; close the cassette and allow the film to remain in the cassette for five minutes; then develop the film in the same manner as a normally exposed radiograph. If the image of the part exposed is imparted to the film, then the screens have lag, which produces a supplementary density that degrades the scale of contrast in the radiographic image.

Chapter 3. **PROCESSING**

THE PROCESSING ROOM

In our experience the processing room is the most important single room in the department of radiology; yet it is the one room most often neglected by both radiologic technologists and radiologists. A technologist can never hope to be a really good technologist unless he is *master* of the darkroom and processing technique. The best and most expensive radiographic equipment is of no avail if one tolerates carelessness or does not have a rigid time-temperature developing routine set up for processing x-ray films. The processing room can make or break a department as far as quality of radiographic films is concerned.

Because of the special importance of this room in the handling, processing, and even flow of work, both the general and detailed features should be most thoughtfully worked out.

Arrangement of equipment

The three major elements of equipment—loading bench, processing tanks, and dryer—should be arranged so that the number of steps taken can be kept at a minimum. Automatic processing has eliminated many of the problems heretofore encountered.

Light-tight entrance

An entrance that is easily accessible while providing complete protection from outside white light is an essential to the x-ray processing room.

Figure 3.1. A photographic example of postexposure fog.

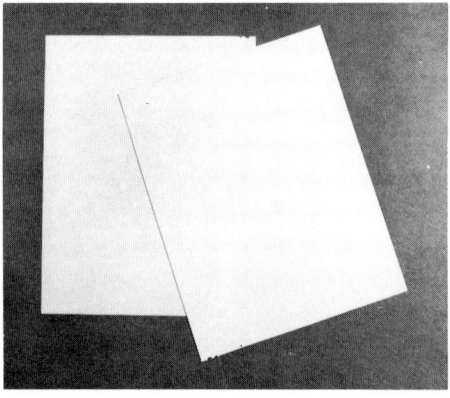
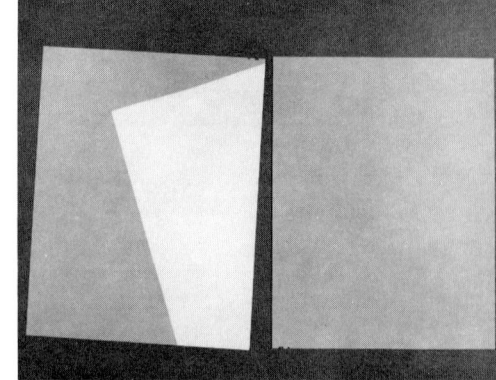

Processing

Ventilation

Satisfactory ventilation of an x-ray processing room requires more consideration than the ventilation of other rooms. The processing room contains certain elements that directly affect the air in it. If hand processing is used, open tanks of developer, acetic-acid solution, and water increase the humidity and create slight odors. Automatic processing eliminates the problems of humidity and chemical odor.

When improperly controlled, the temperature and humidity of the air have adverse physiological effects on the technologists as well as physical effects on film handling and storage. For example, excessive humidity causes the body to perspire, and damp fingers readily mark dry films and screens. If the air is too dry, film is susceptible to static accumulations.

Color

It is not necessary for the processing room to be a drab, all-black room. It is neither necessary from a technical standpoint nor desirable from a psychological one. If the *quality* of the light from a safelight lamp is *safe*, the illumination from any surface is also "safe" regardless of color.

The best processing-room illumination is that transmitted by a Kodak Safelight Filter, Wratten Series 6-B, using a 10-watt tungsten light source, directly over the manual-processing tank. The light transmitted is in the yellow and yellow-red portion of the spectrum. Therefore, maximum reflec-

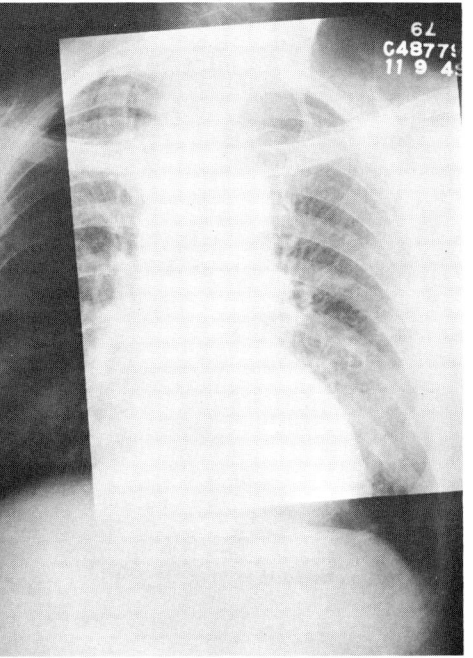

Figure 3.2. Postexposure fog. The lighter portion of this radiograph was protected by a sheet of cardboard during the safelight test which fogged the rest of the film.

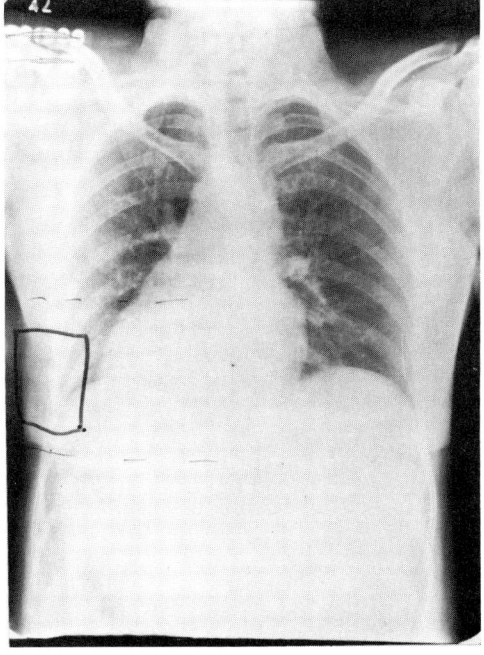

Figure 3.3. A simulated rib fracture due to postexposure fog.

tion under safelight illumination is achieved if the wall finish is either a color within the same spectral range or a light enough shade of any other color.

The color of the loading-bench top should be chosen with the thought that film, interleaving paper, and other objects must be readily distinguished.

One of the most durable materials used for the loading-bench top is sheet plastic.

Effect of safelight illumination

With present-day safelights (Wratten 6-B), it is possible to see clearly in the processing room. When the safelight lamps are fitted with a 10-watt bulb and a filter recommended for the light-sensitive film being used, the exposed films can be exposed, without fogging, for one minute at three feet from the safelight, or for one-half minute at two feet.

Exposed radiographic films are more sensitive to safelight illumination than unexposed films, in fact, *eight times more sensitive* to fog than are unexposed films. The effect on x-ray film of exposure to the illumination from safelight lamps is referred to as *postexposure*. The quality of a radiograph may be impaired by unnecessary exposure to safelight illumination, which is the reason for variations in density encountered in routine radiographs and for the lack of brilliancy that is frequently attributed to scattered radiation (Figures 3.1–3.3).

With respect to films exposed to *direct x-radiation* (exposed with a cardboard holder), the effect is very slight and may be disregarded. This is largely true, also, with respect to films that have received relatively heavy x-ray exposures employing calcium tungstate intensifying screens, although radiographic contrast is slightly impaired. However, in radiography of light density, as of the chest or gallbladder, the radiographic contrast may be seriously affected.

When radiographs have been *unprotected* from postexposure and we begin to protect them from postexposure, the contrast will increase to such a degree as to permit an increase in exposure thereafter.

To eliminate undesirable postexposure, we may reduce the intensity of the safelight illumination in one of three ways: (1) by employing bulbs of lower wattage; (2) by increasing the distance between the safelight lamps and the top of the film-loading bench; (3) by reducing the number of safelight lamps.

Safelight test. In testing a darkroom light for safety, one should subject part of an exposed x-ray film to the illumination of the safelights under the conditions used during normal processing and compare with a portion similarly exposed to x-rays but developed in total darkness.

Cleanliness

Owing to the sensitivity of x-ray film emulsions, cleanliness is essential in processing procedures. It is imperative that the processing room, as well as the accessories and equipment, be kept scrupulously clean (Figure 3.4). Solutions that are spilled should be wiped up at once; otherwise, upon evaporation, the chemicals may get into the air and later settle on film surfaces, causing spots.

Films should be handled with care in the processing room; permitting them to become wrinkled or bent will result in small marks called "crinkle

Processing

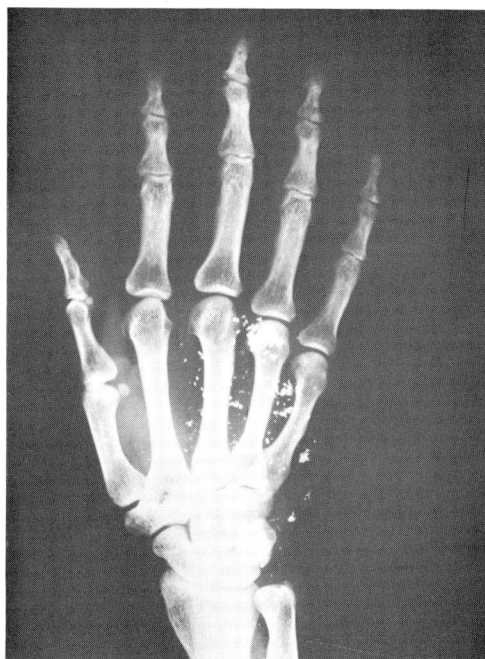

Figure 3.4. Cigarette ashes in the cassette.

marks." Rubbing films together before processing will cause static marks resembling the branches of a tree. If two films come in contact with each other during the developing process, an area of nondevelopment will appear in the area of film contact. This also occurs if the film is allowed to touch the side of the developing tank (Figures 3.5 and 3.6).

Excessive exposure of a film to light during development may result in *reversal of the image;* the "blacks" will be white and the "whites" will be black (Figure 3.7). A greasy appearance on the surface of the film is due to improper washing after fixing.

SILVER RECOVERY

Recovery of silver from used radiographic processing solutions, in addition to being economically profitable, conserves a natural resource essential to the radiographic and photographic industry. This desirable practice leads to a cleaner environment, since silver is classified as a water pollutant. It is also a significant source of revenue for the department of radiology.

Basically, there are three methods of recovering silver from spent photographic-processing solutions: metallic replacement, electrolytic plating, and chemical precipitation. The Kodak silver recovery system, which the author has had the most experience with, is based on metallic replacement. It involves the use of two simple, non-moving pieces of equipment: the Kodak Chemical Recovery Cartridge, Type P, and the Kodak Circulating Unit, Type B. The system is designed to efficiently remove valuable silver from used fixing baths. Although the equipment is particularly designed to remove silver from the overflow streams of automatic replenishing systems, it is

FORMULATING X-RAY TECHNIQUES

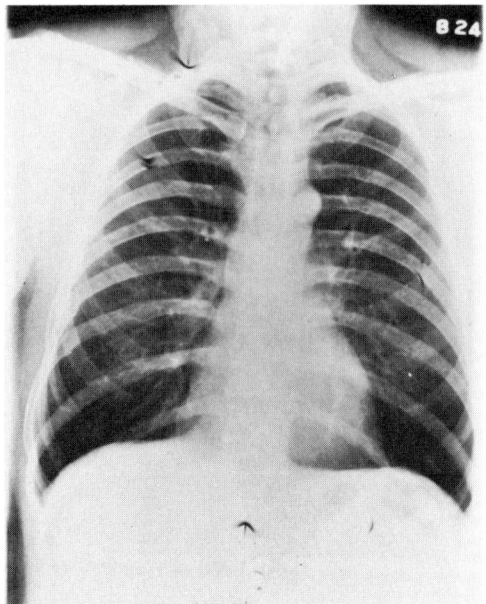

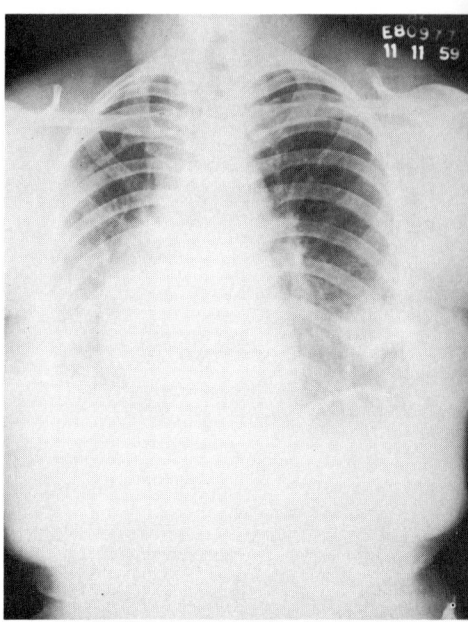

Figure 3.5. Crinkle marks due to bending the film before exposure.

Figure 3.6. An area of underdevelopment that has resulted from contact with another film during development.

equally adaptable for use with hand processing systems. Since the recovery cartridge functions by chemically replacing the silver in solution with another metal, the system has several advantages over electrolytic or chemical precipitation methods. These advantages include low initial cost of the equipment, simple non-electrical installation, high efficiency and no required maintenance. The Chemical Recovery Cartridge unlike some metallic-replacement recovery systems, does not generate combustible or explosive gases such as hydrogen during the recovery process.

AUTOMATIC PROCESSING

In automatic processing, film is transported at *high* temperatures through developing, fixing, and washing stages prior to hot-air drying. The wet-to-dry cycle is made possible by drastically reducing the time required for washing and drying. In order to achieve this, the film must be conditioned chemically in the wet section. To minimize film swelling and to prevent the emulsion from adhering to the rollers, a hardening agent is incorporated in the developer.

The key to the best in film quality in automatic processing is *uniform replenishment*. Careless or improper film feeding results in a wasteful increase in the amount of solution used. If a 14 x 17-inch film is fed the 17-inch way instead of the 14-inch way, the replenisher microswitch is activated by 17 inches of film travel, instead of 14 inches. This results in overreplenishment by a factor of 22 per cent. It is of utmost importance that films be fed the proper way in order to avoid overreplenishment, which results in excessive density.

Processing

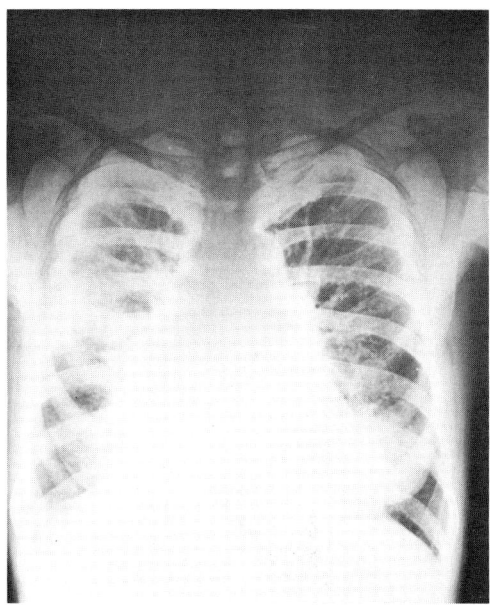

Figure 3.7. Reversal action.

The replenishment rates for medical screen-type film will vary depending on the *type* and *brand* of film and the *exposure* employed.

FILM-FEEDING PROCEDURE

Figure 3.8 shows the proper film-feeding procedures. The arrows indicate the direction in which film is fed into the processor.

To avoid overreplenishment, it is advisable to feed all narrower films side by side. Feed films into the processor square with the edge of the side guide. Feed multiple films simultaneously.

For occlusal film or roll film, in order to provide proper transport, use a leader of sheet film (Figure 3.9). The leader should be as wide as or wider than the roll film and at least 7 inches long. Using a 1-inch-wide tape, such as Scotch brand Electrical Tape No. 3, butt-splice the film to the leader, making sure that the adhesive side of the tape is not exposed. Most other types of tape are not suitable, owing to the solubility of their bases in the processing solution.

SOME QUESTIONS ON 90-SECOND PROCESSING (AUTOMATIC)

Is there any reason, apart from the value of acid in neutralizing the developer, why a fixer should be acid in pH?

Yes. The aluminum sulfate and chloride hardeners are effective only in an acid solution. Wetness or tackiness in film coming out of a processor may be caused by a fixer with a pH that is not acid enough. But there are many other reasons why wet films are produced—for example, inadequate replenishment of the fixer, and a dryer that is set too low.

FORMULATING X-RAY TECHNIQUES

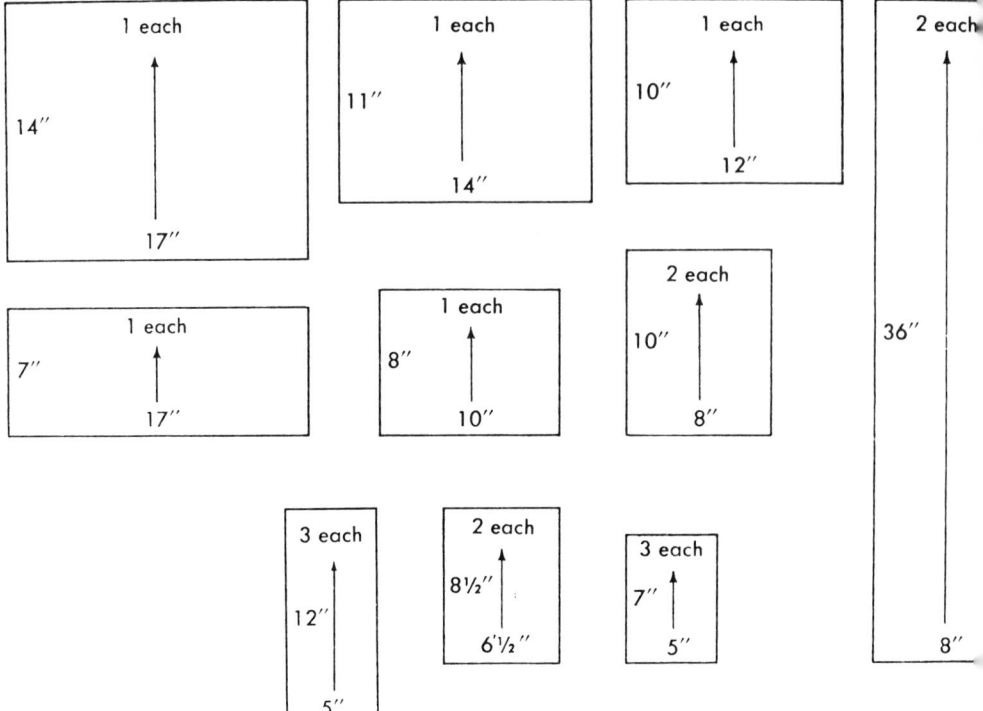

Figure 3.8. Film-feeding chart for automatic processing.

What is clearing time?

Clearing time is the length of time needed to completely remove the undeveloped silver bromide from the film.

Why do 90-second films fix so rapidly?

The 90-second films have a lower gelatin content than other films. The lower the ratio of gelatin to silver bromide in a film, the easier it is for the developing agents to get into the emulsion and convert the exposed silver crystal to black metallic silver. In other words, a man can run through a doorway faster alone than when three men hit it together. The same is true in washing. The less gelatin, the less thiosulfate it holds. Then the wash water has an easier job to do, since it can get into the emulsion easier because of the lower gelatin content and since there is less thiosulfate (hypo) to remove. Another factor in speed is the fast flow of water (2 to 4 gallons per minute) in an automatic processor. This flow prevents water, laden with thiosulfate, from remaining in proximity to the films. The higher temperature of wash water in 90-second processing makes washing more efficient, and the agitation caused by the rollers and by incoming water hastens the action.

Processing

Figure 3.9. A leader for film feeding of occlusal film or 35-mm copy film.

Suppose one shut down the processor with a film in the fixer tank. What would happen overnight?

The fixer would bleach out the developed black silver image. This, of course, rarely occurs, but in manual operation there have been cases in which the technologist has pulled a film out of a fixer tank after a night of immersion and found it blank. Figure 3.10 shows the result of improper washing.

What causes the blotchiness on films which is made visible by reflected light?

This effect, which is often described as random shiny and dull areas on the film, is caused by *variation in the rate of drying*. The drive rollers, while in contact with the film, momentarily prevent the forced air that is circulating through the chamber from reaching the contact areas. This effect can be reduced by lowering the dryer temperature to the lowest safe setting. Lower the temperature until films show some dampness; then increase the temperature until this condition disappears.

What effect can be expected from temperature variations in the developer?

Higher temperature will cause an increase in speed, density, and fog. Temperatures lower than normal will have the opposite effect. Higher temperatures in the developer will cause more emulsion swell and an increase in the carry-over into the fixer. At times, even properly replenished fixer will be affected, and the result will be wet films (Figures 3.11 and 3.12).

FORMULATING X-RAY TECHNIQUES

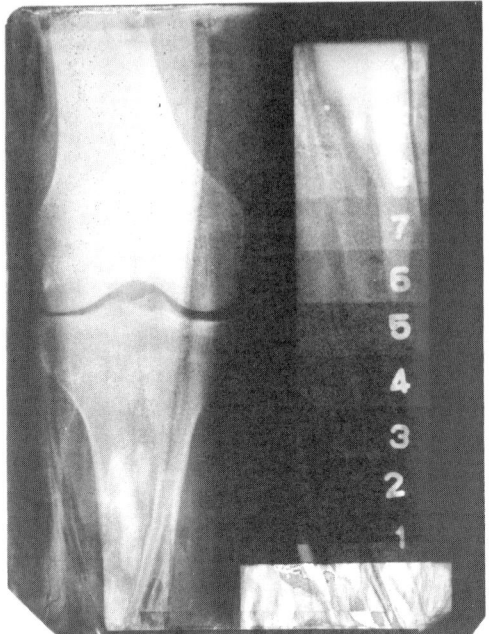
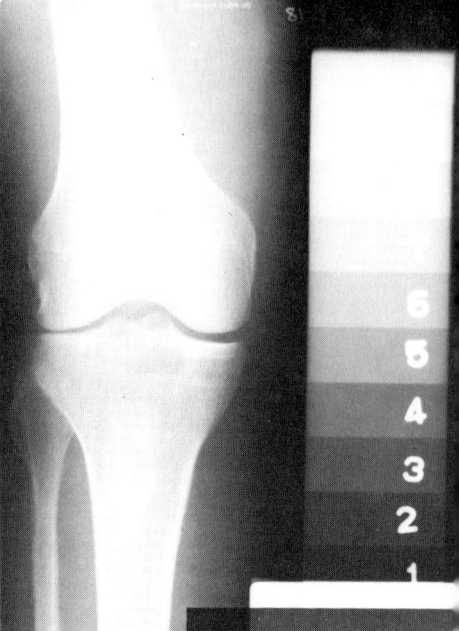

Figure 3.10. Improper washing in automatic processing. Development and fixing have been correct. Note the build-up of silver.

Figure 3.11. The result of cold chemicals in automatic processing. Note the loss in density.

What effect can be expected when the developer-recirculating system is not functioning?

Light films and generally lower density.

What causes grayed-out films of insufficient contrast and density?

Assuming that the x-ray equipment is functioning properly, the main reason is usually exhausted developer caused by underreplenishment, or improper mixing (usually overdilution). Replenishment rates may be set too low or there is probably a mechanical problem, e.g.:

(a) The microswitch is not operable;
(b) The pump is not operable;
(c) Air has gained entry into replenishment lines;
(d) There is a kink or blockage of the replenishment lines.

One clue to underreplenishment is a gelatin coating on the downpath rollers in the developer tank. This coating is sometimes green to grayish in color, an indication of lack of hardening.

Ninety-second processing allows increased utilization of examination rooms and equipment and also the handling of more patients, with no expansion of facilities or staff. It means significant speeding up of fluoroscopic and other serial examinations that require processed films during the course of the examination.

The patient benefits by the greater efficiency of the radiologic team through better care. Nearly immediate delivery of processed films means greater patient comfort, through shortened serial examinations, and elimination of patient callbacks. The radiologist can often start treatment sooner, and anesthesia time doing special procedures can be significantly reduced.

Processing

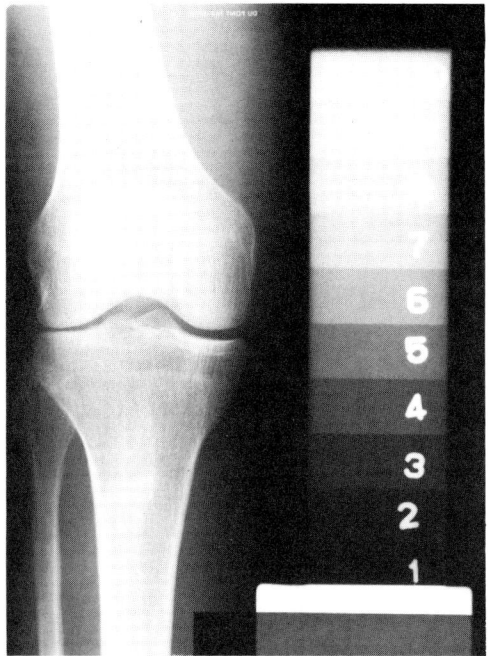

Figure 3.12. A result of automatic processing with solutions at the correct temperatures. Compare with Figure 3.11.

The technologist becomes more efficient working with the 90-second processing system. Immediate film access reduces film loss or misplacement. Quality improves because technique can be checked before the patient leaves the room. Finished radiographs can be correlated with the technique used.

MISCELLANEOUS ARTIFACTS

Dirt deposits

Irregular deposit, often light in color, generally elongated in direction of film travel (see Figure 3.13), is caused by dirt or precipitate in water supplied to washing section. If condition is temporary, clean wash rack and replace wash water in processor; drain wash tank when shutting processor down. If condition persists, use filters in incoming water lines. (Some dirt deposits can be removed from the dry radiograph by gentle rubbing with dry cotton or a soft cloth.)

Pi lines, so called because they occur 3.14 times the diameter of a roller away from the leading edge of a film (see Figure 3.14), are most common in newly installed or freshly cleaned processors. They tend to disappear with use of processor. Some processors are equipped with buffer rollers at the exit of the wash rack, which remove the deposit before the radiograph enters the dryer.

Guide marks, regularly spaced scratches or high-density lines (see Figure 3.15), are due to improperly adjusted guides in processor. Check clearances between guide devices and adjacent rollers or other components.

FORMULATING X-RAY TECHNIQUES

Figure 3.13. Surface deposits can be caused by dirt in the wash water supplied to an automatic processor. [Courtesy, Radio Markets Division, Eastman Kodak Company.]

Figure 3.14. "Pi line," thought to be caused by minute deposit left on a roller by the leading edge of film. The deposit is then carried around and transferred to the film. [Courtesy, Radio Markets Division, Eastman Kodak Company.]

Figure 3.15. Guide marks are caused by improperly adjusted film guides in automatic processors. They are regularly spaced and in the direction of film travel. [Courtesy, Radio Markets Division, Eastman Kodak Company.]

Processing

Table 3.1. FILM TROUBLE CHART

Condition	Cause	Correction
Light film	Underexposure	Increase Ma.-time or Kv.P. Decrease distance
	Bucky cut-off	Check tube center and distance
	Equipment—	
	1. Valve tube failure	Replace valve tube
	2. Line voltage too low	Adjust compensator
	3. Gassy x-ray tube	Replace x-ray tube
	4. Incorrect technique	Check technique chart and control adjustments
	5. Increased filtration	1. Check added filters
		2. If inherent filter has increased because of melting copper or tungsten, increase Kv.P. or replace tube
	6. Wrong type of film	Check type of film
Dark film	1. Overexposure	Reduce Ma.-time-Kv.P. Increase distance. Check for two exposures on one film
	2. Incorrect technique	Check technique chart and control adjustment
	3. Fog	Check for radiation or light leaks
Blank film	1. No x-ray	1. Check all fuses
		2. Check circuit breaker
		3. Check voltage selection for dead buttons
		4. Check interlock switches
		5. Check hand-foot-switch selector
		6. Check under- or over-table tube selection
		7. Check tube overload protection
		8. Check meter readings. If above does not correct trouble, call service man
	2. Cassette placement	If cassette is lead-backed, check whether or not it was placed in holder backwards
	3. X-ray tube alignment	Correctly center x-ray tube to film
Grey film	Fog	1. Use Bucky or grid
		2. Use collimation or cone
		3. Reduce Kv.P.
		4. Check for light or radiation leaks

FORMULATING X-RAY TECHNIQUES

Table 3.2. AUTOMATIC PROCESSING TROUBLES AND REMEDIES

Trouble	Cause	Remedy
Incorrect film density	Incorrect developer starting mix	Replace with correct solution.
	Developer reaching exhaustion	Replace developer with a starting mix and check replenishment.
Incorrect film density, continued	Over or underreplenishment due to: a. Valve shut off or line clogged b. Microswitch not properly adjusted or not functioning properly c. Flow not correct d. Flowmeter inaccurate e. Air in the lines f. Incorrect film feeding methods g. Leak in system h. Replenisher pump failure	a. Open valve or clean line. b. Check and adjust. c. Adjust flowmeter knob. d. Replace tube and ball. e. Bleed air out. f. See film feeding diagrams. g. Stop leak. h. Replace pump.
	Developer contaminated with fixer (fixer rack used in developer tank by mistake)	Replace developer with starting mix. Be sure fixer rack is in fixer tank. Keep splash guard over developer tanks when removing or replacing fixer rack. Add chemicals through replenisher pump housings.
	Developer temperature too low	Check heaters. Adjust thermostat.
	Inadequate wash-water flow	a. Be sure the stop valves in the water-mixing valves are completely open. b. Be sure all valves in the supply lines are open. c. Check the supply pressure. d. Clean the strainer screens. e. Check that there is not an accumulation of lime deposits within the mixing valve or in the strainers and check valves.
Increase in film density	Developer temperature too high Developer replenishment rate too high	Adjust thermostat. Feed small films in pairs and larger films with long dimension parallel to feed rollers. Check that replenishment rate is correct on flowmeter, then measure overflow from developer tanks to verify this rate.
	Concentration of developer too high	If replenishment rate is correct, remix developer replenisher to proper concentration.
Films stick in dryer	Solution temperatures too high	Adjust thermostat.

Processing

Table 3.2, continued

Trouble	Cause	Remedy
Films stick in dryer, continued	Incorrect developer starter mix (hardener not added)	Remix solution.
	Developer dilution or under-replenishment	Replace developer with starting mix. Check replenishment flow. If not controllable with flowmeter, clear possible restriction or air lock in lines.
	Fixer exhaustion or under-replenishment	Replace fixer. Check replenishment flow. If not controllable by flowmeter, clear possible restriction or air lock in lines.
	Solutions improperly mixed or contaminated	Replace with correctly mixed solutions.
	Foam in solution tanks	Check for air leaking into replenisher lines, recirculating pumps, etc., or clogged drain tube or fitting.
	Recirculation rate of solutions low	Check pumps. Check for clogged or air-locked lines.

	Improper washing	If flow is less than 4 gpm (15 liters/min.):
		a. See "Incorrect Film Density" above.
		b. Clear possible restriction in solenoid valves.
		c. If water flow is completely shut off:
		  1) Be sure the stop valves in the water mixing valve are open.
		  2) Be sure all valves in the supply line are open.
		  3) Check for failure of cold water supply pressure.
		d. If water temperature varies:
		  1) Check for lime deposits around the piston of the water mixing valve, causing it to bind in the piston cylinder.
		  2) Test the thermostatic motor.
		e. If water flow is untempered hot or cold water, replace the thermostatic motor in the water mixing valve.

Drying streaks on film	Dirty air tubes	Clean.

FORMULATING X-RAY TECHNIQUES

Table 3.2, continued

Trouble	Cause	Remedy
Drying streaks on film, continued	Air tubes out of position	Readjust.
Dirty film	Dirty water	Install filter in supply lines.
Scratched film	Improperly seated rollers	Realign and seat properly.
Pi line on films	Fresh chemicals	Lines will disappear after short run.
	Developer contaminated with fixer	Replace developer with starting mix.
Films not drying	Dryer motor running backwards (at installation)	Interchange 2 or 3 power wires.
	Clogged air filter	Replace if necessary.
	Dryer temperature too low	Check thermostat setting.
	Heater burned out	Replace.
	No exhaust air flow	Repair the exhaust blower or clear clogged vent pipe.
	Chemical imbalance	Check replenishment. Replace fixer and/or developer if suspect.
Fogged film	Light leaking into darkroom	Caulk openings.
	Cover on wet section of processor not fastened properly	Refasten.
	Developer contaminated with fixer	Replace developer with starting mix.
	Chemical imbalance	Replace chemicals.
Other film processing problems	Streaking	Weak developer.
	Mottling	Excessive developer concentration.
	Yellow smudges	Fixer exhausted.
	Lack of clearing	Excessive fixer concentration.
Solids separate out of developer during mixing	Mixing at incorrect temperature	All liquids should be 100–120° F. (38–49° C.) when mixing.
	Pouring additive in too rapidly	Follow mixture exactly.

Processing

Table 3.2, continued

Trouble	Cause	Remedy
Solids separate out of developer during mixing, continued	Excessive hardener	Use with caution.
Water flows when mixing valve is shut off	Faulty shut-off disc	Replace the shut-off disc.
	Faulty piston cylinder	Replace the piston cylinder.
Maximum water temperature specified is not attainable	Hot water supply to mixing valve not hot enough	Be sure temperature of hot water supply to mixing valve is at least 30° F. (18° C.) above the temperature setting.
Leak occurs around temperature adjustment handle of mixing valve	Packing gland nut not tight	Tighten.
	Faulty packing	Replace packing.

Chapter 4. CONES, DIAPHRAGMS, COLLIMATORS, FILTERS, GRIDS, AND STEREORADIOGRAPHY

One of the most important factors in the production of good quality radiographs is the use of *cones, lead diaphragms,* or *collimators.*

CONES

The value of a cone is far greater than most technologists realize. Cones are most important in the control of secondary-radiation fog. By limiting the port of entry of the primary beam, less tissue is irradiated and less secondary radiation is emitted to fog the film. The greatest benefit derived from the use of cones is the increase in contrast (Figure 4.1); contrast makes *detail* more plainly visible. Radiographic *density* is also affected, since the total density is reduced in proportion to the amount of secondary-radiation fog that is eliminated. See Figures 8.38 and 8.39 (in Chapter 8), radiography of the gallbladder, and Figures 4.2–4.7.

COLLIMATORS

Collimators are devices for shaping the x-ray beam and centering it on a part, usually more flexible and sophisticated than cones and diaphragms.

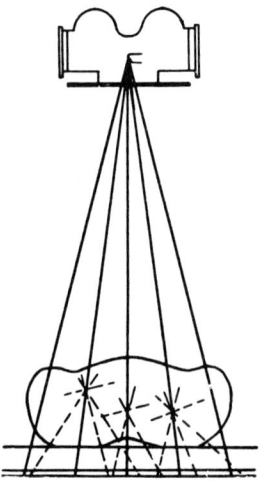
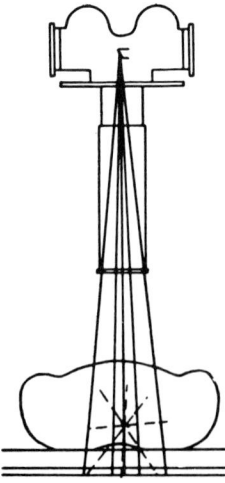

Figure 4.1. Effect of the cone upon density and contrast. In the diagrams at left, it is to be assumed that only the central portion of the body section shown is of diagnostic interest. In the first diagram, without cone, it will be seen that secondary radiation set up in portions of the body outside the area of interest but within the area irradiated by the x-ray tube can reach the film: the resulting secondary-radiation fog will increase density and reduce contrast in the radiograph. The second diagram demonstrates the use of a cone to restrict radiation to the area of interest. Since the area in which secondary radiation can be set up is reduced, secondary-radiation fog density in the resulting radiograph will be reduced and contrast will be improved.

Cones, Grids, Stereoradiography

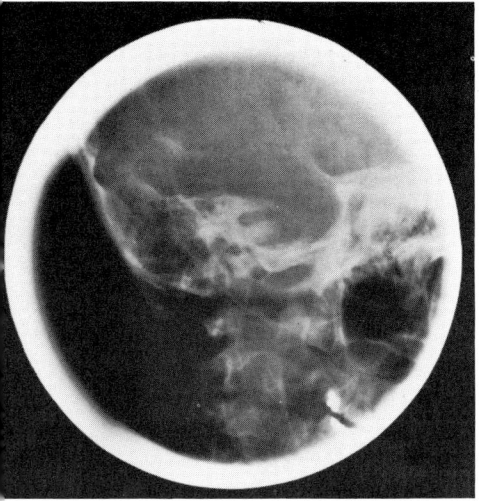

Figure 4.2. Radiograph showing the use of a cylinder cone: Stenvers view.

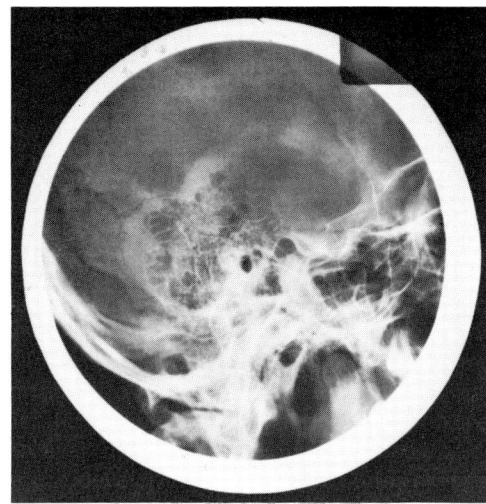

Figure 4.3. Radiograph of the lateral mastoid, with a cylinder cone.

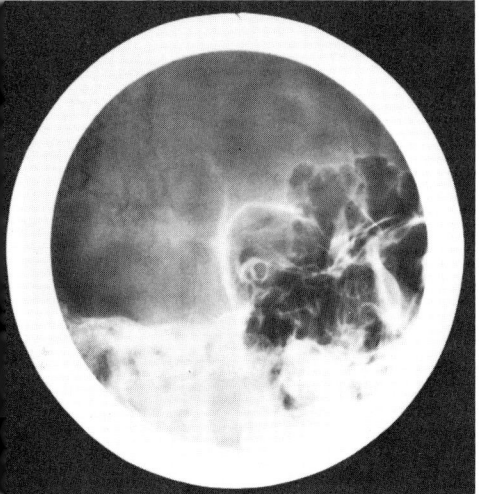

Figure 4.4. Radiograph of the optic foramen, with a cylinder cone.

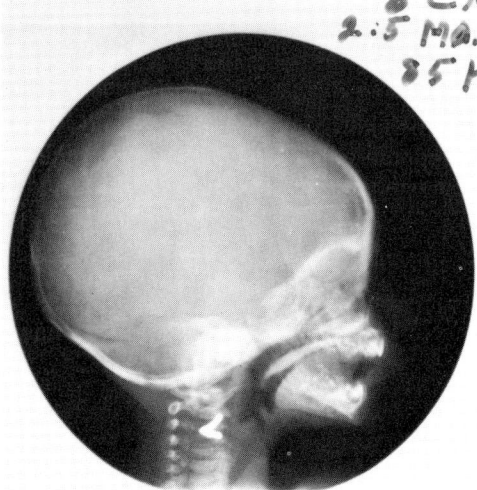

Figure 4.5. Radiograph of an infant skull, with a cylinder cone.

The modern collimator uses light to center the x-ray beam and produces openings by means of several sets of adjustable shutters. Thanks to exact positioning and limiting of the beam area, the patient need not be exposed unnecessarily to x-radiation, and the off-focus radiation that may fog the film is avoided. Available beam shapes vary from near-circular polygons, large and small, to rectangular slots with choice of axis (Figure 4.8). The collimator often allows for the insertion of filters and measuring tapes.

More than seventy years ago, in the April 4, 1903, issue of *The Electrical Review,* an article on "The Form of the Opening in the Diaphragm Plate of

FORMULATING X-RAY TECHNIQUES

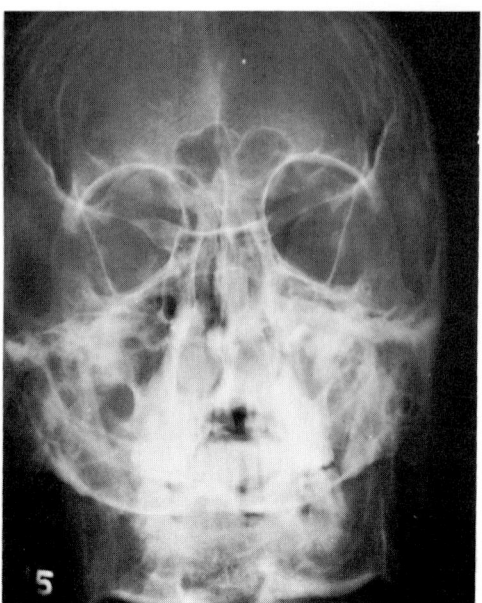 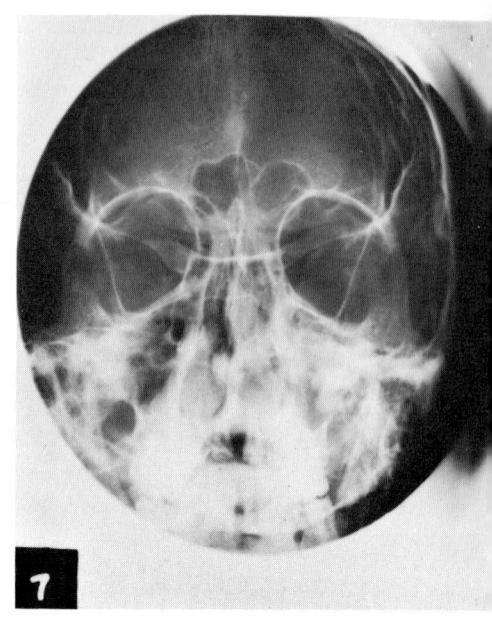

Figure 4.6. A radiograph taken without a cone. Note the lack of contrast and increased fog density.

Figure 4.7. The same area as in Figure 4.6, taken with a cone.

the X-Light Tube Box and on a Means of Adjusting the Size of the Beam of X-Light" made a statement that holds good today:

> The opening in the diaphragm plate of the X-light tube box should be rectangular for diagnostic and photographic work because this is the form of the fluorescent screen and photographic plate. If we use a round opening, the section of the cone of X-light escaping from the tube box is a circle. [See Figure 4.9.] It is evident the only part of the illumination which will be useful will be that included in the rectangular area of the largest plate or screen. All the X-light (radiation) which strikes the patient outside the rectangular area *PS* is objectionable, for it is unwise to expose a patient unnecessarily; besides the excessive illumination fogs the plate.

The collimator takes the guesswork out of localizing and centering the part to the film. Scattered radiation is controlled, producing better radiographic contrast; and there is a reduction of radiation to the patient. The collimator shows exactly the body area to be exposed *before* the exposure is made.

FILTERS

The filters normally used in radiography are sheets of aluminum placed between the x-ray tube and the part to be exposed. The thickness of the filter will depend upon the kilovoltage employed, but external filtration of *at least* 2 mm. of aluminum is recommended.

It has long been customary to use a 2-mm. aluminum filter in medical radiography. Such a filter is known to remove some of the *softer* x-rays, which would be almost completely absorbed in the patient and would be of

Cones, Grids, Stereoradiography

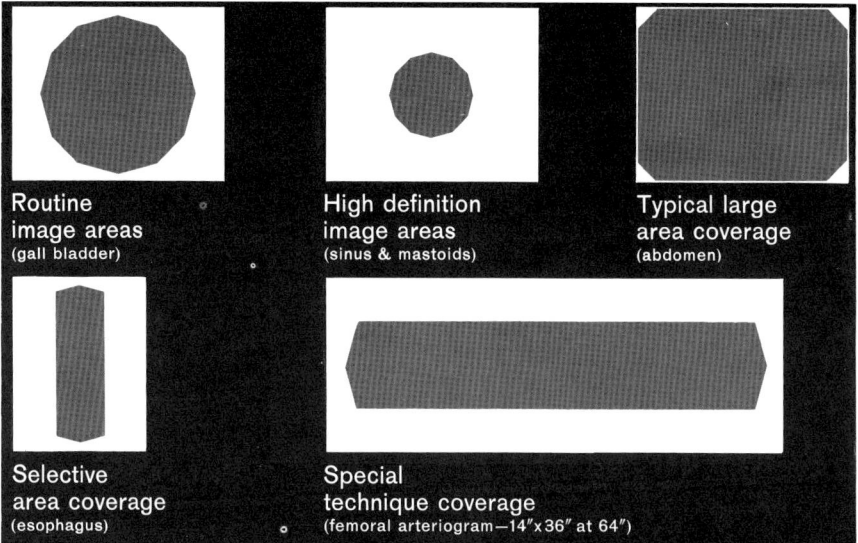

Figure 4.8. Some examples of beam shapes ("geometry") available from the shutter systems of a modern collimator.

no value to the radiographic image. Radiation of this nature, absorbed by the patient, contributes to his radiation dosage. Trout and his co-workers studied the effect on radiographic contrast of various amounts of filtration and the corresponding reduction in the patient dosage. They found that from 1 to 3 mm. of aluminum could be used, depending on the body part, without detrimentally affecting the radiographic image quality.

Gianturco, Miller, and Wenks use 2 mm. of aluminum up to 50 Kv.P., 4 mm. between 50 and 90 Kv.P., and 6 mm. between 100 and 120 Kv.P.

Figure 4.9. How the rectangular diaphragm improved the shape of the x-ray beam.

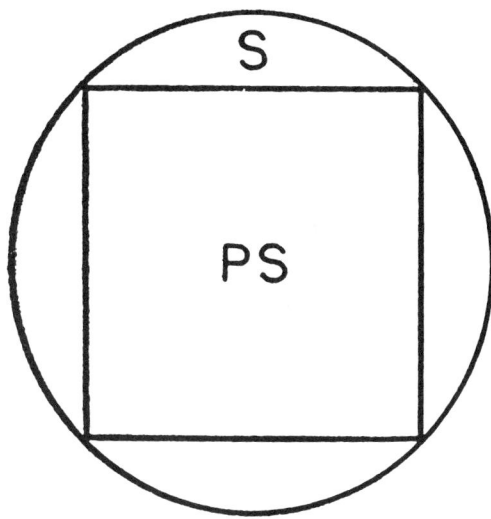

FORMULATING X-RAY TECHNIQUES

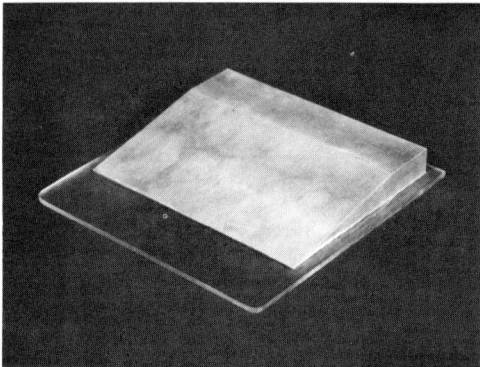

Figure 4.10. A wedge filter.   Figure 4.11. A trough filter.

The author has found 3 mm. total filtration to be adequate up to 100 Kv.P.; the resulting radiographs are of superior quality to those in which 1 or 1½ mm. of aluminum was used. No additional adjustments in milliampere-seconds were required except in chest radiography at 80 Kv.P., for regular film in a cardboard holder for extremities, and low-voltage infant extremity techniques.

According to Trout, Kelley, and Cathey, added filtrations of up to 2 mm. of aluminum at voltages up to 70 Kv.P., and above 70 Kv.P. 3 mm. or 0.1 mm. of copper, produce no significant changes in the radiograph. They state further, that at 130 Kv.P. and thick parts, even 0.25 mm. of copper does not alter the radiograph.

WEDGE AND TROUGH ALUMINUM ADAPTER FILTERS

The wedge and trough adapter filters provide uniform density throughout the radiograph in certain examinations where body parts vary widely in opacity. The filters *hold back* radiation where body parts transmit too much radiation and *increase* it where body parts transmit too little. Thus, one radiograph of uniform density serves where two were required previously.

The DuPont Company offers two types of compensating filters, the wedge and trough filters, made of machined wrought aluminum. Each filter is designed for a specific examination.

THE POTTER-BUCKY DIAPHRAGM

The grid diaphragm was invented by Gustav Bucky of Germany in 1913; however, it was not very practical, since it was used in a stationary position. Dr. Hollis Potter of Chicago made the Bucky practical by moving the grid during the radiographic exposure, a procedure that blurred the grid lines out of the image. The grid has since been known as the Potter-Bucky diaphragm.

A series of articles published in the early thirties by R. B. Wilsey presented the results of quantitative determinations of the proportion of scattered radiation in the radiography of a water phantom, under a variety of combinations of thickness, kilovoltage, and field size. These papers, which are con-

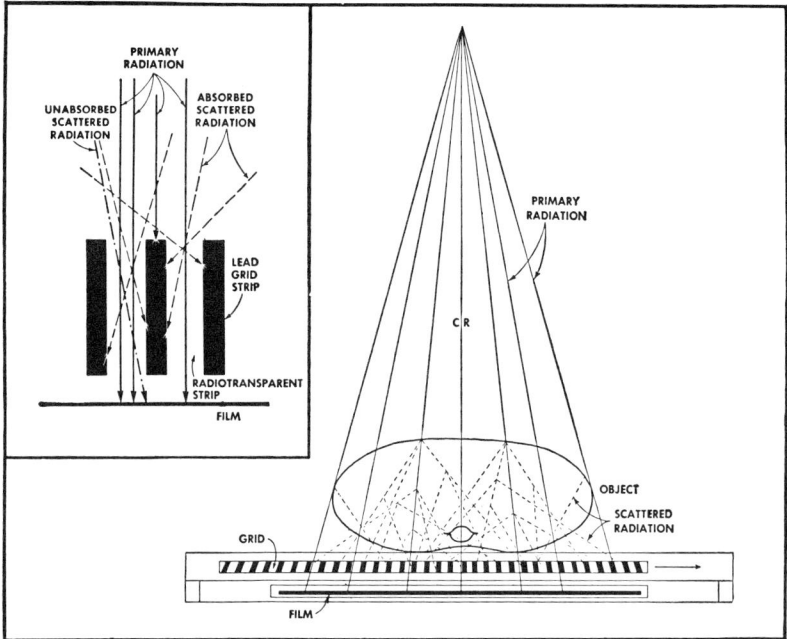

Figure 4.12. Left, detail of a grid. Note how a large portion of the scattered radiation is absorbed, but image-forming radiation passes through. Right, diagram of a Potter-Bucky diaphragm.

sidered classics in their field, showed an increase in scatter with increase in each of these three variables.

In 1949 Trout, Graves, and Slauson published a paper in which they showed the effect of the use of high-ratio grids on radiographic contrast at the higher kilovoltages. This work was undertaken because of the increasing interest in extending the kilovoltage range up to 130 Kv.P. Because of their greater efficiency in the removal of the scattered radiation, the use of high-ratio grids made possible the production of radiographs of satisfactory contrast at high kilovoltage, and at the same time reduced tube loads and radiation dosages to the patient.

There is, however, a limit to the advantages gained by grids and the use of higher kilovoltages. Wilsey showed that the exposure of the normal adult chest of medium size is formed by about 45 per cent primary radiation and 55 per cent scattered radiation. This fact led Seemann and Splettstosser to do research on subject contrast employing an 8-to-1 and a 16-to-1 grid. They found by employing a 5.7 cm. phantom which approximated the normal chest, that in subject contrast, and with such relatively small amounts of scattered radiation, an 8-to-1 grid is almost as useful as a 16-to-1 grid. The 16-to-1 grid should be employed only when it offers a significant advantage by increasing subject contrast. Several types of examinations in which higher kilovoltage (120–150 Kv.P.) and 16-to-1 grids have been widely accepted are pregnancy studies and gastrointestinal, colon, and lateral lumbar spine radiography. The 12-to-1 grid now seems to be the most popular grid for general radiography.

FORMULATING X-RAY TECHNIQUES

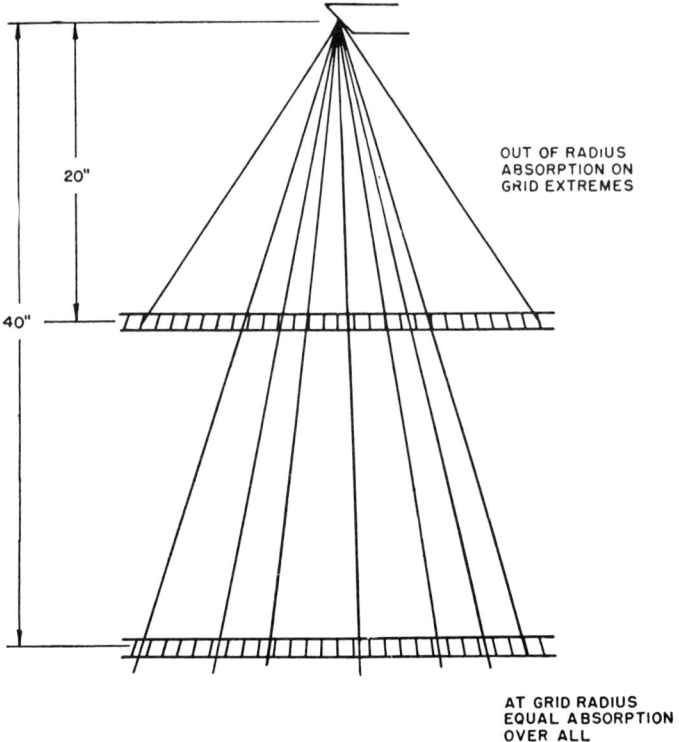

Figure 4.13. The effect of grid radius and distance on absorption.

Since the first grid was built in 1913, Bucky's principle of *lead foil* strips standing on edge separated by x-ray-transparent interspacers has remained the only known way to trap the secondary or scattered radiation.

Crossed grid for Potter-Bucky diaphragm

The Liebel-Flarsheim Company is now manufacturing a cross-hatch grid for use in its Recipromatic Potter-Bucky Diaphragm. This cross-hatch grid equals the 16-to-1 linear grid for clean-up and freedom from grid pattern, yet allows generous positioning latitude. It is especially good for high kilovoltage work. Its only *contra-indication* is for *angled techniques.* This is the first full size cross-hatch grid for Bucky radiography and is available in focus-film distance ranges of 34 to 44 inches, and 48 to 72 inches, at 80 lines per inch. The actual ratio is 8 to 1 with an *effective* ratio of 16 to 1 plus.

Grid cut-off

There are certain restrictions one must observe when employing a grid. These restrictions concern the *centering* of the x-ray tube, *direction* of stereoshift, direction and degree of *tilt* of the x-ray beam, and the choice of *focus-film distance.*

All of these factors are involved with the direction of the primary beam in its passage through the grid. Ratio governs the amount of restriction placed on the technologist. A low-ratio grid is easy to work with because some off-

Cones, Grids, Stereoradiography

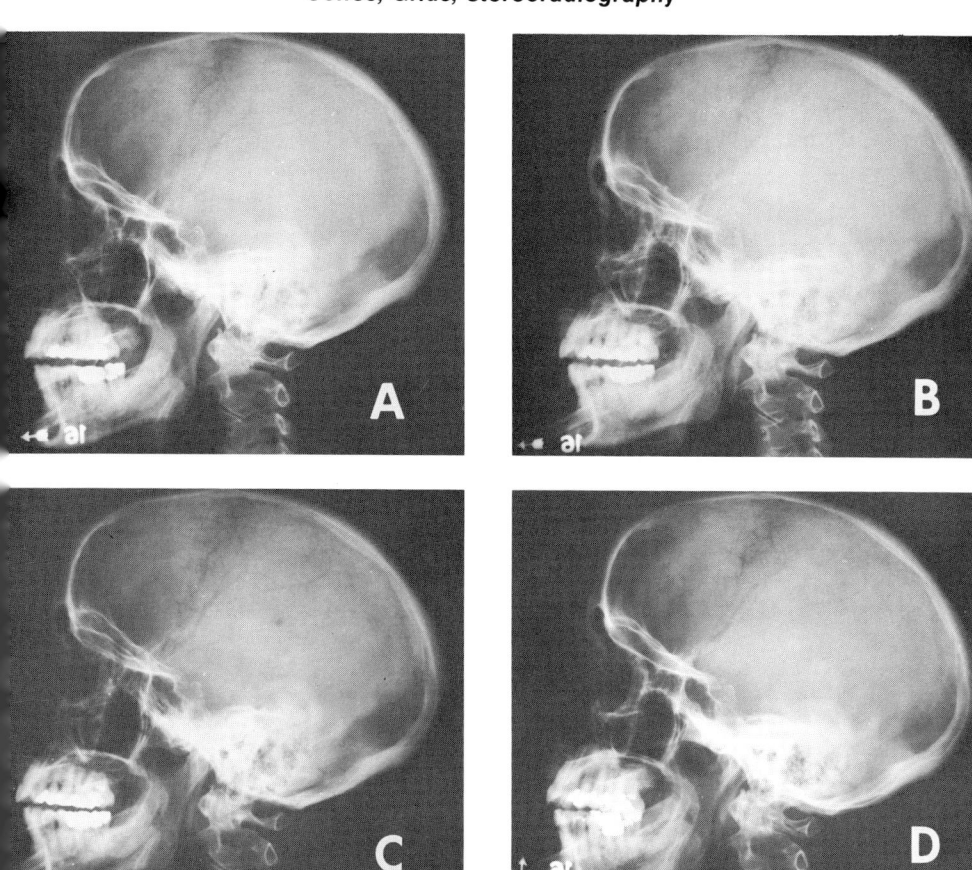

Figure 4.14. Radiographs of a skull made in stereo with a 16-to-1 grid. A and B are made with a crosswise (horizontal) shift; C and D with an up-and-down (vertical) shift.

centering and distance change can be tolerated, while a high-ratio grid requires very precise centering and operation only at the focal distance of the grid.

The ratio of a grid is defined as the *relation of the height of the lead strips to the width between them.* Thus, with interspacers 8 times as high as they are wide, a grid is said to be 8-to-1 ratio or "8-to-1."

STEREORADIOGRAPHY

An ordinary photograph made with a camera shows perspective: the relative positions and sizes of the various objects shown in the photograph are readily apparent. This is not true of a radiograph because it is a shadow picture of overlying parts having various opacities to x-ray. The single radiograph does not necessarily show the depth in the structures.

Stereoradiography is relatively simple for all modern x-ray machines and almost any region of the body may be stereoradiographed with little effort; however, two requirements must be kept in mind: namely, perfect position-

FORMULATING X-RAY TECHNIQUES

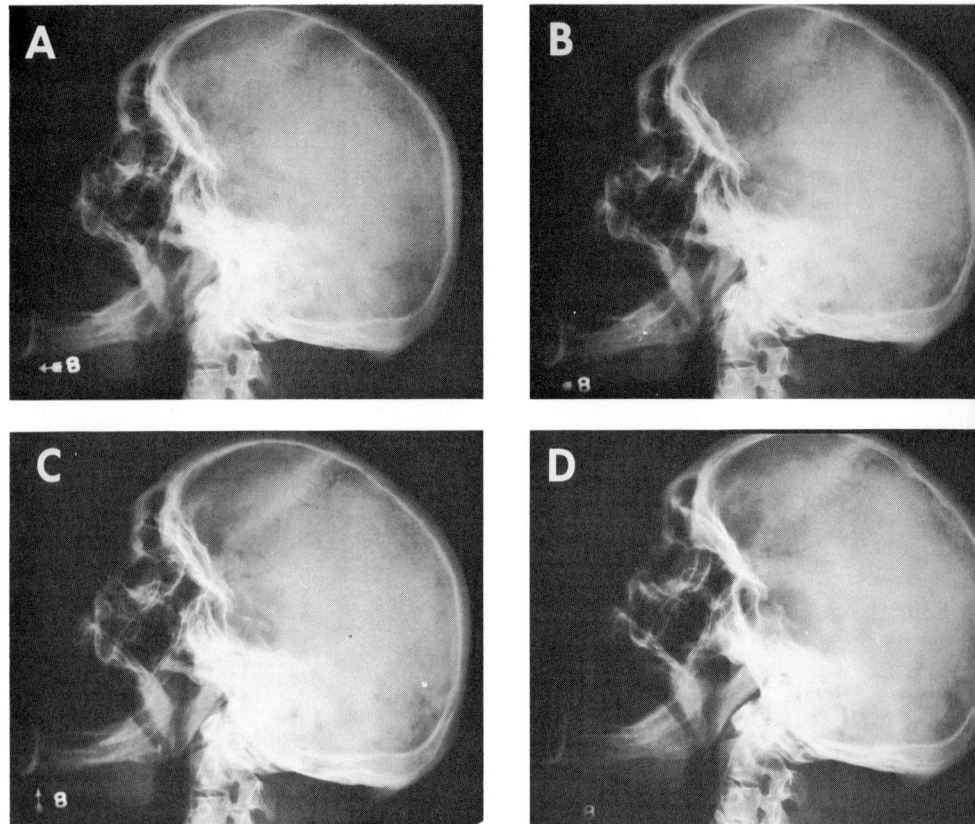

Figure 4.15. Radiographs of the skull made with an 8-to-1 grid. A and B have a crosswise (horizontal) shift; C and an up-and-down (vertical) shift.

ing and complete immobilization. Stereoscopic vision is directly dependent upon the definition in the radiographic images as well as the degree of stereoscopic shift and a moderately long anode-film distance (36 inches) for creating a greater depth of focus.

Stereoscopic films are made by exposing two films; the part of the body and the film are in exactly the same position, but with a different position of the anode of the tube for each exposure. In stereoscopic views of the chest the plate must be changed without disturbing the part, and this is provided for by the use of a cassette changer.

In exposing stereoscopic films, the distance and direction of the shift of the tube between the two exposures are both of considerable importance. Normally the distance of the tube is controlled by the construction of the stereoscope in which the films are to be examined; using a stereoscope with a 25-inch distance between the mirrors and the view boxes, a $2^{1}/_{2}$-inch stereo shift would be required. *Generally speaking, the tube shift in stereoscopic radiography should be 10 per cent of the anode-film distance.*

The direction of the tube shift in exposing stereoscopic film is controlled by the direction of the predominating lines in the parts being radiographed. The tube shift should be as nearly as possible at right angles to the line. In the thorax the predominating lines are the borders of the ribs; therefore

Cones, Grids, Stereoradiography

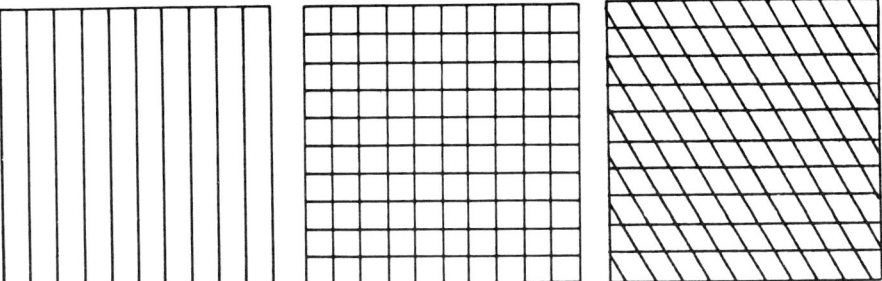

Figure 4.16. Three common grid patterns: linear (left), crossed (middle), and rhombic (right).

the tube shift should be along the vertebral column. In making films of the long bones, the shift should be across the bones; for those of the skull it may be in either direction, depending on which structures are to be investigated. In exposing stereoscopic films, the parts to be radiographed are placed in position as for a normal single radiograph. For the first film from the center position, the tube is moved in the proper direction one-half of the distance of the shift. It is now in position for the exposure of the first film, and when this has been made, the tube should be moved past the center position an equal distance and the second film exposed.

Stereo shift and grids

With a 5-to-1 or 6.5-to-1 Bucky grid, one may stereo-shift across the grid strips. Tube centering is not critical, and the focus-film distance can be changed through a reasonable range. As grid ratio increases, cross-shift stereoscopic exposures become difficult. The difficulty is in *matching* the density of the two films of the stereo pair. It is recommended that cross-table stereo-shifting be abandoned when using an 8-to-1 grid. When a 16-to-1 grid is used, cross-shift stereoscopic radiography is impossible. The radiographic tube must be centered precisely over the midline of the table and focus-film distance must be fixed at the focal distance of the grid. Whenever an underexposed radiograph results from a technique that has been giving consistent results with a 16-to-1 grid, always check the *tube centering.* The tube may have been "off center" to account for the underexposure.

Linear grids vs. cross-hatch. The term "linear" refers to a grid that has lead lines running in only one direction. Linear grids are very popular and versatile.

If cross-hatch grids are used, it is impossible to tilt the tube more than just enough to accomplish a stereo-shift in either direction. Cross-hatch grids are normally used for high kilovoltage at a fixed distance and the central ray aligned at 90° to the grid surface.

Off-distance cut-off. Off-distance cut-off occurs when a grid is used at a focus-film distance greater or less than the focus distance of the grid. It appears on the radiograph as areas of *decreased* density along the outside edges of the film or on the fluoroscopic image (Figures 4.17 and 4.18).

Stereoradiography: accessory nasal sinuses

Caldwell projection. In the posteroanterior projections of the sinuses, it

FORMULATING X-RAY TECHNIQUES

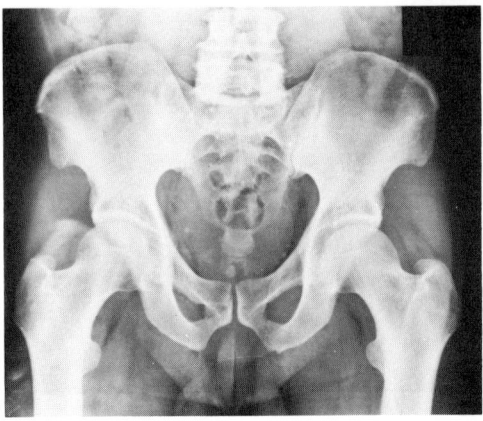

Figure 4.17. An example of grid cut-off.

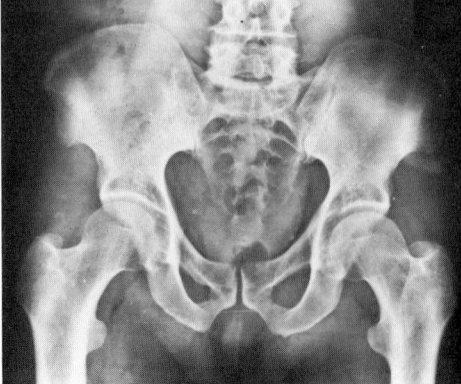

Figure 4.18. The grid cut-off of Figure 4.17 corrected.

is important that the stereoscopic shift be made vertical and *front to back* and *never crosswise,* in order to prevent overshadowing of the anatomy of interest by the oblique projection of adjacent structures.

The normal Caldwell projection should throw the shadow of the petrous portion of the temporal bone in the upper portion of the maxillary sinuses.

Waters projection. When using the Waters projection for the maxillary sinuses, the shadow of the petrous portions of the temporal bone should be thrown below, or caudad to the antra. The tube shift should be made toward the top of the head (cephalad), so the antra will be free of superimposed structures.

Lateral projection. In the lateral projections, the tube shift may be horizontal or vertical.

Sphenoid, open-mouth projection. The tube shift should be horizontal (cephalad).

STATIONARY GRID

The stationary grid is a modern application of the original Bucky principle — elimination of secondary radiation by means of a mechanical grid placed between the film and the body part being examined. There are numerous applications where there is need for elimination of secondary x-ray but where the Potter-Bucky diaphragm cannot be employed. The stationary grid is used for fluoroscopy, portable radiography, spot-film radiography, and unusual techniques, such as large chest radiography (Figures 4.19 and 4.20), and oblique cervical spine radiography which require target-to-film distances above the limits of regular Potter-Bucky diaphragms.

Stationary grids are of two types, *parallel* and *focused* (Figure 4.21). In the parallel grid the lead strips are not angulated; it is used where the film is of limited width or where the target-to-film distance is great. Any application requiring the use of a wide film at moderate target-to-film distance calls for the use of a focused grid in which angulation of the lead strips is present. The focused grids are aligned for either 30- or 36-inch focus-film distance.

Cones, Grids, Stereoradiography

Table 4.1 STEREOSCOPIC TUBE SHIFTS FOR COMMON FOCUS-FILM DISTANCES UNDER PRACTICAL VIEWING CONDITIONS

	For eye-image distance of		
	25 inches	28 inches	30 inches
Focus-film distances (inches)	Use tube shift (inches) of:	Use tube shift (inches) of:	Use tube shift (inches) of:
25	2 9/16	2 1/4	2 1/16
30	3 3/16	2 3/4	2 9/16
36	3 7/8	3 7/16	3 1/8
42	4 5/8	4 1/16	3 3/4
48	5 3/8	4 11/16	4 5/16
60	6 13/16	6	5 1/2
72	8 5/16	7 1/4	6 11/16
84	9 3/4	8 1/2	7 7/8
96	11 3/16	9 13/16	9 1/16

SELECTION OF A GRID

The selection of a grid to be used for a particular radiograph will be primarily dependent on the following considerations:

1. Relative quantity of secondary radiation produced by subject being radiographed;
2. Kilovoltage technique to be used;
3. Capacity of x-ray generator.

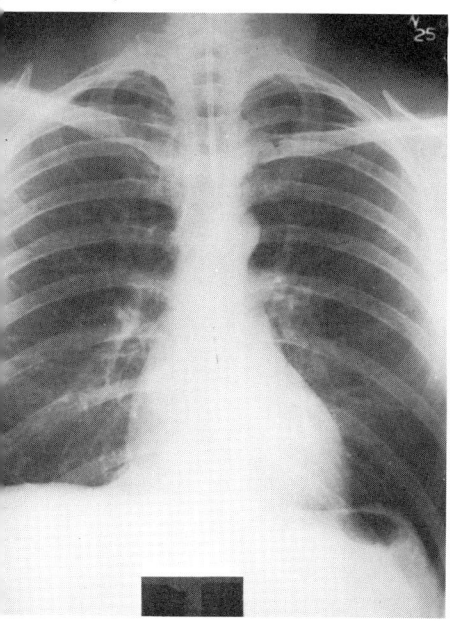

Figure 4.19. Chest radiograph of a large patient, made without a grid.

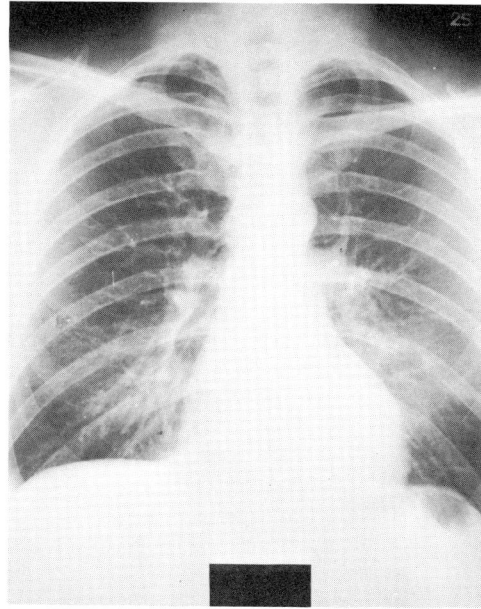

Figure 4.20. Radiograph of the patient of Figure 4.19, made with a grid cassette.

FORMULATING X-RAY TECHNIQUES

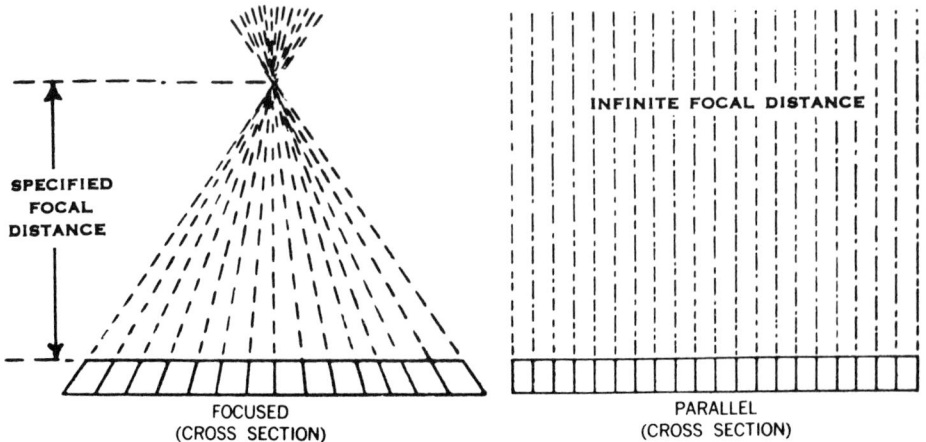

Figure 4.21. Cross sections of two grid arrangements: left, a focused grid with progressively angled leads; right, a parallel grid.

The quantity of secondary radiation produced is dependent on the thickness and relative density of the body volume being radiographed. A non-grid exposure of the chest will consist of about one-half secondary radiation, while a non-grid exposure of the abdomen may consist of more than 90 per cent secondary radiation. From this, it is apparent that for dense body sections the more effective remover of secondary radiation will provide the most striking improvement in the radiograph, and this suggests the use of a high-ratio grid or a crossed grid. The choice between these two grids depends on the ease of aligning the grid correctly relative to the x-ray tube, and whether a high- or low-kilovoltage technique is to be used. If there is any question of the possibility of proper centering and leveling, or if low kilovoltages are to be used, the crossed grid of 5-to-1 ratio will present much greater advantages from the standpoint of positioning latitude and cleanup. For high-kilovoltage techniques, particularly if the grid can be accurately aligned or if it is mounted in a Potter-Bucky diaphragm, greater advantages will be gained with the high-ratio linear grid or an 8-to-1 rhombic grid. (Crossed grids are not recommended for the techniques that require angling of the x-ray tube.)

At kilovoltages of the order of 100 Kv.P. or more, comparable photographic effect requires lower Ma.S. values than at low kilovoltages to keep the radiation dosage to the patient low. However, in order to maintain the same contrast range at the higher kilovoltage, it is necessary to use a grid of higher ratio. The exposure factors are not the same for all ratios, and the increased exposure required for a high-ratio grid may to some extent reduce the patient-dosage advantage gained by going to high-kilovoltage techniques. In general, in spite of the higher exposure factors involved, the use of high kilovoltage and high-ratio grids will result in somewhat lower radiation dosage to the patient.

All technologists must work within the limitations of the physical characteristics of the x-ray equipment at their disposal. While this may not be as important a consideration in the selection of a grid as some others, it is a

Cones, Grids, Stereoradiography

factor to be considered. For instance, the maximum benefits to be derived from a 16-to-1 grid will not be realized with a unit whose top limit is 90 Kv.P., although there will be some advantages over a lower-ratio grid. In general, a 16-to-1 grid will do the most good with equipment which can be used at kilovoltages above 100 Kv.P. This applies also, to a lesser extent, to the 12-to-1 grid. With a bedside or portable unit, where the likelihood of near-perfect alignment of the grid relative to the primary beam is poor, the use of the high-ratio grids is practically impossible, and difficulties may be encountered even with the 8-to-1 grids. For such use, where wide latitude in distance, centering, and leveling is necessary, the 5-to-1 grid is advisable, and for maximum cleanup under these conditions the 5-to-1 crossed grid is ideal.

Table 4.2 GRID CHARACTERISTICS

Type of grid	Features and uses
4:1 ratio, linear (low dose)	Special grid for use in image intensification and spot-filming. It offers adequate cleanup for small coned-down areas, combined with relatively small patient dosage.
5:1 ratio, linear	Moderate cleanup. Extreme latitude in use. Use at lower kilovoltages (up to 80 Kv.P.) wherever wide latitude is desired. Very easy to use.
5:1 ratio, crossed	Very high cleanup, especially at lower kilovoltages. Extreme latitude in use. Use up to 100 Kv.P. wherever wide latitude and excellent cleanup are desired. Very easy to use. Not recommended for tilted-tube techniques.
6:1 ratio, linear	Moderate cleanup. Good positioning latitude. Easy to use.
8:1 ratio, linear	Better cleanup than 5:1 linear. Fair distance latitude. Little centering and leveling latitude. Use up to 100 Kv.P. where wide latitude is not required.
12:1 ratio, linear	Better cleanup than 8:1. Very little positioning latitude. Use for both low and high kilovoltage techniques (up to 110 Kv.P. or slightly higher). Extra care is required for proper alignment in use. Usually used in a fixed mount or Potter-Bucky diaphragm.
16:1 ratio, linear	Very high cleanup. Practically no positioning latitude. Intended primarily for use above 100 Kv.P. in a Potter-Bucky diaphragm. Excellent for high-kilovoltage radiographs of thick body sections.
8:1 ratio, crossed	Extremely high cleanup. Superior to 16:1 ratio linear grid at kilovoltages up to 125. Positioning latitude equivalent to 8:1 ratio linear. Not usable for tilted-tube techniques.
10:1 ratio, 133 line, linear	Special grid for maximum line invisibility. Cleanup similar to 8:1 linear. Very little positioning latitude. Extra care is required for proper alignment in use. Best grid to use stationary in a table to replace the moving Bucky grid.

FORMULATING X-RAY TECHNIQUES

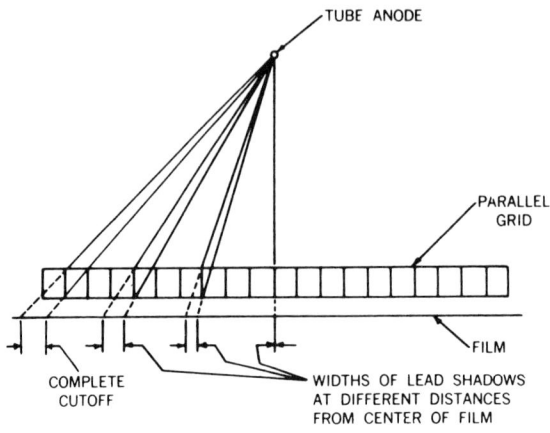

Figure 4.22. Primary cutoff in a parallel grid.

Faulty use of grids

A primary cutoff can easily occur with a parallel grid. As may be seen in Figure 4.22, only the leads directly under the tube anode in a parallel grid throw shadows no wider than themselves on the film. All other leads in the grid make shadows which are wider than the thickness of the lead by amounts proportionate to their distances from the centerline. This cutoff of primary radiation results in progressively decreased density as the edge of the film is approached. Compensation through tapering grid thickness toward the edges (prismatic focus) is undesirable because grid ratio decreases and effectiveness is lost beyond the center portion of the film.

In off-distance cutoff in a focused grid (Figure 4.23) the effect is much the same as when a parallel grid is used; i.e., there is a progressive decrease in density as the edge of the film is approached. However, if the grid is used within its specified focus range this effect should not be objectionable.

In off-center and off-level cutoff (Figure 4.24) the effect is somewhat different than with tube off-distance. Since all the leads are out of correct

Figure 4.23. Off-distance cutoff in a focused grid.

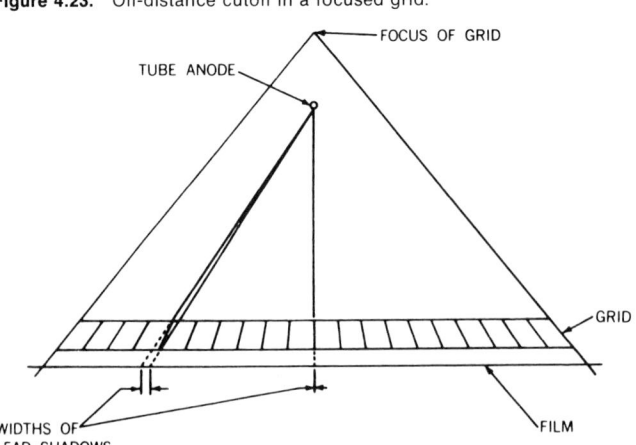

Cones, Grids, Stereoradiography

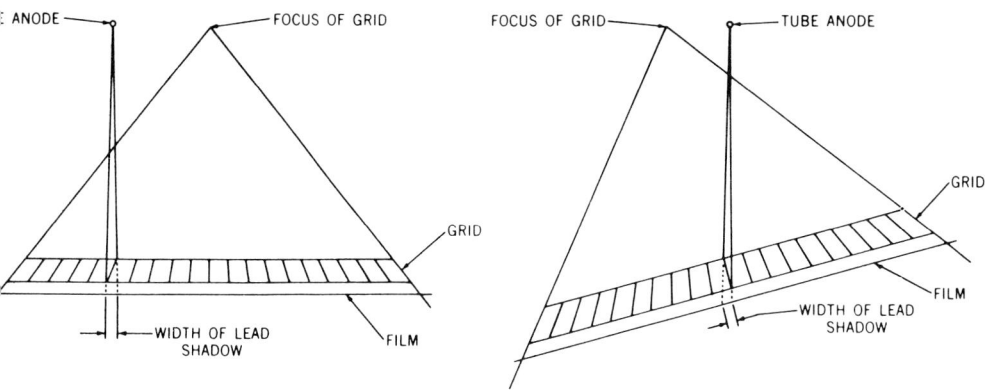

Figure 4.24. Off-center and off-level cutoff in a focused grid.

alignment with the primary rays, the entire film will show a lighter density than it should with proper alignment of the grid. Local misangulations in the grid are also much more apparent when it is used off-center or off-level. These conditions should be carefully avoided with grids of 8-to-1 ratio or higher.

Care is also worth taking to compensate for the effect of grid ratio. In Figure 4.25 radiation at angle X will be more attenuated by passing through more leads in the high-ratio grid than in the low-ratio. The maximum angle of fully transmitted secondary radiation will also be smaller for a high-ratio grid than for a low-ratio grid. This clearly indicates why high-ratio grids remove more scatter and require increased exposure.

The Potter-Bucky diaphragm

When a Potter-Bucky diaphragm is used, the exposure must be increased enough to compensate for:

1. A reduction of about 85 per cent (depending on grid ratio) in the intensity of the *secondary radiation* reaching the film.
2. A slight reduction in the intensity of the *primary radiation* reaching the film, due to the filtration of the table top and the Bucky grid. Under average

Figure 4.25. The effect of ratio on cleanup.

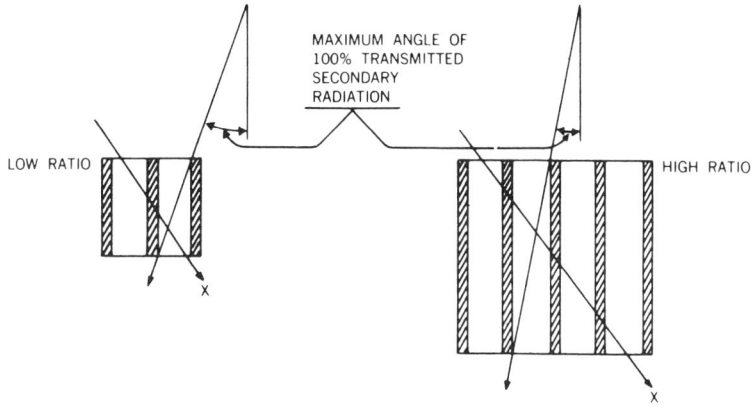

FORMULATING X-RAY TECHNIQUES

circumstances, a Bucky technique requires at least *3 times as much exposure as non-Bucky technique* or an increase in Kv.P. — approximately 20 Kv.P. for an 8-to-1 grid. Stationary grids require slightly less exposure than that required for a Potter-Bucky diaphragm.

The smallest cone possible should be used for *every part.* A grid should be used for any part which is solid and not air-contained, or where there is edema or accumulation of fluid. In *general,* a grid should be considered for any part 12 centimeters and above except some small parts, sinuses, lateral mandible, etc.

In converting a non-grid technique to a grid technique, we must increase either the *Ma.S.* or the *kilovoltage* because of the absorption of the grid. Tables 4.3 and 4.4 may be used as guides in determining the conversion factor.

Table 4.3 GRID CONVERSION FACTORS IN Ma.S.

From No-Grid	To	Ma.S.
	5-1	Use $1\frac{1}{2}$ times the Ma.S.
	6-1	Use 2 " " "
	8-1	Use 3 " " "
	12-1	Use $3\frac{1}{2}$ " " "
	16-1	Use 4 " " "

Table 4.4 GRID CONVERSION FACTORS IN Kv.P.

From No-Grid	To	Kv.P.
	5-1	add 8 Kv.P.
	6-1	add 12 Kv.P.
	8-1	add 20 Kv.P.
	12-1	add 23 Kv.P.
	16-1	add 25 Kv.P.

Note: To change from an 8-to-1 grid to a 16-to-1 grid, add 6 Kv.P. or increase Ma.S. by 30 per cent.

Example: A non-grid technique for the A.P. knee calls for:

 36-inch focus-film distance
 100 Ma.
 $\frac{1}{10}$ second
 screens
 60 Kv.P.

If it is desired to increase the contrast scale by employing the 8-to-1 grid, we would then use: 36-inch focus-film distance

 100 Ma.
 $\frac{3}{10}$ second
 screens
 8-1 grid
 60 Kv.P.

If we wanted to use Kv.P. for our conversion, we would use 80 Kv.P. and all other factors constant. See Figures 10.31 and 10.32.

GRID ABSORPTION

The approximate percentages of secondary radiation absorbed by grids of various ratios are: 5-to-1, 75 per cent; 6-to-1, 85 per cent; 8-to-1, 90 per cent; 12-to-1, 95 per cent.

A large part of the density produced on a film by an exposure made without a grid is due to secondary radiation, and because the grid itself absorbs some primary radiation, it is necessary to increase the exposure when a grid is used. The amount of increased Ma.S. or Kv.P. is dependent upon the *grid ratio* and the *kilovoltage* being used. See Tables 4.3 and 4.4 for conversion factors.

THE ANODE HEEL EFFECT

Various investigators have drawn attention to the angular distribution of radiation intensity from the anode face. Experiments have been described in which ionization measurements were made of the intensities emitted at various angles. The results were illuminating: a wide range of intensities that could have positive radiographic effect was demonstrated. But little more than academic interest has been awakened for applying this inherent characteristic of all x-ray tubes—the "heel effect"—to influence balanced radiographic densities in the image. It must be understood that evidence of the heel effect does not signify a tube fault, for it is an advantageous characteristic of all x-ray tubes and is an invaluable means toward producing balanced radiographic densities (Figure 4.26).

Unexplainable radiographic density differences which could not always be attributed to the incorrect use of exposure factors have annoyingly occurred on radiographs in many x-ray departments. These annoyances have been largely attributable to improper alignment of the tube to the part so that the heel effect could not be properly employed.

The heel effect is a variation in x-ray intensity output (depending upon the angle of x-ray emission from the focal spot) along the longitudinal tube axis and in relation to the long axis of a film. The intensity diminishes fairly rapidly from the central ray toward the *anode* side of the x-ray beam; on the cathode side of the beam, intensity increases slightly over that of the central ray. Generally the heel effect is limited in its application at long focus-film distances. When average or short distances are used on large film areas, its effect is most advantageous, particularly where decided differences in tissue densities require balancing of radiographic densities to avoid over- and underexposures within the same image.

The approximate percentage of x-ray intensity emitted by a tube at various angles of emission may be determined directly from photometric measurements of the radiographic blackening of an x-ray film. For radiographic purposes, this procedure is adequate and gives an indication of the approximate percentage of quantity variation to be expected when the x-ray beam falls on specific areas of different sizes of x-ray films at various focus-film distances. Figure 4.26 graphically represents the mean values of radiographic density measurements obtained from many intensities emitted by various x-ray tubes. This diagram, drawn to scale, shows radii emanating from the target face, drawn at 4° intervals from 0° to 40° and intercepting horizontal lines representing various focus-film distances. At the termination of the

FORMULATING X-RAY TECHNIQUES

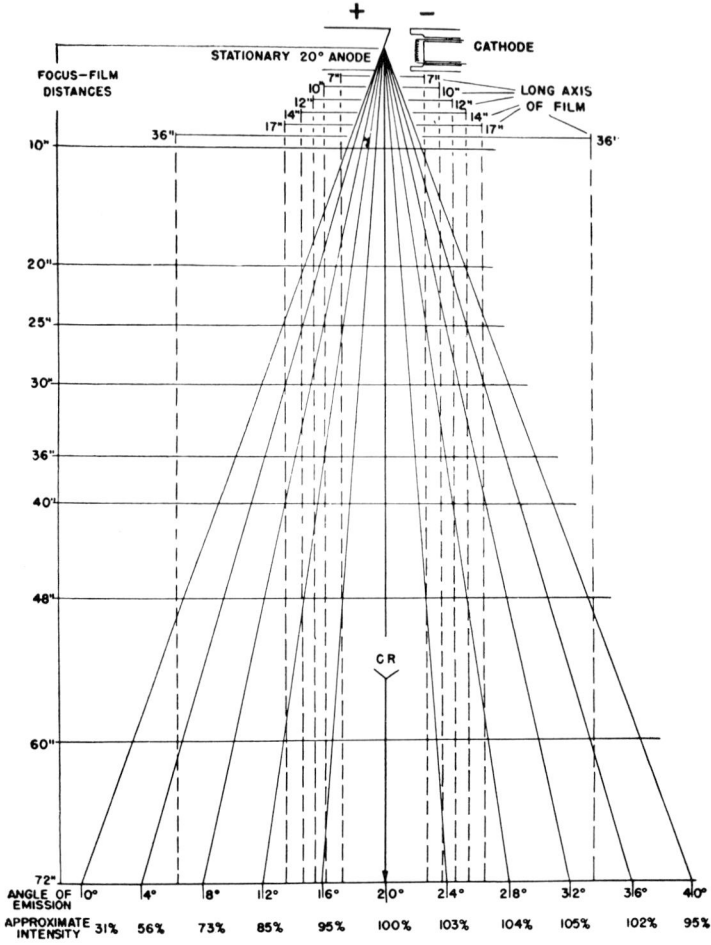

Figure 4.26. The anode heel effect. [Courtesy, Eastman Kodak Co.]

radii at the bottom of the chart, the mean density values in percentages are indicated. For convenience, the radiographic density caused by the central ray (CR) is figured as 100 per cent. To the left or anode side of the central ray, the densities diminish in value, while those to the right or cathode side increase moderately and then decrease slightly.

The spaces between the vertical dotted lines beginning just below the diagram of the anode and terminating at the 72-inch focus-film distance line, when approximately paired, indicate the length of each size of film and the approximate location at various focus-film distances of the respective density values created by the intensities of radiation at various angles of x-ray emission. For example, on the 48-inch focus-film distance line the outermost pair of vertical lines representing the 36-inch length of film passes outside the limits of the x-ray beam. In order to make use of the entire range of intensities on this length of film, it would be necessary to employ a focus-film distance of 49 inches. All intensity radii would intercept at this distance;

Cones, Grids, Stereoradiography

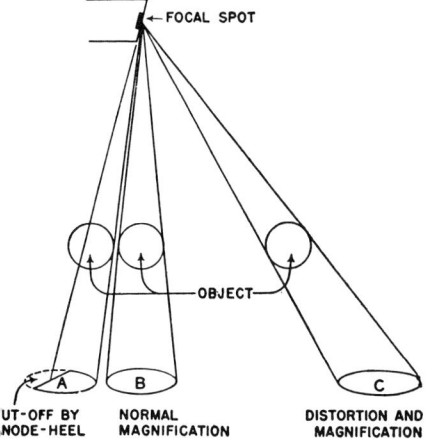

Figure 4.27. Limiting factors in short-focus radiography on large film sizes.

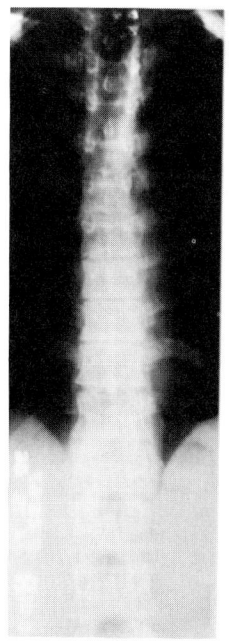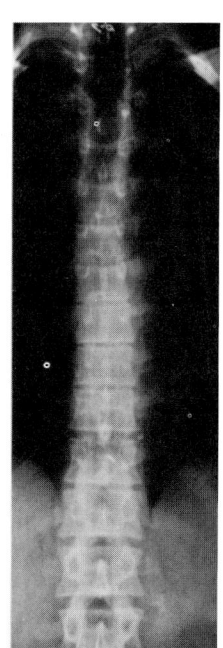

Figure 4.28. Anteroposterior screen-grid radiographs of thoracic vertebrae that demonstrate the density variation caused by the anode heel effect. Left, cathode portion of x-ray beam directed cephalad. Right, cathode portion directed caudad (toward greater body thickness). Note more favorably balanced densities over entire image in the righthand radiograph.

consequently, if an exposure were made, the entire range of intensities would be expected to become evident, let us say, on a radiograph of an entire spine. Since the minimal intensity in the anode portion of the beam, approximately 31 per cent, is emitted in advance to the angle indicated as 0°, it is obvious that the portion of the spine having least tissue density (the neck) should be exposed by this portion of the beam and the heavier portion (the lumbar vertebrae) by the cathode portion of the beam.

When radiographs on large film are made at relatively short focus-film distances, a knowledge of the distribution of the intensity in approximate percentages delivered to a particular size of film at a known focus-film distance is indispensable to correct alignment of the tube and part to the film at the most favorable focus-film distance. Radiographic densities cannot be balanced if only the intensity of the central ray is considered (Figure 4.27).

Radiographs are often secured in which a certain area of the image is definitely underexposed while another is overexposed, even though the factors seemed adequate for the tissue-density traversed by the central ray. This condition usually occurs when improper alignment of the tube relative to the part takes place. This lack of balance between radiographic densities is typical of the heel effect of the anode when it is improperly applied (Fig. 4.28).

The general rule for utilizing the heel effect is as follows: *Align the long axis of the tube parallel with the long axis of the part to be examined and direct the cathode portion of the beam toward the anatomic area of greatest tissue density.*

Chapter 5. SIMPLIFIED MATHEMATICS IN RADIOGRAPHY

A great many problems in radiography can be reduced to mathematics. Technique problems and conversions can be quite accurately calculated. Such calculation represents a much more scientific approach to radiographic technique than the old "hunch method" of radiography. This chapter of simple arithmetic is intended to refresh the student's mind on the fundamentals that are essential for the proper understanding of the modern physical principles of radiography. It is taken for granted that the student technologist has had an elementary course in high school mathematics.

FRACTIONS

A. A fraction has a numerator and a denominator. The number above the line is called the numerator and the number below the line, the denominator.

Example: In the fraction $3/4$, the number 3 is the numerator, and the number 4 below the line is the denominator. This fraction, $3/4$, indicates that 3 is being divided by 4.

B. In multiplying fractions, take the product of the numerators and place it over the product of the denominators and then simplify this new fraction.

Example:

$$\frac{3}{4} \times \frac{4}{5} = \frac{3 \times 4}{4 \times 5} = \frac{12}{20}$$

C. To reduce, simply divide the numerator and the denominator by the same number.

Example:

$$\frac{12}{20} = \frac{6}{10} = \frac{3}{5}$$

D. In computing Ma.S. values, it is often convenient to use the decimal equivalent of the fractional exposure.

Example:

$5/8$ second would be: .625. See Table 7.7 in Chapter 7.

E. The word "of" is often used to mean "multiply."

Example:

$$1/2 \text{ of } 1/2 = 1/2 \times 1/2 = 1/4$$

Mathematics in Radiography

EQUATIONS

In solving equations we place the unknown on the left and solve for the unknown first.

Example:

$$\frac{a}{b} = \frac{c}{d} \qquad \text{Find } a$$

$$a = \frac{bc}{d}$$

This means *a* is equal to *b* times *c*, divided by *d*.

If a letter or number from the right is taken, we place it on the lower left and the letter or number on the bottom left goes to the upper right.

Example:

$$d = \frac{bc}{a} \qquad c = \frac{ad}{b}$$

DECIMALS

A decimal, which is a number with a decimal point (.), is actually a fraction, the denominator of which is understood to be 10 or some power of 10.

A. The number of digits, or places, after a decimal point determines which power of 10 the denominator is. If there is one digit, the denominator is understood to be 10, etc.

Example:

$$.7 = {}^{7}/_{10}, \quad .39 = {}^{39}/_{100}, \quad .727 = {}^{727}/_{1000}.$$

B. The addition of zeros after a decimal point does not change the value of the decimal.

Example:

$$.9 = .90 = .900 \text{ and vice versa,}$$
$$.900 = .90 = .9$$

C. Since a decimal point is understood to exist after any whole number, the addition of any number of zeros after such a decimal point is written in does not change the value of the number.

Example:

$$6 = 6.0 = 6.00, \text{ etc.}$$

PERCENTAGES

The per cent sign (%) is a symbol used to indicate percentage, but no operations can be performed with the number to which it is attached. For convenience, then, it is sometimes required to attach a per cent sign, but to perform operations with the number, it is necessary to remove the sign.

FORMULATING X-RAY TECHNIQUES

A. In general, to remove a per cent sign, divide the number by 100.

Example:

$$900\% = 9$$

B. A per cent may be expressed as a decimal or a fraction by dividing it by 100.

Example:

$$43\% = .43$$
$$7\% = \tfrac{7}{100} \text{ or } .07$$

C. A decimal may be expressed as a per cent by multiplying it by 100.

Example:

$$.39 = 39\%$$

RATIO

A. A ratio expresses the relationship between two (or more) quantities in terms of numbers. The mark used to indicate ratio is the colon (:) and is read as "is to."

Example:

The ratio 6:7 is read "6 is to 7."

B. A ratio represents the function of division. Therefore, any ratio of two terms may be written as a fraction, and any fraction may be written as a ratio.

Example:

$$7:8 = \tfrac{7}{8}$$
$$\tfrac{2}{5} = 2:5$$

C. To simplify any complicated ratio of two terms containing fractions, decimals, or per cents:

1. Divide the first term by the second.
2. Convert to a ratio.

Example:

Simplify the ratio $\tfrac{5}{6} : \tfrac{7}{8}$

Solution:

$$\tfrac{5}{6} \div \tfrac{7}{8} = \tfrac{5}{6} \times \tfrac{8}{7} = \tfrac{20}{21}$$
$$\tfrac{20}{21} = 20:21$$

D. There are two main types of ratio problems:

1. Problems in which the ratio is given.
2. Problems in which the ratio is implied, but not given.

E. To solve problems in which the ratio is given:

1. Add the terms in the ratio.
2. Divide the total by this sum.
3. Multiply each term in the ratio by this quotient.

Mathematics in Radiography

Example: A man bought three X-ray machines. The first one cost $1/4$ more than the second, and the third $1/2$ more than the second. He paid $30,000 for the three machines. How much did he pay for each?

Solution: The basic machine is the second one, which has the ratio value of 1. The first machine cost $1/4$ more than the second; therefore its ratio value is $1\frac{1}{4}$. The third machine cost $1/2$ more than the second, therefore its ratio value is $1\frac{1}{2}$.

Ratio of the costs = $1\frac{1}{4} : 1 : 1\frac{1}{2}$
$1\frac{1}{4} + 1 + 1\frac{1}{2} = \frac{15}{4}$
$\$30,000 \div \frac{15}{4} = \$8,000$
$\$8,000 \times 1\frac{1}{4} = \$10,000$
$\$8,000 \times 1 = \$8,000$
$\$8,000 \times 1\frac{1}{2} = \$12,000$
The first machine cost $10,000
The second machine cost $8,000
The third machine cost $12,000

PROPORTION

A. A proportion indicates the equality of two (or more) ratios, often expressed by the symbol ::.

Example

2:4 = 5:10 = 6:12 is a proportion. The meaning of 2:4::5:10::6:12 is the same.

B. If a proportion contains only four terms, the two outside terms are called the *extremes,* and the two inside terms are called *the means.*

Example: In the proportion 2:3 = 4:6, 2 and 6 are the extremes, and 3 and 4 are the means.

C. In any proportion of four terms, the product of the means equals the product of the extremes.

Example: Relation between milliamperage and time.

1. *Rule:* The milliamperage (M) required for a given exposure is inversely proportional to the time (T).
2. *Problem:* Suppose that 30 milliamperes (M_1) and an exposure time of $1/2$ second (T_1) have been employed, and it is desired to decrease the exposure time to $1/20$ second (T_2). What milliamperage (M_2) would be required?
3. *Solution:*

$M_1 : M_2 :: T_2 : T_1$ $\qquad \frac{x}{20} = \frac{15}{1}$

$30 : x :: 1/20 : 1/2$

$\frac{1}{20} x = 15$ $\qquad x = 15 \times 20$

$\qquad\qquad\qquad x = 300$

$\qquad\qquad\qquad x = 300$ milliamperes

65

Chapter 6. BASIC EXPOSURE EXPERIMENTS

The following experiments may be done on phantoms in order to give a better understanding of the basic principles of radiography. The experiments may be made by the instructor and a wealth of teaching material accumulated, or they may be made with each class in attendance.

By repeating these experiments, the technologist will acquire a knowledge of radiographic technique that cannot be gained in any other way.

Experiment 1: Focus-film density relation

Purpose. To demonstrate the relation between focus-film distance and radiographic density.

Theory. Any change in focus-film distance influences the intensity of radiation. The intensity varies inversely as the square of the focus-film distance. Since changes in distance produce changes in intensity, radiographic density changes.

Procedure 1. Make a series of three lateral radiographs of the skull using the following factors.

Film: Regular 10 x 12
Screens: Medium 10 x 12
Grid: 8 to 1
Distance: Variable factor
Filter: 2-mm. aluminum
Cone: To film
Ma.S.: 15
Time: $1/10$ sec.
Ma.: 150
Kv.P.: 85
Development: Automatic

Variable factors:
  Exposure 1: 25-inch FFD
  Exposure 2: 36-inch FFD
  Exposure 3: 48-inch FFD

Comment. It may be observed that as the FFD increased, the radiographic density decreased.

Procedure 2. Follow the same routine as in procedure No. 1, but radiograph a postero-anterior hand.

Film: Regular 8 x 10
Cardboard holder: 8 x 10

Basic Exposure Experiments

Grid:	None
Distance:	Variable factor
Filter:	2-mm. aluminum
Cone:	To film
Ma.S.:	70
Time:	$7/10$ sec.
Ma.:	100
Kv.P.:	50
Development:	Automatic

Variable factors:
  Exposure 1: 25-inch FFD
  Exposure 2: 36-inch FFD
  Exposure 3: 48-inch FFD

Experiment 2: Time-FFD density relation

Purpose. To demonstrate the interrelation of time of exposure and focus-film distance to radiographic density when all other factors are constant.

Theory. The time required for a given radiographic density is directly proportional to the square of the FFD when all other factors are constant.

Procedure. Make these postero-anterior radiographs of the hand employing the following factors.

Film:	Regular 8 x 10
Cardboard holder:	8 x 10
Grid:	None
Distance:	Variable factor
Filter:	2-mm. aluminum
Cone:	To film
Ma.S.:	Variable factor
Time:	Variable factor
Ma.:	50
Kv.P.:	50
Development:	Automatic

Variable factors:	FFD	Time	Ma.S.
Exposure 1:	25 inches	$1/2$ sec.	25
Exposure 2:	36 inches	1 sec.	50
Exposure 3:	48 inches	$1^{8}/_{10}$	90

Comment. The densities of these radiographs are approximately the same, because suitable exposure-time compensation has been made for each FFD change in accordance with the inverse square law.

It is recommended that once an FFD is established for a given projection, it should be considered a constant.

Experiment 3: Milliamperage—FFD density

Purpose. To demonstrate the interrelation of milliamperage and focus-film distance to radiographic density.

FORMULATING X-RAY TECHNIQUES

Theory. When all other factors are constant, the milliamperage required for a given exposure is directly proportional to the square of the FFD.

Procedure. Make a series of three postero-anterior exposures of the hand, employing the following factors.

Film:	Regular 8 x 10
Cardboard holder:	8 x 10
Grid:	None
Distance:	Variable factor
Filter:	2-mm. aluminum
Cone:	To film
Ma.S.:	Variable factor
Time:	Variable factor
Ma.:	Variable factor
Kv.P.:	50
Development:	Automatic

Variable factors:	Ma.	FFD	Time	Ma.S.
Exposure 1:	10	25 in.	2 sec.	20
Exposure 2:	30	40 in.	$1^{3}/_{4}$ sec.	52.5
Exposure 3:	100	60 in.	$1^{2}/_{10}$ sec.	120

If the exact Ma. station listed is not available, use any combination of Ma. and Time to give correct Ma.S.

Comment. As the FFD changes, the Ma. and/or Ma.S. may be used to compensate for the normal loss in density. In routine radiography, however, Ma. should be established as a constant for a given projection whenever possible.

Experiment 4: Influence of Ma.S. on density

Theory. No practical amount of Ma.S. will compensate for inadequate kilovoltage.

Procedure. Make a series of eight radiographs of the hand phantom in the postero-anterior projection.

Film:	Regular 8 x 10
Cardboard holder:	8 x 10
Grid:	None
Distance:	36-in. FFD
Filter:	2-mm. aluminum
Cone:	To film
Ma.S.:	Variable factor
Time:	Variable factor
Ma.:	Variable factor
Kv.P.	30
Development:	Automatic

Exposure:	Ma.S.:
1	15
2	30
3	60

Basic Exposure Experiments

4	120
5	240
6	480
7	960
8	70 but use 50 Kv.P.

Be sure to check the tube-rating chart before making this experiment.

Comment. Only in radiograph No. 8 exposed for 70 Ma.S. at 50 Kv.P. do we have a *practical amount* of Ma.S. and *sufficient* kilovoltage to penetrate the part.

Experiment 5: Kv.P.–density relation

Procedure. Expose a series of four postero-anterior radiographs of the hand employing the following factors:

Film:	Regular 8 x 10
Cardboard holder:	8 x 10
Grid:	None
Distance:	36-in. FFD
Filter:	2-mm. aluminum
Cone:	To film
Ma.S.:	40
Time:	$4/10$ sec.
Ma.:	100
Kv.P.:	Variable factor
Development:	Automatic

Variable factors:
Exposure 1:	40 Kv.P.
Exposure 2:	50 Kv.P.
Exposure 3:	60 Kv.P.
Exposure 4:	70 Kv.P.

Comment. The overall density of the radiographs increases with the Kv.P. Successive increases in kilovoltage cause corresponding increases in density because of greater tissue penetration, since less radiation is absorbed by the tissues and more reaches the film.

Experiment 6: Testing film of two different manufacturers

Purpose. To find whether film A and film B of different manufacture may or may not be used interchangeably.

Procedure. A series of two radiographs of the skull in the lateral projections for each of the films should be made employing (1) low Kv.P. technique, and (2) higher Kv.P. technique.

Film:	Regular 10 x 12
Screens:	Medium 10 x 12
Grid:	8 to 1
Distance:	36-in. FFD
Filter:	2-mm. aluminum

FORMULATING X-RAY TECHNIQUES

Cone: To film
Ma.S.: Variable factor
Time: Variable factor
Ma.: 100 or 150
Kv.P.: Variable factor
Development: Automatic

Variable factors:	Kv.P.	Ma.S.
Film A Exposure 1:	62	70
Film A Exposure 2:	85	15
Film B Exposure 3:	62	70
Film B Exposure 4:	85	15

Constant factor:
All films should be exposed employing the same cassette.

Comment. In order to show that films A and B may be used interchangeably, the contrast and density should remain the same for each set of radiographs.

Experiment 7: Kv.P.-Ma.S.–density relation

Purpose. To prove that satisfactory overall density can be made comparable by using Ma.S. to compensate for the density effect of changing kilo voltage, provided the radiation penetrates the structure.

Procedure 1. A series of four lateral radiographs of the skull should be made employing the following factors:

Film: Regular 10 x 12
Screens: Medium 10 x 12
Grid: 8 to 1
Distance: 36-in. FFD
Filter: 2-mm. aluminum
Cone: To film
Ma.S.: Variable factor
Time: Variable factor
Ma.: Variable factor
Kv.P.: Variable factor
Development: Automatic

Variable factors:	Kv.P.	Ma.S.
Exposure 1:	65	60
Exposure 2:	75	30
Exposure 3:	85	15
Exposure 4:	95	7.5

Procedure 2. Postero-anterior radiograph of the hand.

Film: Regular 8 x 10
Cardboard holder: 8 x 10
Grid: None
Distance: 36-in. FFD
Filter: 2-mm. aluminum
Cone: To film

Basic Exposure Experiments

Ma.S.:	Variable factor	
Time:	Variable factor	
Ma.:	Variable factor	
Kv.P.:	Variable factor	
Development:	Automatic	
Variable factors:	Kv.P.	Ma.S.
Exposure 1:	50	70
Exposure 2:	60	30
Exposure 3:	70	20
Exposure 4:	80	10

Experiment 8: Effect of development and density

Purpose. To demonstrate that as development time increases, density increases.

Procedure. A series of 10 radiographs of the postero-anterior chest are made with the following factors:

Film:	Regular 14 x 17
Screen:	Medium 14 x 17
Grid:	None
Distance:	72-in. FFD
Filter:	2-mm. aluminum
Cone:	To film
Ma.S.:	3.3
Time:	$1/30$ sec.
Ma.:	100
Kv.P.:	80
Development:	Variable factor
Measurement of patient:	22 cm.

Variable factors:
  Exposure 1: Develop 1 min. at 68°
  Exposure 2: Develop 2 min. at 68°
  Exposure 3: Develop 3 min. at 68°
  Exposure 4: Develop 4 min. at 68°
  Exposure 5: Develop 5 min. at 68°
  Exposure 6: Develop 6 min. at 68°
  Exposure 7: Develop 7 min. at 68°
  Exposure 8: Develop 8 min. at 68°
  Exposure 9: Develop 9 min. at 68°
  Exposure 10: Develop 10 min. at 68°
  Manual processing

Experiment 9: Effect of temperature of developer on density

Purpose. To demonstrate the fact that as temperature increases, development time must be decreased to compensate for increased activity.

Procedure. Expose 4 postero-anterior radiographs of the chest with the following factors:

Film:	Regular 14 x 17

FORMULATING X-RAY TECHNIQUES

Screens: Medium 14 x 17
Grid: None
Distance: 72-in. FFD
Filter: 2-mm. aluminum
Cone: To film
Ma.S.: 3.3
Time: $1/30$ sec.
Ma.: 100
Kv.P.: 80
Development: Variable factor
Measurement of patient: 22 cm.

Variable factors:
Exposure 1: Develop $8\frac{1}{2}$ min. at 60°
Exposure 2: Develop 5 min. at 68°
Exposure 3: Develop $3\frac{1}{2}$ min. at 75°
Exposure 4: Develop 2 min. at 80°
Manual processing

Experiment 10: Compensation of density by Ma.S. with increased kilovoltage

No.	Region	Proj.	Cm.	Kv.	D.	Ma.	S.	Ma.S.	Scr.	Dev.	Fil.
1	Elbow	A.P.	7	40	36	100	$2\frac{3}{4}$	275	0	Automatic	Regular
2				50			$1\frac{1}{4}$	125			
3				60			.8	80			
4				70		50	.9	45			
5				80			.7	35			
6				90			.5	25			
7				100			.3	15			
8	Hand	P.A.		40		100	$1\frac{1}{2}$	150			
9				50		100	.4	40			
10				60		100	.2	20			
11				70		30	.4	12			
12				80		30	.25	7.5			
13				90		50	.1	5			
14				100		50	$3/40$	3.75			
15	Chest	P.A.	23	40	72	100	$7/10$	70	Average speed		Regular
16				50			$2/10$	20			

Basic Exposure Experiments

No.	Region	Proj.	Cm.	Kv.	D.	Ma.	S.	Ma.S.	Scr.	Dev.	Film	P-B
17				60			$1/12$	8.3				
18				70			$1/20$	5				
19				80			$1/30$	3.33				
20				90			$1/20$	2.5				
21				100		50	$1/30$	1.66				

Experiment 11: Increase in density with increase in kilovoltage

No.	Region	Proj.	Cm.	Kv.	D.	Ma.	S.	Ma.S.	Scr.	Dev.	Film	P-B
1	Chest	P.A.	23	50	72	100	$1/30$	3.3	Average speed	Automatic	Regular	0
2				60								
3				70								
4				80								
5				90								
6				100								

Experiment 12: Use of inverse square law in compensating density with increase in distance

As distance increases, density is compensated for by inverse square law.

No.	Region	Proj.	Cm.	Kv.	D.	Ma.	S.	Ma.S.	Scr.	Dev.	Film	P-B
1	Hand	P.A.	3	50	25	100	$2/10$	20	0	Automatic	Regular	0
2					30		$3/10$	30				
3					36		$4/10$	40				
4					40		$5/10$	50				
5					48		$7/10$	70				

FORMULATING X-RAY TECHNIQUES

Experiment 13: Decrease in density with increase in distance

As distance increases, density decreases, provided all other factors are constant.

No.	Region	Proj.	Cm.	Kv.	D.	Ma.	S.	Ma.S.	Scr.	Dev.	Film	P-B
1	Hand	P.A.	3	50	25	100	$4/_{10}$	40	0	Automatic	Regular	0
2					30							
3					36							
4					40							
5					48							

Experiment 14: Effect of small changes in Kilovoltage on density

Small changes in kilovoltage on direct exposure cause no readily discernible change in density.

No.	Region	Proj.	Cm.	Kv.	D.	Ma.	S.	Ma.S.	Scr.	Dev.	Film	P-B
1	Hand	P.A.	3	45	36	100	4	40	0	Automatic	Regular	0
2				46								
3				47								
4				48								
5				49								
6				50								
7				51								
8				52								
9				53								
10				54								
11				55								
12	Chest	P.A.	23	75	72	100	$1/_{20}$	3.3		Average speed	Regular	0
13				76								
14				77								
15				78								

Basic Exposure Experiments

No.	Region	Proj.	Cm.	Kv.	D.	Ma.	S.	Ma.S.	Scr.	Dev.	Film	P-B
16				79								
17				80								
18				81								
19				82								
20				83								
21				84								
22				85								

Experiment 15: Limited assistance of Ma.S. in removing secondary radiation fog

No.	Region	Proj.	Cm.	Kv.	D.	Ma.	S.	Ma.S.	Scr.	Dev.	Film	P-B
1	Chest	P.A.	23	80	72	100	$1/15$	6.66	Average speed	Automatic	Regular	0
2				90			$1/20$	5.				
3				100			$1/30$	3.33				
4				80			$1/30$	3.33				
5				90			$1/40$	2.5				
6				100			$1/60$	1.66				

Experiment 16: Rule of thumb—halving or doubling Ma.S. to balance densities when Kv.P. is fixed

No.	Region	Proj.	Cm.	Kv.	D.	Ma.	S.	Ma.S.	Scr.	Dev.	Film	P-B
1	Skull	Lat.	16	85	36	100	$1/20$	5	Average speed	Automatic	Regular	8-1
2							$1/10$	10				
3							9 imp.	7.5				
4	Skull	P.A.	18	80	36	100	$3/10$	30				
5						100	$3/20$	15				
6						50	$3/20$	7.5				
7				100		50	$2/10$	10				

FORMULATING X-RAY TECHNIQUES

Experiment 16, continued:

No.	Region	Proj.	Cm.	Kv.	D.	Ma.	S.	Ma.S.	Scr.	Dev.	Film	P-B
8							$1/10$	5				
9							$1/20$	2.5				
10	Shoulder	P.A.	14	60	36	50	$1/20$	2.5				0
11						50	$1/10$	5				0
12						50	$2/10$	10				0
13						100	$1/30$	3.3				0
14						100	$1/24$	4.125				0
15	1–7 Cervical vert.	Lat.	10.5	85	72	100	$1/20$	5				0
16						50	$1/20$	2.5				0
17						50	$3/40$	3.75				0
18	Chest	R. obl.	31.5	85	72	100	$1/10$	10				0
19							$1/20$	5				
20	Leg	Lat.	8.5	60	36	25	$1/30$	.83				0
21							$1/15$	1.66				0
22	Chest	P.A.	23	80	72	100	$1/15$	6.6				0
23						100	$1/30$	3.3				0
24						100	$1/60$	1.66				0
25	Lumbar	A.P.	20	70	36	100	$1/10$	10				8-1
26							.2	20				8-1
27							.3	30				8-1
28	Use immobilization						.4	40				8-1

Experiment 17: Influence of a grid in removing secondary radiation fog

No.	Region	Proj.	Cm.	Kv.	D.	Ma.	S.	Ma.S.	Scr.	Dev.	Film	P-B
1	Chest	P.A.	25	80	72	100	$1/24$	4.16	Average speed	Automatic	Regular	0

Basic Exposure Experiments

No.	Region	Proj.	Cm.	Kv.	D.	Ma.	S.	Ma.S.	Scr.	Dev.	Film	P-B
2	Chest			100	72	100	$1/24$	4.16				Lysholm
3	Chest	Lat.	35	90	72	200	$3/40$	15				0
4	Chest			100	72	200	$2/10$	40				Lysholm

Experiment 18: Influence of cones and presence or absence P-B grid in elimination of secondary radiation fog

No.	Region	Proj.	Cm.	Kv.	D.	Ma.	S.	Ma.S.	Scr.	Dev.	Film	P-B
1	Skull	P.A.	19	70	36	100	$6/10$	60	Average speed	Automatic	Regular	8-1
2	Skull											
3	Skull											
4	Skull											
5	Skull											
6	Skull	P.A.	19	70	36	100	$2/10$	20				0
7	Skull											
8	Skull											
9	Skull											

Nos. 1 and 6 — no cone
Nos. 2 and 7 — 13-in. cone
Nos. 3 and 8 — 8-in. cone
Nos. 4 and 9 — 6-in. cone
Or collimation equivalent

Experiment 19: Wide exposure latitude

Procedure 1.

Absorber:	Step Wedge
Film:	Regular 8 x 10
Cardboard holder:	8 x 10
Grid	None
Distance:	36-in. FFD
Filter:	2-mm. aluminum
Cone:	To film
Ma.S.:	10
Time:	$1/10$ sec.
Ma.:	100
Kv.P.:	Variable factor
Development:	Automatic

FORMULATING X-RAY TECHNIQUES

	Ma.S.	Kv.P.
Exposure 1:	10	60
Exposure 2:	10	70
Exposure 3:	10	80
Exposure 4:	10	90
Exposure 5:	10	100

Procedure 2.

Part:	AP elbow
Film:	Regular 8 x 10
Cardboard holder:	8 x 10
Grid:	None
Distance:	36-in. FFD
Filter:	2-mm. aluminum
Cone:	To film
Ma.S.:	Variable factor
Time:	Variable factor
Ma.:	100
Kv.P.:	60
Development:	Automatic

	Ma.S.	Kv.P.
Exposure 1:	50	60
Exposure 2:	70	60
Exposure 3:	90	60
Exposure 4:	120	60
Exposure 5:	140	60

Experiment 20: Narrow exposure latitude

Procedure 1.

Part:	PA chest
Film:	Regular 14 x 17
Screens:	Medium 14 x 17
Grid:	None
Distance:	72-in. FFD
Filter:	2-mm. aluminum
Cone:	To film
Ma.S.:	Variable factor
Time:	Variable factor
Ma.:	100
Kv.P.:	60
Development:	Automatic

	Ma.S
Exposure 1:	2.5
Exposure 2:	5
Exposure 3:	10
Exposure 4:	15
Exposure 5:	20

Basic Exposure Experiments

Procedure 2.

Part:	Lateral skull
Film:	Regular 10 x 12
Screens:	Medium 10 x 12
Grid:	8 to 1
Distance:	36-in. FFD
Filter:	2-mm. aluminum
Cone:	To film
Ma.S.:	Variable factor
Time:	Variable factor
Ma.:	100
Kv.P.:	60
Development:	Automatic

	Ma.S.
Exposure 1:	50
Exposure 2:	100
Exposure 3:	150

Comment. When the kilovoltage is insufficient to penetrate the part, no practical amount of Ma.S. will compensate for density.

Experiment 21: Effect of voltage on exposure

Purpose. To study the effect of voltage on x-ray exposures and prove the law that, other factors remaining constant, the intensity of an x-ray exposure, measured photographically, varies as the square of the voltage.

Procedure. Use a non-screen film in a cardboard holder. Set and keep the milliamperes constant at 20 and the distance at 36 inches. Expose the different areas, using the voltages and times given in the following table:

Area No.	Kv.P.	Time in seconds	Area No.	Kv.P.	Time in seconds
1	40	4.0	5	40	2.0
2	50	2.6	6	50	2.0
3	60	1.75	7	60	2.0
4	70	1.3	8	70	2.0

Develop the film until the lightest area, no. 5, shows some blackening. Rinse, fix, wash, and dry the film.

Discussion. The first four areas will exhibit approximately the same degree of blackening, while areas 5 to 8 will increase progressively in density. In exposing the first four areas, the voltage is changed 10 kilovolts for each area, but there is a corresponding decrease in the time to compensate for the increased voltage. The exposure times used have about the same ratio to each other as the numbers 1600, 2500, 3600, and 4900, which are the same as the squares of the voltages. This part of the experiment shows that the intensity of the exposure does vary directly as the square of the voltages measured in peak kilovolts.

In the areas 5 to 8 the exposure time is kept constant so that an increase in the density of the film from areas 5 to 8 would be expected.

The effects of voltage changes on x-ray exposures are influenced by a

FORMULATING X-RAY TECHNIQUES

number of factors. Most important of these is the original voltage or the voltage appropriate for the part to be radiographed. Voltage changes will have a more pronounced effect if the original voltage is low than if it is high, because a voltage change *will add or subtract a greater proportion of shorter wavelengths from those produced* by a lower voltage than from *those produced by a higher original voltage.* See Chapter 7, Tables 7.3 and 7.4.

Experiment 22: Photographic effect

Purpose. To demonstrate the laws that if other factors remain constant, the intensity of an x-ray exposure, as measured by its photographic effect, varies directly as the milliamperes through the tube and directly as the time of the exposure.

Procedure. Mark off with a pencil six equal areas on an 8 x 10-inch film in a cardboard holder, three squares on each side of a line that divides the film lengthwise into equal parts. Beginning at the upper left corner and extending downward, number the areas on the left half from 1 to 3 and those on the right half from 4 to 6.

Use a small cone, 50 Kv.P., and a 30-inch anode-film distance and the milliampere-seconds given in the following table.

Area	Ma.	Time	Ma.S.
1	10 Ma.	3 seconds	30 Ma.S.
2	20 Ma.	1½ seconds	30 Ma.S.
3	30 Ma.	1 second	30 Ma.S.
4	20 Ma.	½ second	10 Ma.S.
5	20 Ma.	1 second	20 Ma.S.
6	20 Ma.	1½ seconds	30 Ma.S.

When the exposures have been completed, develop the film until the lightest area shows some blackening, disregarding the density of the other areas. Fix, wash, and dry the film.

Discussion. The finished film will show areas 1 to 3 of nearly the same density. Areas 4 to 6 will show a progressive increase in the density of the different areas. In the areas 1 to 3 the milliamperes through the tube have been increased from 10 to 30, but the time has been correspondingly decreased. For each of these areas, a quantity of x-rays equal to 30 Ma.S. (milliampere seconds) has been used. For areas 4 to 6 the quantity of x-rays has been increased from 10 Ma.S. to 30 Ma.S. This graded increase in quantity should cause a definite and regular increase in the density of these areas. The density of area 5 should be twice that of area 4; that of area 6, three times that of 4.

This experiment shows, therefore, that with voltage and distance constant, the photographic effect of x-ray exposures varies directly as the number of milliampere seconds used. If the milliamperage is kept constant, it varies directly as the variations in the time of the exposure; if the time is kept constant, the photographic effect varies directly as the variations in milliamperage. Thus if an exposure is made with any milliamperage for a certain number of seconds, doubling the time will double the photographic effect; halving the time will reduce the effect to one-half.

Chapter 7. PRODUCING A RADIOGRAPH: TECHNICAL CONVERSIONS

The production of a radiograph involves *four* so-called primary factors. Three of these, *milliamperage, time* (Ma.S.) and *kilovoltage* (Kv.P.) are usually considered the factors controlled by the x-ray machine. The fourth factor is the *distance* from the focal spot of the x-ray tube to the film (focus-film distance).

The term milliampere-seconds (Ma.S.) is descriptive of the milliamperage or *amount* of current passing through the tube for a given period of *time.* The radiographic density of a film varies directly with the milliampere-seconds, provided the kilovoltage is sufficient to penetrate the part (see in Chapter 8, Figure 8.26).

The kilovoltage, spoken of as kilovolts-peak or Kv.P., is the factor that controls *penetration* and *contrast.*

EXPOSURE

The word *exposure* has different radiographic meanings, depending upon the context. For example, "exposure" may be used to designate the radiographic conditions—kilovoltage, milliamperage, and time used for a certain technique. In somewhat different usage "exposure" may indicate only the milliamperage and time (Ma.S.) or source strength and time. Again, "exposure" is sometimes used to designate radiation exposure to the patient, in terms of roentgens. Exposure may refer to a measure, in absolute or relative units, of the amount of radiation reaching a certain area of the film. Exposure in the latter case means the amount of energy reaching a particular area of film and responsible for producing a particular density on the processed film. The word is thus used in the study of the sensitometric properties of x-ray films (see Appendix B).

THE PRIMARY EXPOSURE FACTORS

1. For any radiographic problem, the "correct exposure" will require a precise combination of the four primary factors:
   (a) Kilovoltage
   (b) Milliamperage
   (c) Exposure time
   (d) Focus-film distance

Provided that no other factors in the radiographic problem are changed, the radiographic density may be altered to a predetermined degree by varying any one of the four primary factors.

2. Since milliamperage is so much a function of tube capacity, it is quite impractical to use it as a variable.

FORMULATING X-RAY TECHNIQUES

3. Time can be used as a variable with excellent results except where motion is a factor. In all moving parts there is a certain optimum exposure time beyond which motion becomes objectionable.

4. Kilovoltage affects both the quality and quantity of x-rays and hence can be used as a variable to compensate for differences in part thickness. This technique is practical only when the autotransformer design permits changes of 1 or 2 kilovolts to be made.

5. Under average conditions, variations in part thickness will require compensations of 2 kilovolts per centimeter thickness (*with variable kilovoltage technique;* Chapter 10).

6. Distance can be used as a variable, but is recommended only when control limitations and motion make kilovoltage or time variations impractical. Distance changes cause changes in image magnification with consequent variations in image detail.

It is good technique to keep three factors constant and vary only the fourth to effect changes in radiographic density (Ma.S.).

THE SECONDARY FACTORS

Intensifying screens

Until non-screen films were introduced, all x-ray film had an emulsion most sensitive to *blue light,* the color of the fluorescence of calcium tungstate intensifying screens.

When intensifying screens are used, about *99 per cent of the total exposure* is effected by "printing the visible image onto the x-ray film." Only about *1 per cent of the total exposure* is produced by the x-rays striking the film.

When intensifying screens are used, the "scale of gradation" of the radiographic image is considerably shortened; hence the radiographic image has more contrast.

Cones

The amount of exposure compensation to be used for cones is governed by:

1. The proportionate decrease in "volume of part" irradiated; this is governed by:
    (a) Thickness of the part
    (b) The size of the cone
    (c) The focus-film distance
2. The structure of the part
3. The kilovoltage

In general, when using a cone we have to add from 3 to 5 Kv.P. in order to compensate for loss in density due to the *absorption* of some of the primary radiation. By limiting the size of the x-ray beam by a cone and/or a collimator, less tissue is irradiated and less secondary radiation is emitted from the part to fog the film.

Grid or non-grid technique?

With few exceptions, a stationary grid or a Bucky mechanism should be used for radiography of all anatomical parts exceeding 12 cm. in thickness.

Producing a Radiograph

Use of a grid in radiography of the heart and lungs, and parts such as the knee, shoulder, and cervical vertebrae, is a matter of choice.

In pediatric radiography, certain body regions, even though they measure less than 12 cm. in thickness, such as the skull, abdomen, pelvis, and vertebral column, set up a considerable amount of secondary radiation when struck by primary radiation. Effective control of the fogging effect can be accomplished only through use of a stationary grid or Bucky.

When converting a non-grid technique to a grid technique, compensation must be made for the grid either by an increase in Kv.P. or Ma.S. It is preferable to make required compensation for adding the grid to a procedure by adding 20 kilovolts. This method of compensating for the grid assures adequate penetration and does not result in a great difference in radiographic contrast between the non-grid and grid radiographs. Twenty kilovolts will provide adequate compensation for any modern grid. If, however, compensation is made in Ma.S., then the required compensation is a function of grid ratio. When a grid is removed from a procedure, compensation in exposure must again be made. In this instance, however, do not reduce kilovoltages. Compensation is more properly made by reducing Ma.S. rather than Kv.P. Obviously the higher the grid ratio, the greater the absorption of primary and secondary radiation. It must also be remembered that grids of identical ratio will not necessarily absorb the same amount of radiation and that thicker parts and anatomical areas greatly affected by secondary radiation require a proportional increase in exposure factors.

Beam restrictor

Radiographic quality is visibly improved through the proper use of some beam-restricting device, provided the device accomplishes restriction of the primary beam at the film to an area no larger than the size of film being used.

Since x-ray film is either square or rectangular in shape, any beam restrictor which leaves a circular field of radiation large enough to cover an entire film contributes little if anything to minimize the effect of secondary-radiation fog. That is one reason for obsoleting the once familiar flare cone. An extension cylinder, used alone or in conjunction with an adjustable diaphragm collimator, is a useful beam restrictor. If used properly it can be extended to confine a circular field of x-radiation inside the limits of even small-size films.

Secondary radiation and fog increase with the amount and type of tissue struck by primary radiation, so by confining the field of primary radiation to only the useful area, secondary radiation emanating from tissue is reduced. Secondary-radiation fog affects visibility of image detail, radiographic contrast, and density. It reduces contrast by a graying effect and as an unpredictable supplemental density added to proper density, it makes this latter film quality uncontrollable.

Conversion factors:
    Extension cylinder collapsed—increase Ma.S. 40 per cent
    Extension cylinder extended—increase Ma.S. 60 per cent

Field size (based on a 14 x 17 field):
    To convert to an 8 x 10 field—increase Ma.S. 60 per cent
    To convert to a 10 x 12 field—increase Ma.S. 40 per cent

FORMULATING X-RAY TECHNIQUES

MILLIAMPERAGE, TIME, DISTANCE, AND KILOVOLTAGE

1. Milliamperage must necessarily depend upon the capacity of the x-ray unit (including the tube capacity) and the requirements of the focal-spot dimensions. High milliamperage imposes the requirements of relatively large focal-spot dimensions, which detract from the sharpness of detail.

2. Time of exposure should be reduced to a minimum to counteract the effects of motion. For all practical considerations, the time of exposure and the milliamperage are interchangeable. The greater the milliamperage, the less will be the time of exposure required and vice versa.

3. Roughly, Kv.P. changes might be interpolated with respect to Ma.S. values as indicated in the two paragraphs below; however these should be used only for Kv.P. ranges from 60 Kv.P. to 80 Kv.P. Above 80 Kv.P. and below 60 Kv.P. the charts on kilovoltage–Ma.S. conversions (Tables 7.1 and 7.2) should be used.

To decrease kilovoltage by:

10 Kv.P. requires twice the amount of Ma.S.
13 Kv.P. requires three times the amount of Ma.S.
15 Kv.P. requires four times the amount of Ma.S.
20 Kv.P. requires five times the amount of Ma.S.

To increase kilovoltage by:

10 Kv.P. requires a reduction to one-half of the Ma.S.
13 Kv.P. requires a reduction to one-third of the Ma.S.
15 Kv.P. requires a reduction to one-fourth of the Ma.S.
20 Kv.P. requires a reduction to one-fifth of the Ma.S.

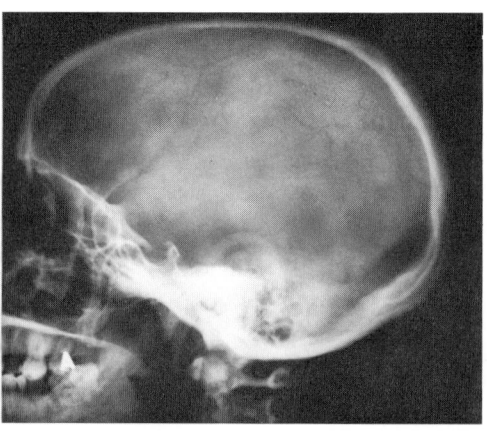

Figure 7.1. Radiograph of lateral skull made at 85 Kv.P. and 15 Ma.S.

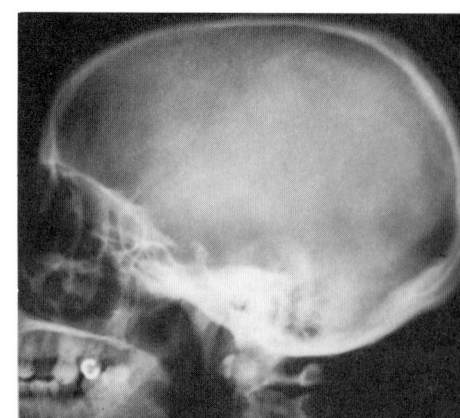

Figure 7.2. Radiograph of lateral skull made at 1⦁ Kv.P. and 10 Ma.S.

Producing a Radiograph

Kilovoltage — distance conversion

When a variation from an established distance is found necessary, the following chart will prove of value. *However, the use of the inverse square law will prove to be more accurate to maintain radiographic density and the contrast scale will remain about the same. The chart below should be used only when it is impossible to vary the Ma. and time values.*

Change in distance (inches)		Change in Kv.P. (kilovolts)
From	To	
36	42	add 5
36	48	add 9
36	54	add 11
36	60	add 13
36	72	add 16
36	30	subtract 6
72	60	subtract 5
72	48	subtract 11
72	36	subtract 20

RELATION OF Kv.P.–Ma.S. AND DENSITY

Theory. Radiographic density varies greatly with the Kv.P. In medical radiography, there is no precise mathematical method for determining Kv.P.–Ma.S. density ratios. Such factors as the thickness and density of the body tissues to be examined, the characteristics of the x-ray apparatus, and whether the film is used with or without intensifying screens exert pertinent influences. Fairly close approximations between Kv.P. and other exposure factors have been of necessity established by empirical means — by trial and error. There are two procedures that may be followed in estimating the Kv.P. required for a given density change or for determining the approximate change in Ma.S. required to compensate a density change in Kv.P. One is for screen exposures and the other for direct exposures.

Tables 7.1 and 7.2 were developed empirically from radiographs of living subjects on screen-type film. By the use of Ma.S. multiplying factors, approximate Ma.S. values may be obtained for changes in the Kv.P. range of 50 to 100 in increments of five. Since the film response to x-ray exposure differs when screens are used and when direct exposure is employed, two tables of values are required. Table 7.1 is for screen exposures and Table 7.2 for direct x-ray exposures. Some Ma.S. values derived from these tables may require the use of a time value that is not within the practical scope of the timer. It is then necessary to employ the *nearest* practical value. The resulting density difference is usually so small that it often is not recognizable. In most instances the derived Ma.S. values are approximations and, if necessary, only slight alterations need be made for a given projection and body tissue. X-ray generators may differ in the manner in which their x-ray outputs vary with Kv.P. and owing to calibration differences. Tables cannot, therefore, be expected to apply accurately to *all* generators but they can provide a close guide to an anticipated value.

FORMULATING X-RAY TECHNIQUES

Table 7.1 SCREEN EXPOSURES TABLE: TO FIND Ma.S. WHEN Kv.P. IS CHANGED

Locate the original Kv.P. in the left-hand vertical column and the new wanted Kv.P. in the bottom horizontal row. The square where the corresponding row and column cross will show the multiplying factor which will yield the new Ma.S. For screen exposures only.

Old Kv.P.	Ma.S. multiplying factor									
50	1.	.5	.42	.33	.25	.21	.17	.13	.1	.08	.06
55	2.	1.	.83	.67	.5	.41	.33	.25	.2	.15	.1
60	2.4	1.2	1.	.8	.6	.5	.4	.3	.25	.2	.15
65	3.	1.5	1.25	1.	.75	.62	.5	.38	.34	.3	.25
70	4.	2.	1.66	1.33	1.	.83	.66	.5	.45	.33	.3
75	4.8	2.4	2.02	1.61	1.21	1.	.81	.61	.5	.4	.35
80	6.	3.	2.5	2.	1.5	1.24	1.	.75	.6	.5	.4
85	7.	3.5	3.	2.5	2.	1.65	1.33	1.	.9	.7	.6
90	8.	4.5	4.	3.	2.5	2.	1.6	1.5	1.	.9	.75
95	12.	6.	5.	4.	3.	2.47	2.	1.6	1.3	1.	.9
100	18.	8.	6.	5.	4.	3.	2.5	1.8	1.6	1.4	1.
New Kv.P.	50	55	60	65	70	75	80	85	90	95	100

Example: Assume that 85 Kv.P. was used to radiograph a lateral skull. The Ma.S. was 15. It is desired to use 100 Kv.P. in order to lengthen the scale of contrast and stop motion (Figures 7.1 and 7.2).
Solution: Locate 85 Kv.P. in the left-hand vertical column and 100 Kv.P. in the horizontal bottom row. In the square where the corresponding row and column cross, we find the Ma.S. multiplying factor to be .6. Thus:

$$\begin{array}{r} 15 \\ \times .6 \\ \hline 9.0 \end{array}$$ Ma.S., the correct Ma.S at 100 Kv.P.

The value 9 is not ordinarily available on modern x-ray control panels, and the nearest practical value should therefore be used. In this example, one would use 10 Ma.S.

Table 7.2 DIRECT EXPOSURES TABLE: TO FIND Ma.S. WHEN Kv.P. IS CHANGED (REGULAR FILM)

Locate the original Kv.P. in the left-hand vertical column and the new wanted Kv.P. in the bottom horizontal row. In the square where the corresponding row and column cross, find the multiplying factor which will yield the new Ma.S. For direct exposures only.

Old Kv.P.	Ma.S. multiplying factor									
50	1.	.69	.5	.39	.3	.29	.19	.14	.12	.1	.09
55	1.45	1.	.73	.56	.43	.34	.27	.21	.18	.15	.13
60	2.	1.37	1.	.77	.6	.47	.37	.29	.25	.21	.19
65	2.58	1.77	1.29	1.	.77	.61	.48	.37	.32	.27	.24
70	3.33	2.29	1.66	1.29	1.	.79	.62	.48	.42	.35	.31
75	4.21	2.89	2.1	1.63	1.26	1.	.79	.6	.52	.44	.39
80	5.33	3.66	2.66	2.06	1.6	1.26	1.	.76	.66	.56	.5
85	6.95	4.78	3.48	2.69	2.	1.65	1.3	1.	.87	.74	.65
90	8.	5.5	4.	3.1	2.4	1.9	1.5	1.15	1.	.85	.75
95	9.41	6.47	4.71	3.64	2.8	2.23	1.76	1.35	1.17	1.	.88
100	10.66	7.33	5.33	4.13	3.2	2.53	2.	1.53	1.33	1.13	1.
New Kv.P.	50	55	60	65	70	75	80	85	90	95	100

Producing a Radiograph

Kilovoltage — Ma.S. conversion factors

The charts in Table 7.3 can be used to increase the Ma.S. from two to ten times and/or decrease the Ma.S. from one-half to one-tenth.

Table 7.3 Kv.P. DECREASE TO BE MADE WHEN Ma.S. IS INCREASED

Initial Kv.P.	2X	3X	4X	5X	10X
40	4	6	7	9	13
45	5	8	9	11	15
50	6	10	11	13	18
55	7	12	13	15	21
60	8	13	15	17	23
65	9	14	17	19	25
70	10	15	19	20	27
75	11	16	20	22	29
80	11	17	21	23	31
85	12	18	22	24	33
90	13	19	23	25	35
95	14	20	24	27	37
100	15	21	25	29	39
105	16	22	27	31	41
110	17	23	29	33	43
115	18	25	31	35	45
120	19	27	33	37	47
125	20	29	35	39	49
130	21	31	37	41	51

Table 7.4 Kv.P. INCREASE TO BE MADE WHEN Ma.S. IS DECREASED

Initial Kv.P.	$1/2$	$1/3$	$1/4$	$1/5$	$1/10$
30	4	6	8	11	16
35	5	8	11	13	20
40	6	11	14	17	25
45	7	12	16	19	29
50	8	13	18	21	33
55	9	15	20	23	36
60	10	17	22	25	39
65	11	18	24	27	42
70	12	19	26	29	45
75	13	20	28	31	
80	14	21	30	33	
85	15	23	32		
90	16	25	34		
95	17	27			
100	18	30			

RELATION BETWEEN KILOVOLTAGE AND TIME

It is often necessary to *estimate* the kilovoltage approximately for a given change in exposure time, or what approximate change in exposure time is necessary to compensate for a desired change in kilovoltage. While it is not possible to give an exact rule for all cases, the table below provides estimates of the corrections that should be applied to kilovoltage or exposure time

FORMULATING X-RAY TECHNIQUES

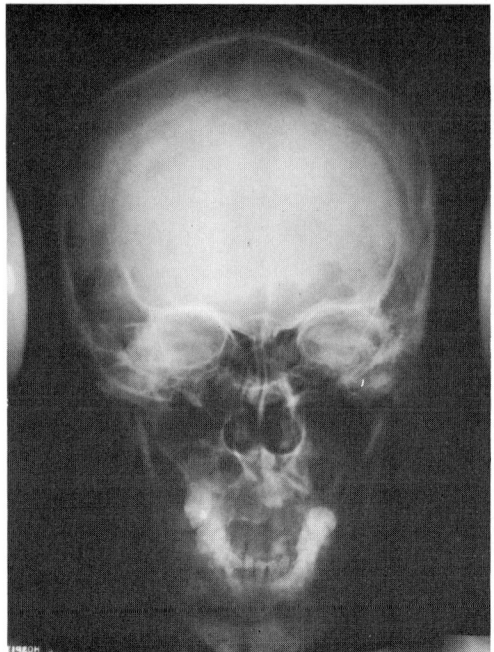 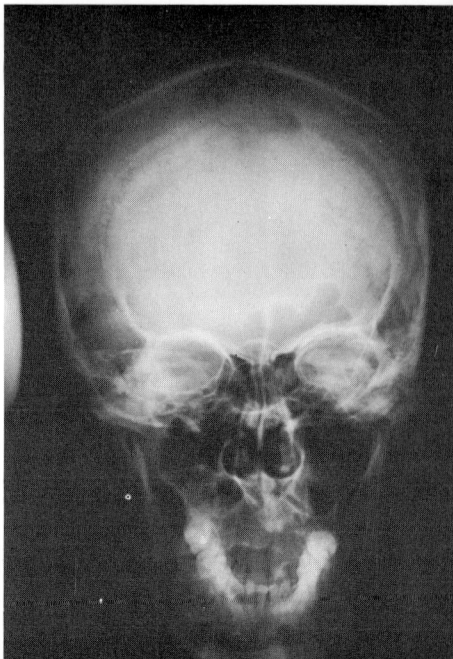

Figure 7.3. Radiograph made at 85 Kv.P. and 30 Ma.S.

Figure 7.4. The skull of Figure 7.3, taken at 76 Kv.P. and 60 Ma.S. Increasing the exposure time 100 per cent demanded a 16 per cent decrease in Kv.P. Compare Table 7.6.

when either is changed. It must be kept in mind that an increase in kilovoltage with the exposure adjusted to maintain the same density will produce lower contrast in the radiograph; and, conversely, a decrease in kilovoltage will produce higher contrast.

Example: Suppose that with intensifying screens a kilovoltage of 80 and an exposure time of 4 seconds have been employed, and it is desired to decrease the exposure time to 2 seconds. What kilovoltage would be required?

According to the table, the decrease in exposure time is 50 per cent, which necessitates a 20 per cent increase in kilovoltage:

$$20\% \text{ of } 80 \text{ Kv.P.} = 16 \text{ Kv.P.}$$

$$80 \text{ Kv.P.} + 16 \text{ Kv.P.} = 96 \text{ Kv.P.}$$

Table 7.5

To decrease exposure time	Increase kilovoltage	
	With double screens	Without screens
25%	7%	15%
50%	20%	40%
75%	50%	100%

Producing a Radiograph

Table 7.6

To increase exposure time	Decrease kilovoltage	
	With double screens	Without screens
25%	5%	10%
50%	10%	18%
75%	13%	25%
100%	16%	30%

Example: Suppose that with intensifying screens a kilovoltage of 80 and an exposure time of 4 seconds have been employed, and it is desired to decrease the kilovoltage to 70. What exposure time would be required?

The decrease in kilovoltage is about 13 per cent, which necessitates a 75 per cent increase in exposure time.

$$75\% \text{ of } 4 \text{ sec.} = 3 \text{ seconds}$$
$$4 \text{ sec.} + 3 \text{ sec.} = 7 \text{ seconds}$$

Kilovoltage–time relation (15 per cent rule)

To reduce the exposure (Ma.S.) to one half *at any level* of kilovoltage, add 15 per cent more kilovoltage.

Examples: We are employing a technique at 100 Ma.S. and 70 Kv.P. and we wish to reduce the time of exposure by one-half our original.

```
    70
   .15
   350
    70
 10.50
```

We would now add 10 or 11 Kv.P. and reduce the Ma.S. by one-half.

We are employing a technique at 10 Ma.S. and 40 Kv.P. and wish to reduce the exposure time to 5 Ma.S.:

```
        40 Kv.P.
      × .15
        2 00
        4 0
        6.00 Kv.P.

        40 Kv.P.
      +  6 Kv.P.
        46 Kv.P.
```

Our technique would now be 46 Kv.P. and 5 Ma.S.

Using a technique of 10 Ma.S. and 60 Kv.P., we wish to reduce exposure time to 5 Ma.S.:

```
        60 Kv.P.
      × .15
        3 00
        6 0
        9 00 Kv.P.

        60 Kv.P.
      +  9 Kv.P.
        69 Kv.P.
```

Our technique would now be 69 Kv.P. and 5 Ma.S.

FORMULATING X-RAY TECHNIQUES

Using a technique of 10 Ma.S. and 80 Kv.P., we again wish to reduce exposure time to 5 Ma.S.:

```
    80 Kv.P.
  × .15
    4 00
    8 0
  12.00 Kv.P.

    80 Kv.P.
  + 12 Kv.P.
    92 Kv.P.
```

Our technique would now be 92 Kv.P. and 5 Ma.S.

DISTANCE

X-ray intensities can be altered by moving the tube from or toward the plane of the image. Fuchs suggests that a light bulb be used to demonstrate this fact. With no other illumination in the room, move a single light toward this printed page. You will find that the closer the light is to the page, the more brightly the page is illuminated. Exactly the same thing occurs with x-rays: as the distance from the object to the source of radiation is decreased, the intensity at the object increases, and vice versa.

Changes in milliamperage and changes in distance are very similar in their effects upon the intensity of the image. It is important to know that these changes in intensity affect the overall image.

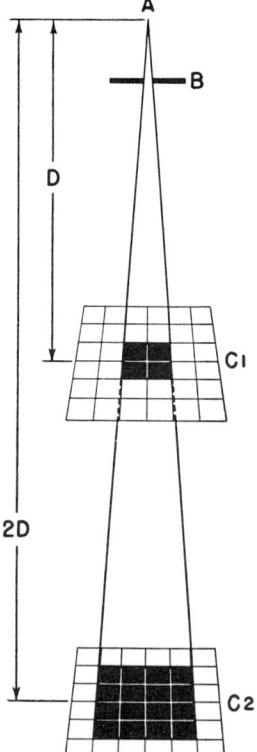

Figure 7.5. The inverse square law.

Producing a Radiograph

When the x-ray tube output is held constant, the x-ray intensity reaching the subject is governed by the distance between the x-ray tube and the subject, varying inversely with the square of this distance. Since x-rays conform to the laws of light, they diverge when they are emitted from the anode and cover an increasingly larger area with lessened intensity as they travel from their source. In Figure 7.5 this principle is illustrated. In this example it is assumed that the intensity of the x-rays emitted at the anode (A) remains constant, and that the x-rays passing through the aperture (B) cover an area of 4 square inches on reaching the recording surface C_1, which is 12 inches (D) from (A). Then, when the recording surface C_1 is moved 12 inches farther from the anode to C_2, so that the distance between A and C_2 is 24 inches (2D), or twice the distance between A and C_1, the x-rays will cover 16 square inches—an area 4 times as great as that at C_1. It follows, therefore, that the radiation *per square inch* on the surface at C_2 is only one quarter that at the level C_1. Thus the exposure that would be adequate at C_1 must be increased 4 times in order to produce at C_2 a radiograph of equal density.

The inverse square law

The inverse square law is one of the most important and most useful laws in standardized radiography, since factors that give a satisfactory radiograph at one distance may be known, and if it is desired to increase or decrease the distance, the voltage and milliamperage may be kept constant and the new milliampere seconds calculated by this formula. The inverse square law may be stated thus:

$$\frac{I_1}{I_2} = \frac{D_2^2}{D_1^2}$$

Where I_1 and I_2 are the intensities at distances D_1 and D_2 respectively. The inverse square law may be stated thus:

The intensity of radiation varies inversely as the square of the distance.

In Figure 7.5 this is demonstrated. The radiation that covers a given area at a distance D from the focal spot must disperse over an area *four times as great at twice the distance*, 2D (4 being the square of 2). This means that the intensity of the radiation at a point in the area at 2D is $1/4$ that at D. To expand the example further, if a distance 3D were shown, representing a distance 3 times the original distance, the area covered by the radiation would be 9 times that of D (9 being the square of 3) and the intensity would be $1/9$ of the intensity at D.

The inverse square law can be used in establishing formulas for calculating various exposure-distance relationships. For example, the Ma.S.–distance formula of the next section can be set up because we know how the intensity of radiation will be affected if the distance between the tube and target is varied. In this case, the Ma.S. *in use* is to the *new* Ma.S. as the *old distance* squared is to the *new distance* squared.

Ma.S.–DISTANCE RELATIONSHIP

The inverse square law is the eventual basis for our formula relating Ma.S.

FORMULATING X-RAY TECHNIQUES

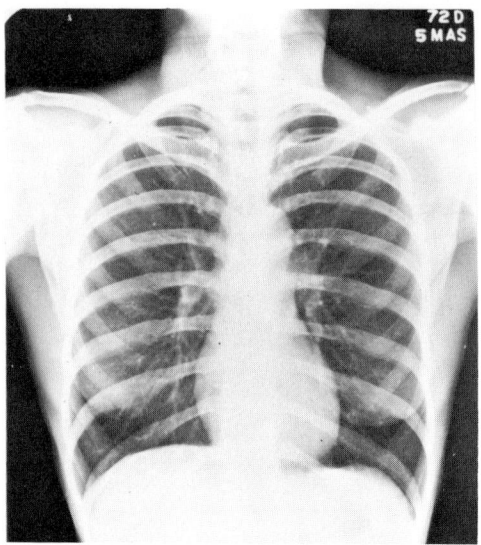

Figure 7.6. Radiograph of the chest at 72-inch focus-film distance.

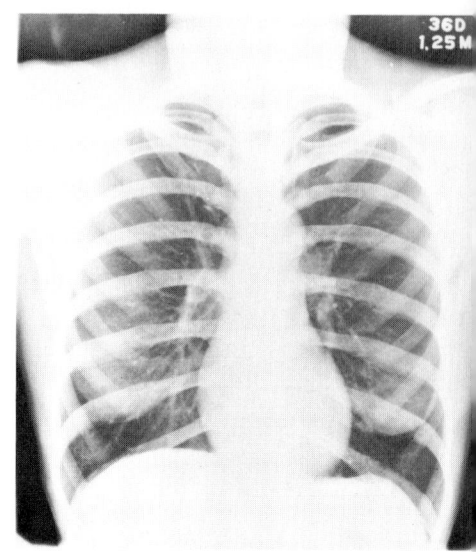

Figure 7.7. The same chest as in Figure 7.6, but taken at a 36-inch focus-film distance.

to the distance between the focus of radiation and the film; but the way that the law applies is not quite direct.

By the inverse square law, two features mark the relation between distance and amount of light. First, the *greater* the distance between focus and film, the *less* the radiation that reaches the film. This is the *inverse* part. But besides that, the amount of light, as the source moves away, reduces in proportion to the *square* of the distance, and not directly with the distance. This is the *square* part:

$$I_1 : I_2 :: D_2^2 : D_1^2$$

In our formulation of Ma.S. and distance, we need the square part but we do not need the inverse part of this formula. That is, though the greater the distance, the less the radiation reaching the film, by the same reasoning, the *greater* the distance, the *more* Ma.S. we need to compensate for the reduced light; and the *shorter* the distance between source and film, the *less* the Ma.S. is that we need to achieve the same exposure. Thus we are back with a direct relationship:

$$\text{Ma.S.}_1 : \text{Ma.S.}_2 :: D_1^2 : D_2^2$$

If factors that give a satisfactory radiograph at one distance are known and we desire to increase or decrease the distance between focus and film, we can keep the same voltage (the same contrast) and calculate a new Ma.S. by using the formula just shown. First, we convert the proportion into an equation (see Chapter 5) by multiplying means and extremes. The *product of the means equals the product of the extremes:*

$$\text{Ma.S.}_1 : \text{Ma.S.}_2 :: D_1^2 : D_2^2$$

i.e., $\quad \text{Ma.S.}_1 \times d_2^2 = \text{Ma.S.}_2 \times D_1^2$

Producing a Radiograph

Example: A technique calls for 80 Kv.P. at a 72-inch focus-film distance and it is desired to decrease the distance to 36 inches. The old technique calls for 10 Ma.S. What would the new Ma.S. be at 36 inches?

$$Ma.S._1 : Ma.S._2 :: d_1^2 : d_2^2$$

$$10 : x :: 72^2 : 36^2$$

$$5184x = 12960$$

$$x = 2.5$$

We then would use 2.5 Ma.S., 80 Kv.P. at a 36-inch focus-film distance.

Figure 7.6 shows a chest radiograph made at 72 inches. Using the above formula, the same subject was then radiographed at a 36-inch focus-film distance: the results are shown in Figure 7.7.

Ma.S.–distance formula (short method). Divide the original distance into the new distance. Square this answer. Multiply the squared answer by the original Ma.S. This will give the new Ma.S. to be used at the new distance.

Example:

Old distance 72 inches
Old Ma.S. 10
New distance 36 inches

```
    .5
72/36.0           .5            10
   36.0           .5            .25
                  .25           2.50
```

2.5 Ma.S. will be the new Ma.S. to be used at 36 inches.

Example:

Old distance 36 inches
Old Ma.S. 10
New distance 72 inches

```
   2.0
36/72            2             10
   72            2              4
                 4             40
```

40 Ma.S. will be the new Ma.S. to be used at 72 inches.

THE RECIPROCITY LAW

Oftentimes in doing very exact radiography or experimental work, one will have the feeling that the inverse square law is invalid, but a very important concept advanced by Bunsen and Roscoe in 1875 states that the reaction of the photographic emulsion to light is equal to the product of the intensity of the light and the duration of exposure. This is known as the reciprocity law. The phenomenon occurs in radiography *only* when *intensifying screens* are used, because exposure of the film under these circumstances is chiefly caused by the fluorescent light emitted by the screens and very little by x-rays. Failure of this law may be observed when the radiographic density produced by short exposure with a large quantity of fluorescent light is greater than is that produced by a long exposure and a small amount of fluorescent light, even though the quantity of radiation exposing the films (measured by Ma.S.) is the same in both cases. In general radiography, it is

FORMULATING X-RAY TECHNIQUES

not necessary to be concerned about this effect. Today it is seldom encountered, because it has been largely compensated by the characteristics of x-ray film emulsions. Therefore, the Ma.S. value may be considered reliable for use as an exposure factor in general medical radiography; for example, approximately the *same radiographic density* will be obtained whether we use 100 Ma for $1/_{10}$ second or 200 Ma for $1/_{20}$ second; either combination will give us 10 Ma.S.

The milliampere-seconds factor, indicated by the symbol Ma.S., directly influences radiographic density with all other factors constant. It is the product of the milliamperage (Ma.) and the duration of the exposure time in seconds (s.). Either factor, Ma. or s., may be changed at will to perform the required radiographic exposures as long as the product—Ma.S.—remains the same.

In standardized radiography, machine calibration becomes a very valuable factor, since it becomes imperative that no matter what Ma. and time increment value we are using, as long as the product, Ma.S., remains the same, the density level should remain the same. This factor holds true on all *direct* x-ray exposures. As we have seen, intensifying screen exposures may show some loss in radiographic density when they are exceedingly long because of failure of the *reciprocity law.* In general radiography, the Ma. factor is seldom changed for a given exposure and may usually be considered a constant. The time of exposure however, can be readily changed and should constitute the available factor in the Ma.S.

It is *highly recommended* that the student become adept at computing Ma.S. values. For example, an extremity technique at 10 Ma. for $1/_2$ second equals 5 Ma.S., however, if a patient has had trauma and cannot hold the extremity still, it would be far better to use 100 Ma. and $1/_{20}$ second, which would equal 5 Ma.S. and the radiograph would be devoid of motion. This certainly would be a more skillful and scientific approach to good radiography.

It requires at least a *30 per cent increase in Ma.S.* to produce a significant increase or decrease in density. To produce a diagnostically acceptable radiograph which requires either an increase or decrease in density, the 30 per cent figure can be employed to affect density changes in a scientific, mathematical manner.

Example: Assuming we had an exposure of 15 Ma.S. at 80 Kv.P., and the radiograph was slightly underexposed, we would multiply 15 by 130 per cent and we now would use 19.5 Ma.S. (or 20 Ma.S.) to correct this condition. When the Kv.P. and processing are constant, serious underexposure or overexposure should be corrected by either doubling or halving the initial Ma.S. value to change density.

DECIMAL EQUIVALENTS OF FRACTIONAL EXPOSURES

In computing milliampere-seconds values, it is often more convenient to use the decimal equivalent of the exposure time fraction. Table 7.7 below lists decimal equivalents of various exposure fractions. The numerators of fractions are listed horizontally at the top of the table; the denominators are listed vertically. The square in which the column and row cross contains the decimal equivalents.

Example: To determine the decimal equivalent of the fraction $3/_5$, find the number 3 in the horizontal row at the top of the table. Then find 5 in the left-hand vertical column; the square in which row and column cross will show .6. The milliamperage may be multiplied by this decimal to obtain the milliampere-seconds value.

If we were using 100 Ma. for $3/_5$ second, we would now have 100 × .6, or 60 Ma.S.

Producing a Radiograph

Table 7.7 DECIMAL EQUIVALENTS OF FRACTIONAL EXPOSURES

Denominators \ Numerators	1	2	3	4	5	6	7	8	9	10	11	12
2	0.5	1.	1.5	2.	2.5	3.	3.5	4.	4.5	5.	5.5	6.
3	.333	.666	1.	1.33	1.666	2.	2.33	2.66	3.	3.33	3.66	4.
4	.25	.5	.75	1.	1.25	1.5	1.75	2.	2.25	2.5	2.75	3.
5	.2	.4	.6	.8	1.	1.2	1.4	1.6	1.8	2.	2.2	2.4
6	.167	.333	.5	.667	.835	1.	1.167	1.333	1.5	1.667	1.833	2.
7	.143	.286	.429	.572	.715	.858	1.	1.143	1.286	1.429	1.57	1.7
8	.125	.25	.375	.5	.625	.75	.875	1.	1.125	1.25	1.375	1.5
9	.111	.222	.333	.444	.555	.666	.777	.888	1.	1.111	1.222	1.333
10	.1	.2	.3	.4	.5	.6	.7	.8	.9	1.	1.1	1.2
11	.09	.18	.27	.363	.455	.545	.636	.727	.818	.090	1.	1.09
12	.083	.167	.25	.333	.415	.5	.583	.667	.75	.833	.917	1.
15	.067	.134	.2	.267	.333	.4	.467	.533	.6	.667	.733	.8
20	.05	.1	.15	.2	.25	.3	.35	.4	.45	.5	.55	.6
24	.042	.083	.125	.167	.208	.25	.292	.333	.375	.416	.458	.5
30	.033	.067	.1	.133	.167	.2	.233	.267	.3	.333	.367	.4
40	.025	.05	.075	.1	.125	.15	.175	.2	.225	.25	.275	.3
60	.017	.033	.05	.067	.083	.1	.117	.133	.15	.167	.183	.2
120	.008	.017	.025	.033	.042	.05	.058	.067	.075	.083	.092	.1

FORMULATING X-RAY TECHNIQUES

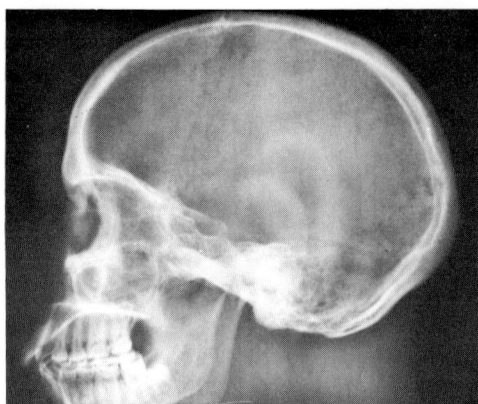

Figure 7.8. A skull radiograph with normal exposure

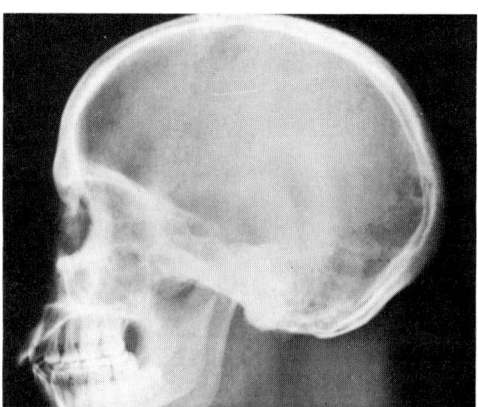

Figure 7.9. The skull of Figure 7.8, but with a decrease of 30 per cent in the Ma.S.

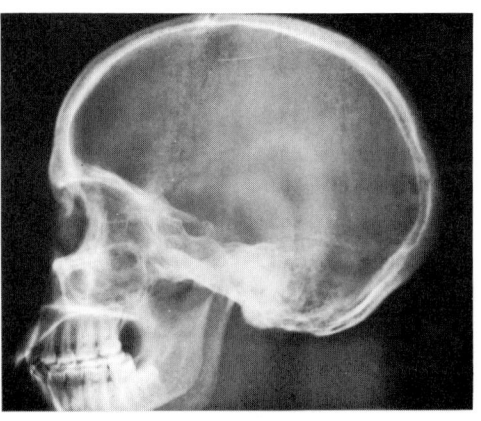

Figure 7.10. The skull of Figure 7.8, but with an increase of 30 per cent in the Ma.S.

Producing a Radiograph

Figure 7.11. Lateral skull, taken with normal exposure.

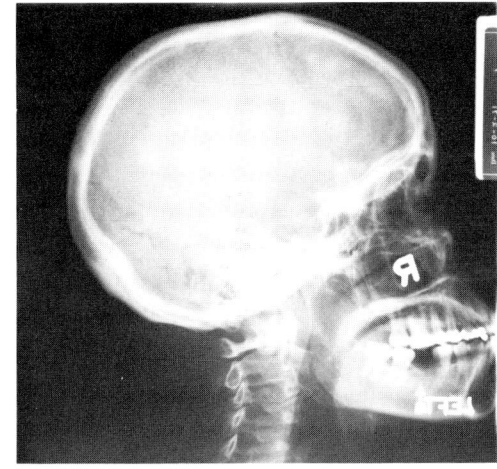

Figure 7.12. The skull of Figure 7.11, but with an increase of 30 per cent in the Ma.S.

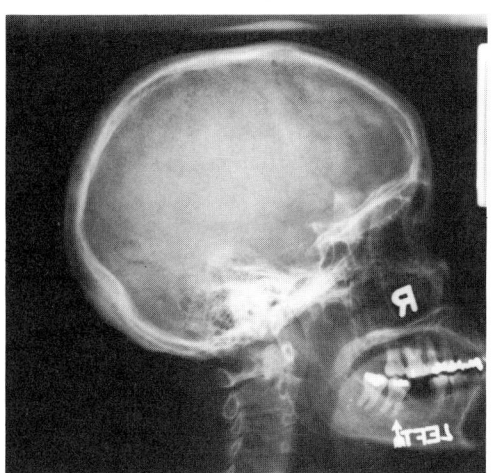

Figure 7.13. The skull of Figure 7.11, but with a decrease of 30 per cent in the Ma.S.

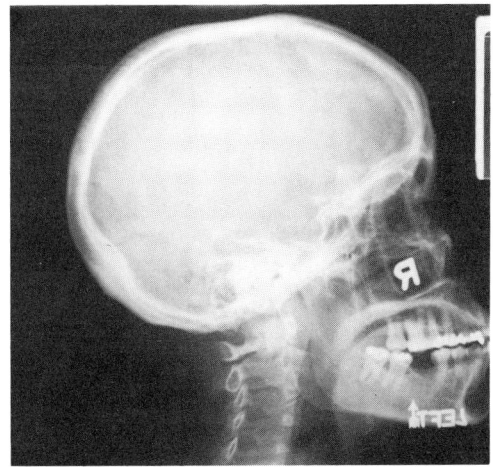

FORMULATING X-RAY TECHNIQUES

THE PHOTOGRAPHIC EFFECT

If other factors remain constant, the intensity of an x-ray exposure, as measured by its photographic effect, varies directly as the milliamperage through the tube and directly as the time of exposure. If the voltage and distance are kept constant, the photographic effect of x-ray exposures varies directly as the number of milliampere-seconds used. If the milliamperage is kept constant, the photographic effect varies directly as the variations in the time of the exposure; if the time is kept constant, the photographic effect varies directly as the variations in milliamperage. Thus, if an exposure is made with any milliamperage for a certain number of seconds, doubling the time will double the photographic effect; halving the time will reduce the effect to one-half.

Photographic effect is *directly proportional* to the milliamperage (Ma.). P.E. $\propto$ Ma. Photographic effect is *directly proportional* to the time of exposure. P.E. $\propto$ T. Photographic effect is *approximately proportional* to the kilovoltage squared. P.E. $\propto$ Kv.P.^{2}.

Photographic effect is *inversely proportional* to the square of the focus-film distance; therefore, with the other exposure factors constant, the intensity of x-ray exposures varies inversely as the square of the focus-film distance.

The relationship of all factors in photographic effect may be expressed in a single equation:

$$\text{P.E.} = \frac{\text{Ma.} \times \text{T} \times (\text{Kv.P.})^2}{\text{D}^2}$$ when T is in seconds and D in inches.

Suppose the following factors produce a good radiograph: Ma., 30; time, 1 second; Kv.P., 60; distance, 30 inches. Then we would have, according to the above formula,

$$\text{P.E.} = \frac{30 \times 1 \times 60^2}{30^2} = \frac{30 \times 1 \times 3600}{900} = \frac{1080}{9}$$

P.E. = 120

Suppose it is necessary to change the technique to the following factors: Ma., 10; time, ?; Kv.P., 60; distance, 30 inches. We substitute in the equation:

$$\frac{10 \times \text{T} \times 60^2}{30^2} = 120$$

and discover the value of T:

$$\frac{10 \times \text{T} \times 3600}{900} = 120$$

$$\frac{36000\,\text{T}}{900} = 120$$

$$40\text{T} = 120$$

$$\text{T} = 3 \text{ seconds,}$$

the new time of exposure.

Producing a Radiograph

RELATION BETWEEN TIME AND DISTANCE

Rule. The exposure time (T) required for a given exposure is directly proportional to the square of the focus-film distance (D).

Example: Suppose that an exposure time of 10 seconds (T_1) and a focus-film distance of 30 inches have been employed. and it is desired to decrease the focus-film distance to 24 inches (D_2); what exposure time (T_2) would be required?

$T_1:T_2::D_1^2:D_2^2$

$10:x::30^2:24^2$

$900x = 5760$

$x = 6.4$ seconds

Example of this problem would apply to radiography of the temporomandibular articulation. where use of close focus-film distance is desired.

Example: Suppose that an exposure time of 2 seconds (T_1) and a focus-film distance of 72 inches (D_1) have been employed. and it is desired to decrease the exposure time to $1/4$ second (T_2); what distance (D_2) would be required?

$T_1:T_2::D_1^2:D_2^2$

$2:1/4::72^2:x^2$

$2x^2 = 1296$

$x = 25.5$ inches

RELATION BETWEEN MILLIAMPERAGE, TIME, AND DISTANCE

Rule. Since the milliamperage (M) and the time (T) required for a given exposure are both directly proportional to the square of the focus-film distance (D), the product of the two, milliampere seconds (Ma.S.) or (MT), is also directly proportional to the square of the focus-film distance (D).

Example: Suppose that 60 Ma.S. (MT_1) and a focus-film distance of 36 inches (D_1) have been employed, and it is desired to increase the focus-film distance to 72 inches (D_2); what milliamperesecond factor (MT_2) would be required?

$MT_1:MT_2::D_1^2:D_2^2$

$60:x::36^2:72^2$

$1296x = 311040$

$x = 240$ milliampere seconds

An easy method for calculating the change in milliampere seconds (Ma.S.) is based on the principle that the *squares* of numbers bear constant mathematical relation to each other. In the above example, the square of the number representing the longer focus-film distance 72^2 (5184), is 4 times the square of the number representing the shorter anode-film distance, 36^2 (1296). Therefore, if the number representing the proper Ma.S. factor at the 36-inch focus-film distance, 60, is multiplied by 4, the proper milliamperage time for the 72-inch distance will be found to be 240 Ma.S. Conversely, 36^2 (1296) is one-fourth (.25) of 72^2 (5184); so, if the number representing the proper Ma.S. factor at 72 inches, 240, is multiplied by .25, the proper milliamperage time for the 36-inch distance will be found to be 60 Ma.S.

The interrelation of all focus-film distances may be similarly expressed by means of a conversion factor. Any change in milliamperage seconds necessitated because of a change in the focus-film distance may then be calculated by multiplying by the proper factor, the initial milliamperage-

FORMULATING X-RAY TECHNIQUES

seconds value. Table 7.11 below lists the factors that apply for focus-film distances commonly employed in radiography.

RELATION BETWEEN MILLIAMPERAGE AND DISTANCE

Rule. The milliamperage (M) required for a given exposure is directly proportional to the square of the focus-film distance (D).

Example: Suppose that 50 Ma. (M_1) and a focus-film distance of 36 inches (D_1) have been employed and it is desired to increase the distance to 72 inches (D_2) in order to obtain sharper detail; what Ma. would be required?

$$M_1:M_2::D_1^2:D_2^2$$

$$50:x::36^2:72^2$$

$$1296x = 259,200$$

$$x = 200 \text{ milliamperes}$$

RELATION BETWEEN MILLIAMPERAGE AND TIME

Rule. The milliamperage (M) required for a given exposure is inversely proportional to the time (T). When radiographing children and nervous patients, it is often necessary to employ high Ma. in order to obtain the advantages of very short exposure.

Example: Suppose that 30 milliamperes (M_1) and an exposure time of $1/2$ second (T_1) have been employed, and it is desired to decrease the exposure time to $1/20$ second (T_2); what milliamperage would be required?

$$M_1:M_2::T_2:T_1 \qquad \frac{x}{20} = \frac{15}{1}$$

$$30:x::1/20:1/2 \qquad x = 15 \times 20$$

$$1/20\, x = 15 \qquad x = 300 \text{ Ma.}$$

Example: Suppose that 30 Ma. (M_1) and an exposure time of 2 seconds (T_1) have been employed, and it is desired to increase the milliamperage to 60 (M_2); what exposure time (T_2) would be required?

$$M_1:M_2::T_2T_1$$

$$30:60::x:2$$

$$60x = 60$$

$$x = \text{one second}$$

MAINTAINING FOCUS-FILM DISTANCE AFTER TUBE IS ANGLED

Table 7.8 determines accurately where to place a tilted x-ray tube so that when the central ray is correct with the regional landmark, the anatomical region will be projected in the center of the film and the desired or original focus-film distance will be maintained.

If an x-ray tube is angled other than 90° and the tube is left in its original position, the resultant radiograph will be *underexposed*.

Producing a Radiograph

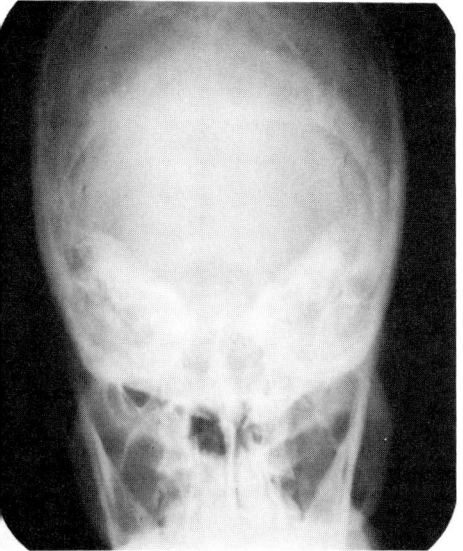

Figure 7.14. Anteroposterior view of the petrous bone.

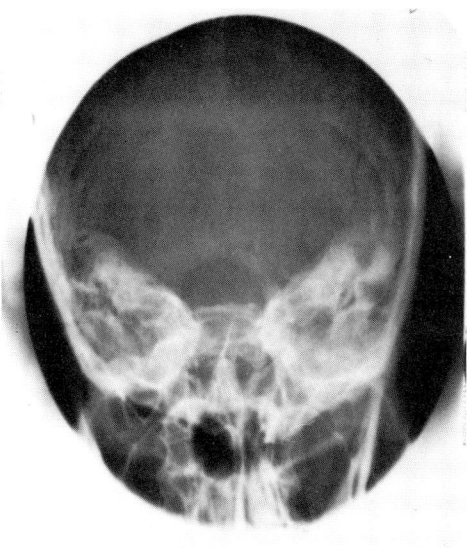

Figure 7.15. A corrected view of the petrous bone of Figure 7.14, according to the Example of Table 7.8.

Table 7.8 DATA FOR TUBE ANGLES USED IN RADIOGRAPHY

	Z 25"			Z 30"			Z 36"			Z 40"	
A	x	y	A	x	y	A	x	y	A	x	y
5°	2.15	24.8	5°	2.6	29.8	5°	2.8	35.8	5°	3.5	39.8
10°	4.3	24.5	10°	5.2	29.6	10°	6.2	35.5	10°	6.9	39.4
13°	5.6	24.25	13°	6.75	29.25	13°	8.0	35.0	13°	9.0	39.0
15°	6.5	24.125	15°	7.75	29.0	15°	9.3	34.8	15°	10.4	38.6
17°	7.3	24.0	17°	8.6	28.6	17°	10.3	34.4	17°	11.6	38.2
20°	8.5	23.5	20°	10.25	28.2	20°	12.6	33.8	20°	13.75	37.6
23°	9.75	23.0	23°	11.7	27.6	23°	14.0	33.0	23°	15.6	36.8
25°	10.5	22.6	25°	12.7	27.2	25°	15.4	32.6	25°	16.8	36.0
30°	12.5	21.5	30°	15.0	26.0	30°	18.0	31.2	30°	20.0	34.6
35°	14.6	20.5	35°	17.25	24.6	35°	20.6	29.5	35°	23.0	32.8
40°	16.0	19.2	40°	19.3	23.0	40°	23.2	27.6	40°	25.75	30.25
45°	17.7	17.7	45°	21.25	21.25	45°	25.4	25.4	45°	28.25	28.25

Z = Focus-film distance   A = Tube angle   x = Tube shift   y = New vertical distance

Courtesy: Ralph Tarrant, R. T.

Example: A. P. view of the petrous bone, at a 36-inch focus-film distance; the tube has to be tilted 35 degrees. What distance should you use at the 35-degree tilt? According to the chart on the 36-inch distance column we have:

Z – 36-inch distance
A – 35-degree tilt
X – tube shift to have central ray to center of film
Y – new vertical distance, which will be 29.5 inches

See Figures 7.14 and 7.15.

FORMULATING X-RAY TECHNIQUES

Table 7.9 IMPULSE–TIME–MILLIAMPERE-SECONDS

Impulses	Time (seconds)	Milliampere seconds										
2	$1/60$	.16	.25	.33	.41	.5	.83	1.66	2.5	3.33	5.	6.66	8.33
3	$1/40$	.25	.37	.5	.62	.75	1.25	2.5	3.75	5.	7.5	10.	12.5
4	$1/30$	.33	.5	.66	.83	1.	1.66	3.33	5.	6.66	10.5	13.33	16.66
5	$1/24$	.41	.62	.83	1.04	1.25	2.08	4.12	6.25	8.33	12.5	16.66	20.83
6	$1/20$	.5	.75	1.	1.25	1.5	2.5	5.	7.5	10.	15.	20.	25.
7		.58	.87	1.16	1.56	1.75	2.91	5.83	8.75	11.66	17.5	23.33	29.16
8	$1/15$	.66	1.	1.33	1.66	2.	3.33	6.66	10.	13.33	20.	26.66	33.33
9	$3/40$	.75	1.12	1.5	1.87	2.25	3.75	7.5	11.25	15.	22.5	30.	37.5
10	$1/2$	.83	1.25	1.66	2.08	2.5	4.16	8.33	12.5	16.66	25.	33.33	41.66
11		.91	1.37	1.83	2.27	2.75	4.58	9.16	13.75	18.33	27.5	36.66	45.83
12	$1/10$	1.	1.5	2.	2.5	3.	5.	10.	15.	20.	30.	40.	50.
13		1.08	1.62	2.16	2.77	3.25	5.41	10.83	16.25	21.66	32.5	43.33	54.16
14		1.16	1.75	2.33	2.91	3.5	5.83	11.66	17.5	23.33	35.	46.66	58.33
15		1.25	1.87	2.5	3.12	3.75	6.25	12.5	18.75	25.	37.5	50.	62.5
16	$2/15$	1.33	2.	2.66	3.33	4.	6.66	13.33	20.	26.66	40.	53.33	66.66
17		1.41	2.12	2.83	3.54	4.25	7.08	14.16	12.25	28.33	42.5	56.66	70.83
18	$3/20$	1.5	2.25	3.	3.75	4.5	7.5	15.	22.5	30.	45.	60.	75.
19		1.58	2.37	3.16	3.95	4.75	7.91	15.83	23.75	31.66	47.5	63.33	79.16
20		1.66	2.5	3.33	4.16	5.	8.33	16.66	25.	33.33	50.	66.66	83.33
21		1.75	2.62	3.5	4.37	5.25	8.75	17.5	26.25	35.	52.2	70.	87.5
22		1.83	2.75	3.66	4.58	5.5	9.16	18.33	27.5	36.66	55.	73.33	91.66
23		1.91	2.87	3.83	4.79	5.75	9.58	19.16	28.75	38.33	57.5	76.66	95.83
24	$1/5$	2.	3.	4.	5.	6.	10.	20.	30.	40.	60.	80.	100.
25		2.08	3.12	4.16	5.20	6.25	10.41	20.83	33.26	41.66	62.5	83.33	104.16
26		2.16	3.25	4.33	5.41	6.5	10.83	21.66	32.5	43.33	65.	86.66	108.33
27		2.25	3.37	4.5	5.62	6.75	11.25	22.5	33.75	45.	67.5	90.	112.5
28		2.33	3.5	4.66	5.83	7.	11.66	23.33	35.	46.66	70.	93.33	116.66
29		2.41	3.62	4.83	6.04	7.25	12.08	24.16	36.25	48.33	72.5	96.66	120.83
30	$1/4$	2.5	3.75	5.	6.25	7.5	12.5	25.	37.5	50.	75.	100.	125.
Milliamperes		10	15	20	25	30	50	100	150	200	300	400	500

Producing a Radiograph

Table 7.10 CONVERSION OF Ma.S. AT VARIOUS MILLIAMPERAGES

Milliampere seconds — across

Time of exposure — read down

Ma. down	1	2	2.5	3	4	5	6	8	10	12	14	15	20	25	30	40	50	60	75	100	150	200	300	500
5	2/10	4/10	1/2	6/10	8/10				2			3	4	5	6	8	10	12						
10	1/10	2/10	1/4	3/10	4/10	1/2	6/10	8/10	1				2		3	4	5	6		10		20		
15				2/10			4/10		7/10	8/10	9/10													
20	1/20	1/10	1/8	3/20	2/10	1/4	3/10	4/10	1/2	6/10	7/10	3/4	1		1½	2	2½	3		5		10		
25		1/15	1/10	1/8		2/10	2/10			4/10		6/10								4	6	8	10	
30	1/30	1/20		1/10			2/10	2/10	1	3/10	9/10			6/10			2		5	2½	5		10	
40	1/40	1/24	1/20	1/10	1/10	1/8		2/10	1/4	1/4	1/3	3/4		6/10	3/4	1		3		2	3	4	5	2
50		1/20	1/24	1/20	1/15	1/10	1/8			1/4		3/10	4/10	1/2	6/10	8/10		1½		2				
60	1/60	1/24		1/20		1/10	1/10		2/10	2/10	2/10	1/4		4/10	1/2	7/10		1						
70											2/10					8/10		9/10						
75		1/40	1/30	1/24		1/15		1/10	1/8	1/8	1/7	1/5	1/4	1/4	4/10	1/2		8/10	1	1¼	2			
80	1/40				1/20		1/15	1/10		3/20	2/10	3/10	1/4	3/10	4/10	1/2		3/4	1	1¼		2	3	
90			1/30						1/8												1½		2	
100		1/40	1/40	1/24	1/20	1/20		1/12	1/10	1/8	1/7	3/20	1/4	1/4	3/10	4/10	1/2	6/10	3/4	1	1½	2	3	5
150			1/60			1/30	1/24		1/15		1/15	1/10	2/10	1/8	2/10	3/10	1/4	4/10	1/2		1		2	
200		1/24				1/40	1/24	1/24	1/20				1/10		3/20	3/20		3/10		1/2	3/4	1		
250						1/60			1/24	1/24				1/8										
300			1/60						1/30	1/30		1/20	1/20		1/10		1/8	2/10	1/4	1/3	1/2	1/2	1	
400									1/40							1/10	1/10	3/20	1/4	1/4			3/4	
500										1/40		1/20	1/20		1/10		1/10	1/8	3/20	1/5	3/10		6/10	1

Example: What time is used at 50 Ma. to obtain 2.5 Ma.S.? Locate 50 Ma. in the left hand column and 2.5 at the top Ma.S. column, read down, find 1/20 second opposite 50 Ma.

FORMULATING X-RAY TECHNIQUES

CORRECTION FACTORS FOR CHANGE IN FOCUS-FILM DISTANCE

Table 7.11 lists the factors that apply for focus-film (anode-film) distances commonly employed in radiography. The initial focus-film distance is located in the left-hand vertical column and the desired distance is located in the horizontal column at the bottom of the chart. The required Ma.S. conversion factor will be found in the entry common to both columns.

Table 7.11 CORRECTION FACTORS FOR FOCUS-FILM DISTANCE

Initial focus-film distance	Ma.S. conversion factors							
20 in.........	1.00—	1.56—	2.25—	3.22—	4.00—	5.76—	9.00—	12.96
25 in.........	.64—	1.00—	1.44—	2.07—	2.56—	3.68—	5.76—	8.29
30 in.........	.44—	.69—	1.00—	1.44—	1.77—	2.56—	4.00—	5.76
36 in.........	.31—	.48—	.69—	1.00—	1.23—	1.77—	2.77—	4.00
40 in.........	.25—	.39—	.56—	.81—	1.00—	1.44—	2.25—	3.24
48 in.........	.17—	.27—	.39—	.59—	.69—	1.00—	1.56—	2.25
60 in.........	.11—	.17—	.25—	.36—	.44—	.64—	1.00—	1.44
72 in.........	.08—	.12—	.17—	.25—	.31—	.44—	.69—	1.00
Desired focus-film distance	20 in.	25 in.	30 in.	36 in.	40 in.	48 in.	60 in.	72 in.

Example: We are employing a technique at a 30-inch distance, and it is desired to decrease the distortion by going to 48 inches. What would we multiply our *original* Ma.S. by? Find 30-inch distance in the left-hand vertical column and 48-inch distance in the horizontal column at the bottom of the chart. The required conversion factor will be 2.56. If we were using 10 Ma.S. at 30 inches, we would multiply 10 by 2.56 to arrive at the correct Ma.S. at 48 inches. The correct Ma.S. would be 25.60 or 26 Ma.S. In this case we would no doubt use 25 Ma.S.

See Figures 7.6 and 7.7, radiographs of the chest at 72 and 36 inches.

CAST RADIOGRAPHY

When using optimum kilovoltage techniques, measure the part and add 10 Kv.P. or 2 x Ma.S.

For lower voltage techniques, measure the part and add 10 Kv.P. for a dry cast and 15 Kv.P. for a wet cast. It is better to alter Kv.P. than Ma.S. If, however, one prefers to use Ma.S., the correction factor would be to double the Ma.S. for a dry cast and triple the Ma.S. for a wet cast.

ADAPTING EXPOSURE TECHNIQUE FROM ONE HOSPITAL TO ANOTHER

From any given technique chart one may adapt the exposure factors to apply to any other machine.

Procedure. Choose a part from any group of parts of similar density. Make three exposures and divide the Ma.S. from the chart being adapted into the Ma.S. producing the most desired density with the new chart. The result obtained serves as the correction factor for all parts of similar density.

Example: A technique from Hospital A for the A.P. skull calls for 85 Kv.P., 20 Ma.S., 36-inch focus-film distance, medium screens, 8-to-1 grid. It is desired to adapt this technique to Hospital B.

Producing a Radiograph

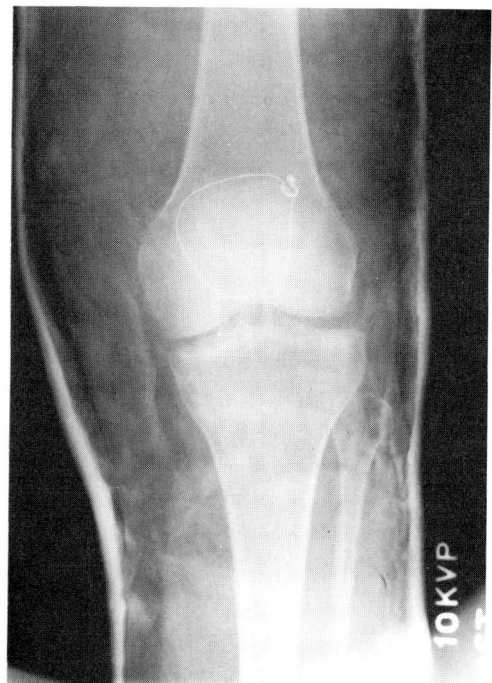

Figure 7.16. Radiograph of the knee in a cast, with a plus of 10 Kv.P.

At Hospital B we make three exposures of the skull, employing all factors as used at Hospital A, except the *milliampere-seconds*. Use the following three exposures:

1. Below the original Ma.S.
2. Equal to the original Ma.S.
3. Above the original Ma.S.

We would use 15, 20, 25 Ma.S. Process all three films at the same time. We now find that the film exposed at 25 Ma.S. produces the desired density, thus:

$$20 \overline{)\begin{array}{c} 1.25 \\ 25.0 \\ \underline{20} \\ 50 \\ \underline{40} \\ 10/20 \end{array}}$$

We would now multiply all Ma.S. values in the S.G. (screen-grid) group by 1.25. All other factors remain constant.

Conversion factors for children when using variable voltage
 Birth to 1 year — use 30% of Ma.S.
 2 to 5 years — use 60% of Ma.S.
 6 to 9 years — use 70% of Ma.S.
 10 to 12 years — use 90% of Ma.S.

Conversion factors for children when using fixed voltage
 Birth to 5 years — use 25% of Ma.S.
 6 to 12 years — use 50% of Ma.S.

Chapter 8. ESSENTIALS OF THE RADIOGRAPH AND IMAGE FORMATION

Every radiologic technologist should have a satisfactory working knowledge of *density, contrast, detail* and *distortion*. He should be able to understand and define the meaning of each; to differentiate each from the other in the finished radiograph; to understand and control each of the various subfactors that enter into the control of each of the main factors; to be able to arrange the four main factors and their subfactors so that any desired results may be obtained. With this knowledge, one may produce any type of radiograph desired.

If we study a good radiograph we know at once that it includes a combination of the above factors. Everyone agrees that there should be a *minimum of distortion, a maximum of detail,* and *sufficient contrast* to make detail more plainly visible. There is a difference of opinion as to what *degree of density* may be most desirable. There are conditions in which *distortion* plays an important part and other conditions in which distortion, within reason, is of little importance.

Radiographically speaking, let us simulate the conditions shown in Figure 8.1. In the radiograph of Figure 8.2 we will use a simulated condition of 10 Ma.S. and 35 Kv.P. In the radiograph of Figure 8.3 we will increase the

Figure 8.1. The penetrating power of x-rays. Scheme A shows x-rays of long wave length being absorbed by the object. In B, x-rays of short wave length penetrate the object and expose the film (remnant radiation). In C, increasing the number of x-rays by the Ma.S. factor increases the number reaching the film, and more silver in the film is exposed than in B.

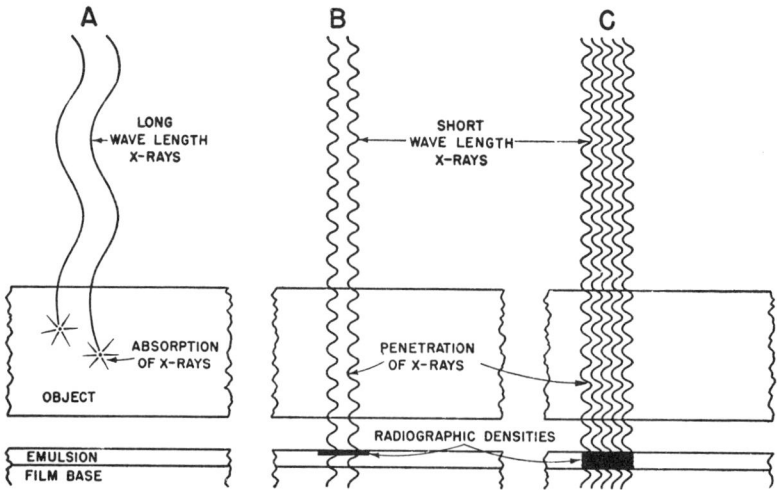

Essentials of the Radiograph

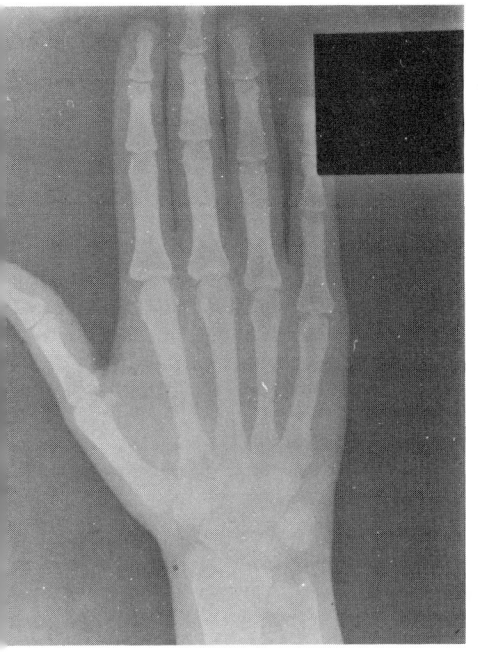

Figure 8.2. Radiograph of the hand: 35 Kv.P. and 10 Ma.S.

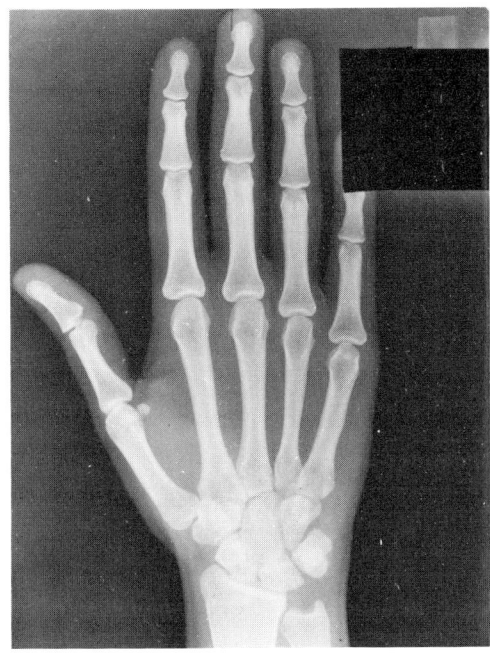

Figure 8.3. Like Figure 8.2: 50 Kv.P. and 10 Ma.S.

Figure 8.4. Like Figure 8.2: 50 Kv.P. and 50 Ma.S.

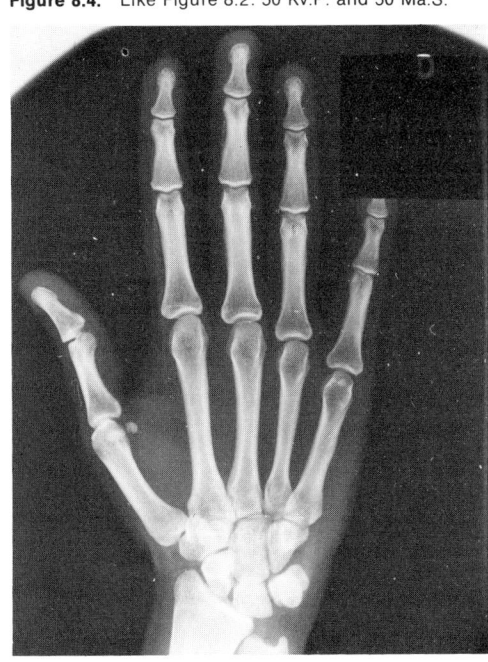

FORMULATING X-RAY TECHNIQUES

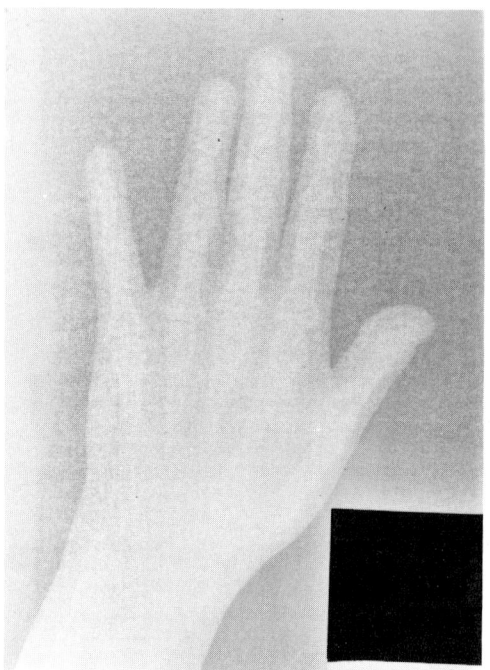

Figure 8.5. 30 Kv.P. and 15 Ma.S.

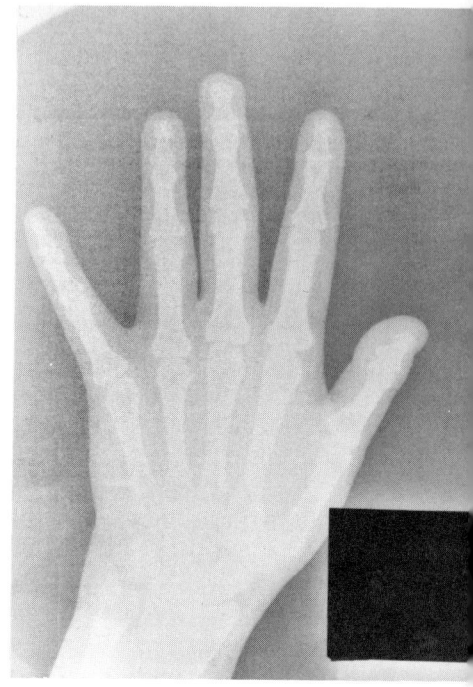

Figure 8.6. 30 Kv.P. and 30 Ma.S.

Figure 8.7. 30 Kv.P. and 60 Ma.S.

Figure 8.8. 30 Kv.P. and 240 Ma.S.

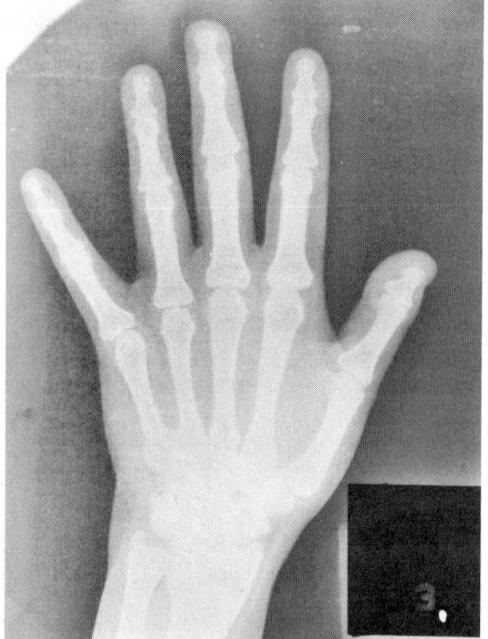

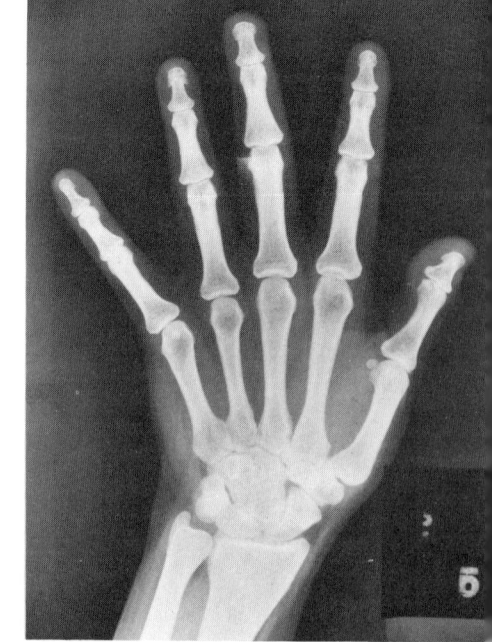

Essentials of the Radiograph

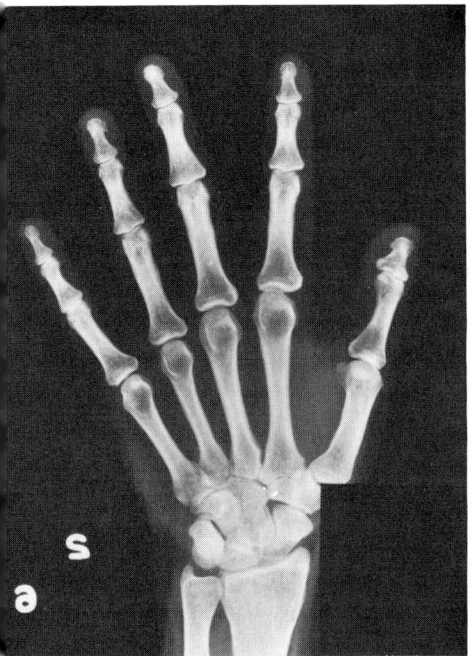

Figure 8.9. 30 Kv.P. and 480 Ma.S.

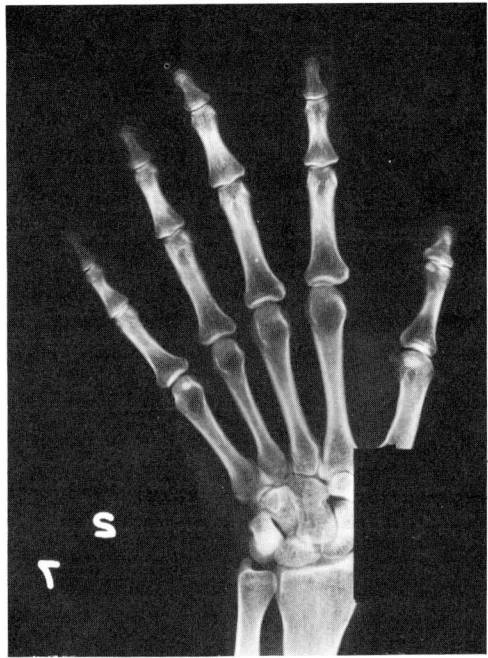

Figure 8.10. 30 Kv.P. and 960 Ma.S.

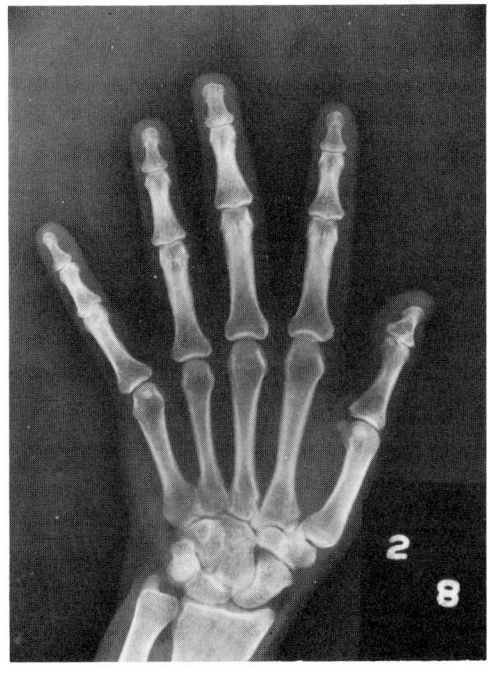

Figure 8.11. 50 Kv.P. and 40 Ma.S. Note the effect of increasing the Kv.P. for adequate penetration, as against increasing Ma.S.

FORMULATING X-RAY TECHNIQUES

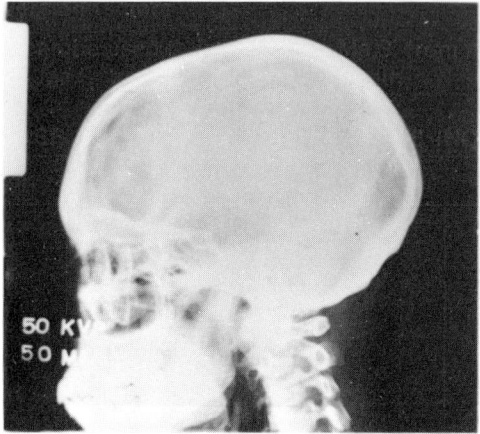

Figure 8.12. 50 Kv.P. and 50 Ma.S.

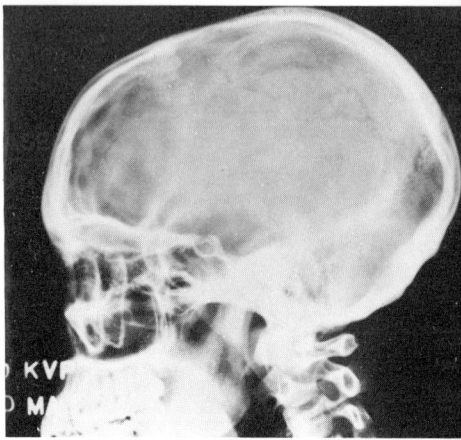

Figure 8.13. 50 Kv.P. and 100 Ma.S.

kilovoltage to 50 Kv.P. and 10 Ma.S., and in Figure 8.4 we will use a kilovoltage of 50 Kv.P. and 50 Ma.S.

In another experiment, let us radiograph the hand using the factors shown in Figures 8.5 to 8.11. This experiment proves that no practical amount of *Ma.S.* will ever compensate for *inadequate kilovoltage or penetration.*

The same experiment done with a skull is shown in Figures 8.12 to 8.16.

DENSITY

Density, which is due to the accumulation of black metallic silver, is the general blackening of the radiograph that appears after exposure by radiation and subsequent processing. Variations in density may exist in a series of radiographs and all of them be of good quality. Correct density is a matter of personal choice; however, all densities of the radiograph should transmit some visible light.

Density is a measure of the *quantity* of radiation absorbed by the film. The quantity is made up of *primary, remnant,* and *secondary* radiation.

Density is affected by a number of things. Among them are thickness of part, tissue opacity, pathology, respiration, distance, secondary radiation fog, old film, screen type or non-screen film, chemicals, cone, stereo shift, Kv.P., filters, compression binders, white light, or any form of radiation, automatic or manual processing, type of grid, and efficiency of equipment.

We can say, in general terms, that density refers to the lighter or darker appearance of the film. Either Ma., time, Kv.P., or distance may be used to control density. The distance factor is rarely used because it introduces the element of distortion. The Ma.S. (Ma. times the time) controls density *provided* we have sufficient penetration (Kv.P.). The Kv.P. factor may also be used to alter density. Increasing the developing time can alter density, but is not recommended. The temperature of the developing solution affects density, but is not considered a practical means of control. Focal-spot damage affects density as well as contrast (Figure 8.17).

Essentials of the Radiograph

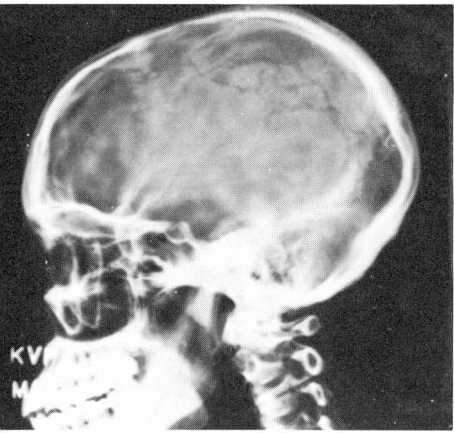

Figure 8.14. 50 Kv.P. and 125 Ma.S.

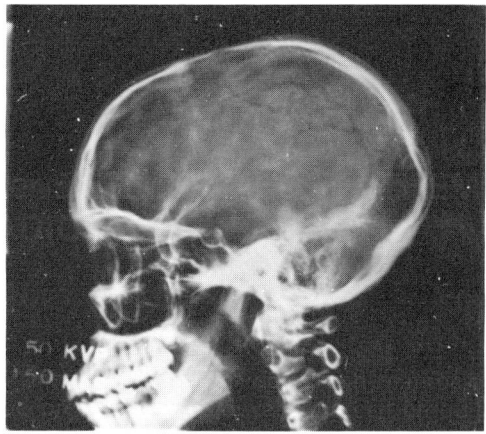

Figure 8.15. 50 Kv.P. and 150 Ma.S.

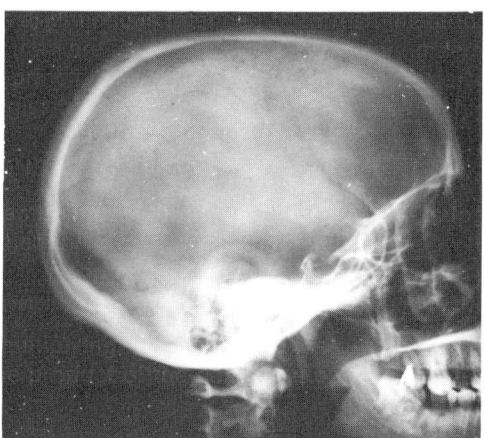

Figure 8.16. 85 Kv.P. and 15 Ma.S. Note the effect of higher Kv.P., as in Figure 8.11.

Primary radiation

The amount of primary radiation is regulated by the quantity of current in milliamperes (Ma.) flowing through the tube for a definite length of time in seconds (s.), usually referred to as Ma.S.

Remnant radiation

Remnant radiation is that radiation which emerges from the part being radiographed to expose the film.

Secondary radiation fog

When a primary beam of x-rays traverses an object, some of the x-rays are absorbed while others pass directly through it; a considerable percentage, however, is scattered in all directions by the atoms of the material struck (Figure 8.18) very much as light is dispersed by a mist. These scattered rays constitute what is known as *secondary radiation* and are radiographically

FORMULATING X-RAY TECHNIQUES

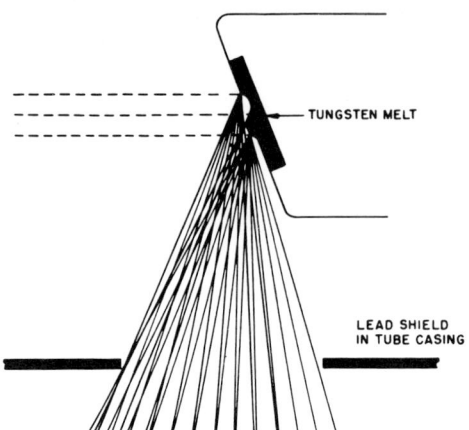

Figure 8.17. The effect of damage to the focal spot. The enlarged source of light and other changes affect density and contrast.

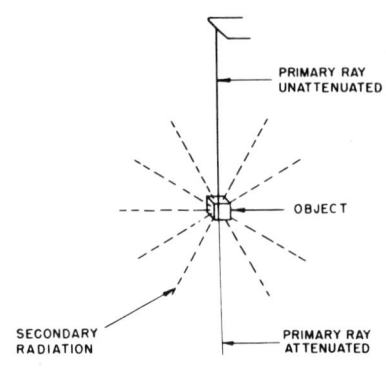

Figure 8.18. How primary radiation cau secondary radiation. The secondary radia is set up in a spherical shape. It is characte tic of the material in which it arises and is longer wave length than the primary radiat The higher the Kv.P., the more the second radiation generated.

non-effective as far as *good radiography* is concerned, but are effective as far as *poor radiography* is concerned. Secondary radiation strikes the film from all directions and produces a fairly uniform deposit of silver (black metallic silver) over the entire image. This veil or haziness of silver overlies the image density produced by the remnant radiation and is, in reality, a supplement density known as *secondary radiation fog.* When fog is present, the effect is as if image details were being viewed through a mist or a cloud. It is like trying to view the ground when flying in an airplane while the visibility of the ground is reduced by thin clouds. Therefore, the quality of the radiographic image is degraded. Secondary radiation fog is characterized by a *dull gray appearance* of the images and the *absence of details* within the radiographic image. Examples of secondary radiation fog are shown in Figures 8.19 and 8.21. Other examples of the secondary radiation fog are shown in Figures 8.38, 8.45A, and 8.55.

In order to understand more fully and graphically the effect of secondary radiation and its influence on the image, we may produce it radiographically with the aid of a coin and paraffin — a material that generates large quantities of secondary radiation and simulates body tissue.

Three principal conditions under which secondary radiation fog may be produced on the radiographic film are illustrated in Figures 8.19A–C.

When a coin is placed on a film, an x-ray exposure will produce a radiograph in which the image of the coin is relatively free of fog (Figure 8.19A). The secondary radiation generated could not undercut the coin enough to fog its image.

When the paraffin block is placed on the film and the coin mounted on its top, the radiograph will show the image of the coin to be fogged by the secondary radiation that undercuts the object. This radiographic example

Essentials of the Radiograph

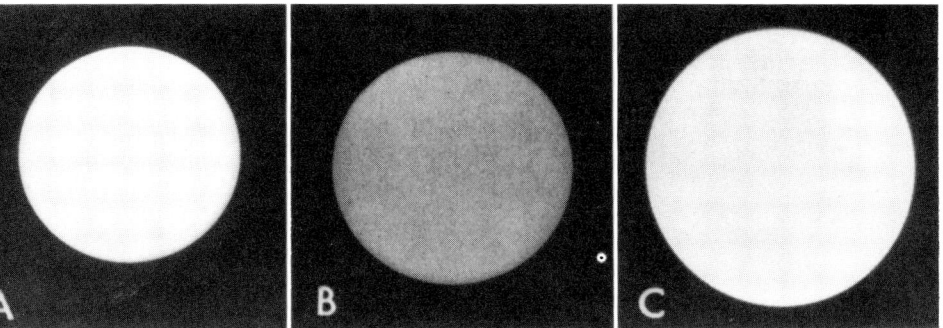

Figure 8.19. Radiographs of a coin. In A, of the coin alone, the radiograph is relatively free of fog. In B, the coin is shown undercut by secondary radiation from the paraffin block on which it is resting. In C, both coin and block have been put at a greater distance from the source of radiation, and secondary radiation is accordingly decreased.

demonstrates that images of objects in or on an emitter, located at a distance from the film, will be fogged when the emitter is adjacent to the film (Figure 8.19B).

When the emitter (paraffin block) together with the coin on its top is moved away from the film (as for Figure 8.19C) the degree of fog in the image will be *less* than that shown in B, since the secondary radiation reaching the film has been diminished by reason of its greater distance from its source. Therefore, by increasing the distance between the emitter/coin combination and the film, the intensity of the secondary radiation reaching the film diminishes. This is true because secondary radiation follows the same laws as primary radiation and the *inverse square law.*

The quantity of secondary radiation emitted by the body thickness depends upon the *tissue thickness* and its density as well as the *kilovoltage* employed. The larger or denser the part, the greater the secondary radiation, and vice

Figure 8.20. Radiograph taken with both cone and

Figure 8.21. Radiograph taken with cone but without grid. Note the fog and the flat-gray film.

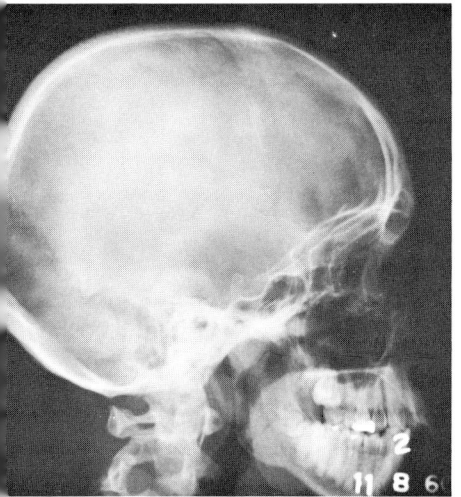
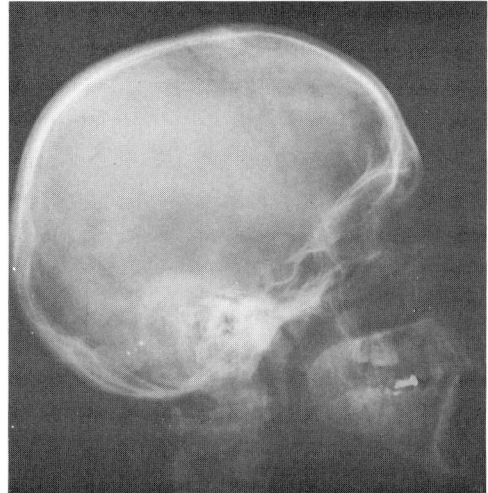

113

FORMULATING X-RAY TECHNIQUES

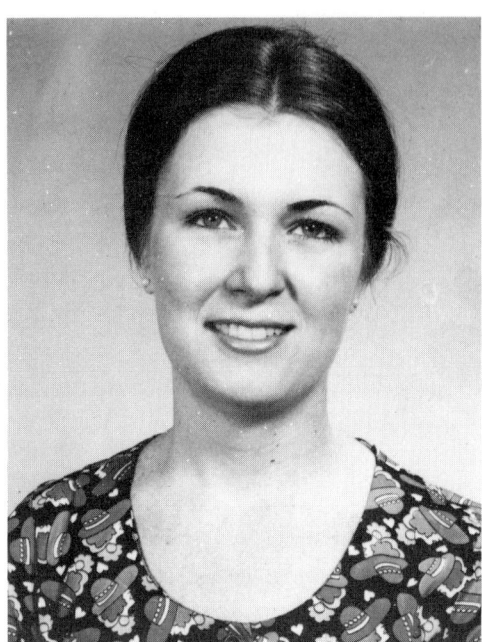

Figure 8.22. Satisfactory contrast in a photograph.

Figure 8.24. Sufficient detail in a photograph.

Figure 8.23. Both insufficient and excessive contrast mark this photograph. There is not enough contrast to distinguish details, yet overall the picture is "contrasty" or "high-contrast," typical of short-scale films and processing.

Figure 8.25. Though the face in this photograph shows good detail note how the detail in jacket and tie have disappeared for lack of contrast.

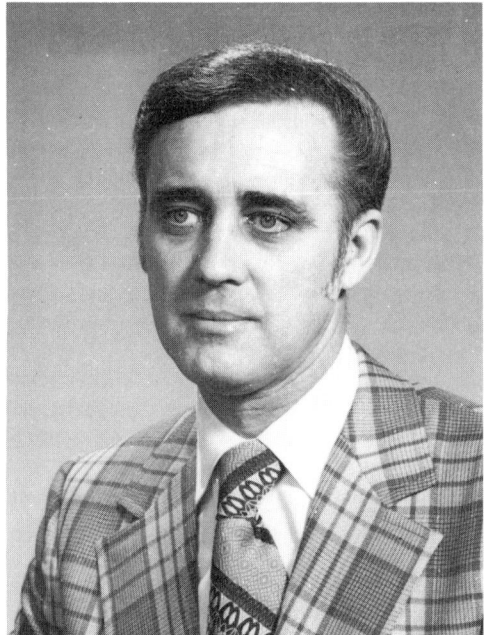
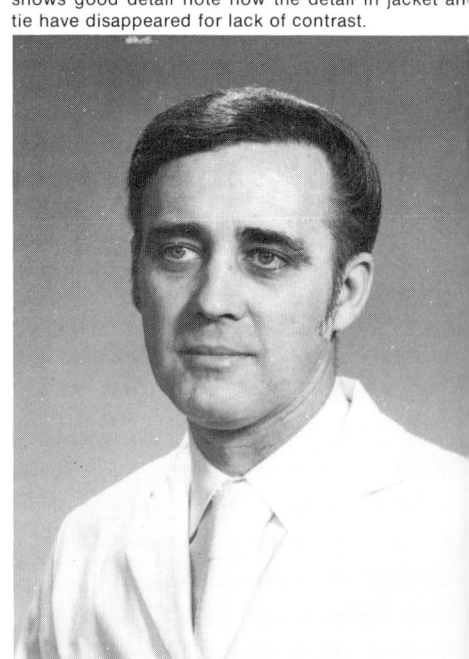

Essentials of the Radiograph

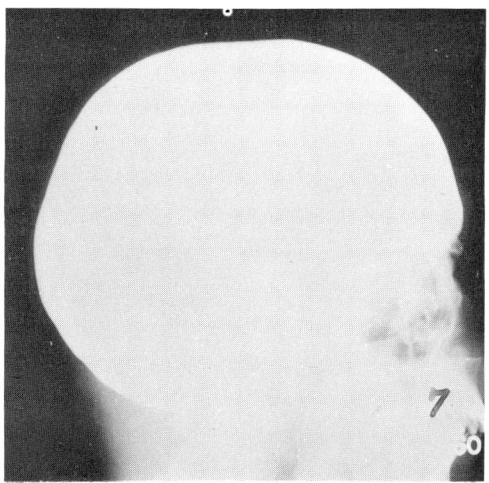

Figure 8.26. Radiograph of lateral skull for which the penetrating power (Kv.P.) has been insufficient.

versa. Bone emits a relatively small amount of secondary radiation, whereas muscle emits large quantities of it and may produce much secondary radiation fog.

The problem of secondary radiation fog increases in proportion to the thickness of the part. Accordingly, the author recommends that the Potter-Bucky diaphragm or grid be used on all parts that are not air-containing which measure 12 cm. or more.

The secondary radiation fog can be eliminated to a great extent by the use of the *smallest cone possible for the part being radiographed,* the use of *grids and/or the Potter-Bucky diaphragm, compression binders, small-sized film for the area being radiographed, and careful selection of a balance between Kv.P. and Ma.S.*

When we control secondary radiation fog, contrast is improved, and so detail of the radiographic image is improved (Figures 8.20 and 8.21).

CONTRAST

Radiographic contrast is defined as the percentage of difference between the extreme *blacks* and *whites* in the radiograph. As contrast is *decreased,* the percentage of difference between various densities on the film is reduced. (This does not refer to the *background* in relation to the *anatomical* part.)

Opinions as to the amount of contrast desired do not seem to vary as much as those concerning radiographic density, yet a considerable range of opinion does exist. For instance, from a photographic standpoint, Figure 8.22 shows sufficient contrast, while Figure 8.23 shows insufficient contrast in the facial features. Again, Figures 8.24 and 8.25 show what effect clothes have on contrast. In Figure 8.24 we have sufficient contrast, while in Figure 8.25, details of the man's clothes blend together because there is too little contrast. For this reason it seems inadvisable to set any definite degree of contrast as a standard.

FORMULATING X-RAY TECHNIQUES

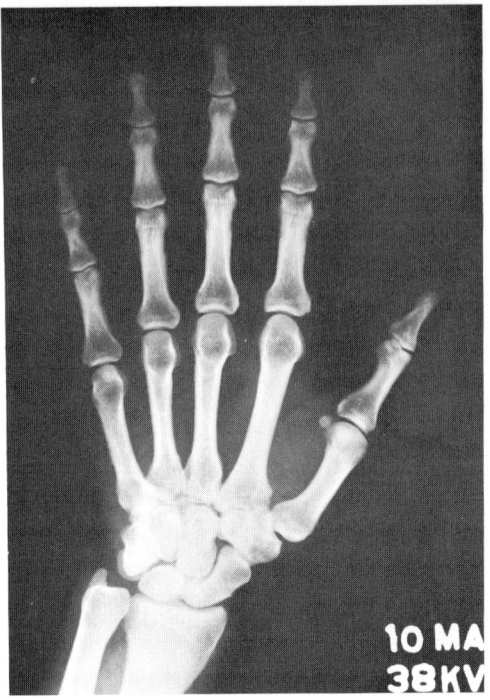

Figure 8.27. Posteroanterior radiograph of the hand an example of short-scale contrast.

The old rule "the lower the kilovoltage and the higher the Ma.S., the greater the contrast" is true only *within certain limits*. For example, the kilovoltage could be so low that we would have *insufficient contrast;* to put it another way, we can say of such a radiograph that the degrees of brightness over the area being examined are too nearly the same for satisfactory discrimination (Figure 8.26). Perhaps a better term here would be *insufficient density,* since we do not have enough black and white in the image to give us contrast and we therefore have no detail.

General differences in tone value may be divided into two arbitrary scales of contrast. As radiographic contrast increases, the difference in tone value between adjacent densities becomes greater or more abrupt. The densities that represent the thinner portions of the part increase and may become opaque. This increase may be carried to excess so that the densities which represent the thick parts become very low, to the extent of not recording detail at all. For example, when low kilovoltage is used for thin parts, *greater contrast* results between radiographic images of the bones and the flesh. However, a point may be reached at which radiographic detail in the thinner portions, such as the subcutaneous tissues and muscles, is obliterated by opaque silver deposits; and some bone detail may be lost because the denser bone tissue absorbs so much radiation that little remnant radiation reaches the film. Visibility of detail in those areas is diminished and *short scale* or *high contrast* results (Figure 8.27). As radiographic contrast decreases, the brightness differences in tone value between densities become less; consequently, a greater number of tones are visualized over the entire

Essentials of the Radiograph

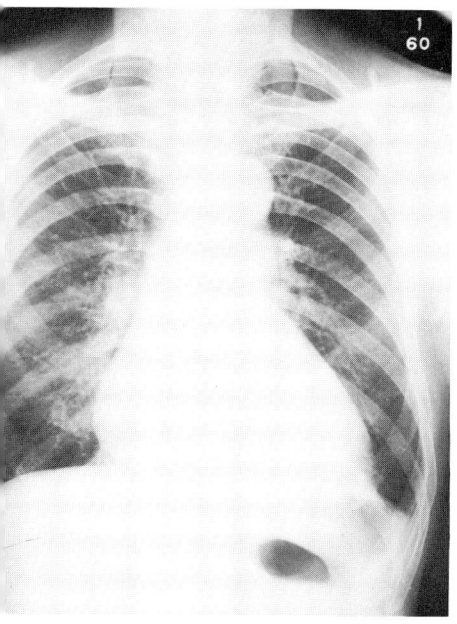

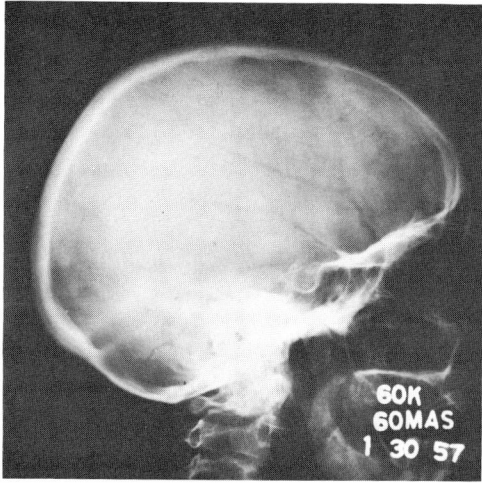

Figure 8.29. An example of short-scale contrast.

Figure 8.28. An example of short-scale contrast.

image. The transition between tones is gradual since only small density differences occur. This type is known as *long-scale* or *low contrast*.

Kilovoltage governs the scale of contrast in the image and influences the production of secondary radiation fog, which is a supplement density.

Radiographic contrast is the product of two factors: (1) *film contrast*, which is inherent in film manufacture and developing process, (2) *subject contrast*, which is the result of the absorption of the radiation by the patient. Radiographic contrast can be controlled by altering either one or both of these contributing factors. Subject contrast can be readily altered by changing the *quality* of radiation or *kilovoltage;* it is good technique to *standardize* the film and development and leave the control of the contrast in the finished radiograph to the single factor—*kilovoltage*.

Short-scale contrast

In a radiograph of a body part with a short range of widely different intermediate translucent densities, short-scale contrast exists. Such radiographs possess instant eye appeal.

On the whole, a radiograph with short-scale contrast (low kilovoltage) is incomplete, for details that represent the thinner and thicker portions of the body are not always shown. Typical radiographic examples of short-scale contrast are shown in Figures 8.28 and 8.29.

Long-scale contrast

Long-scale contrast makes possible the visualization of small image density. The short wavelength (higher kilovoltage) radiation effects greater penetration of the tissues and results in an abundance of remnant radiation of varying intensity which in turn produces a large number of translucent

FORMULATING X-RAY TECHNIQUES

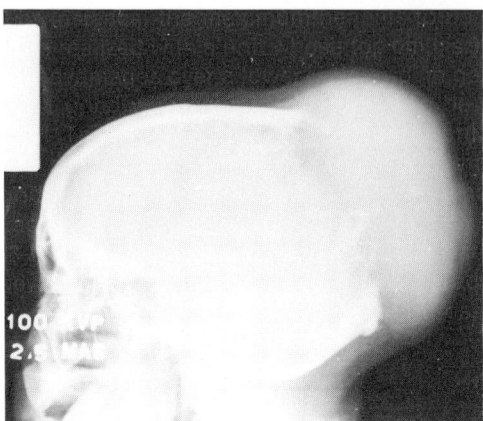

Figure 8.30. Extreme long-scale contrast in order to visualize skin lines. 110 Kv.P. and 2.5 Ma.S.

densities. The contrast scale, however, should never be so long that differentiation between structures is difficult (kilovoltage too high; Figure 8.30). Typical radiographic examples of long-scale contrast are shown in Figures 8.31 to 8.33.

Other factors influencing contrast

A number of factors other than *kilovoltage* influence radiographic contrast. They are (a) developer contrast, (b) film contrast, and (c) tissue contrast. These factors can, however, be regulated so that they can be considered

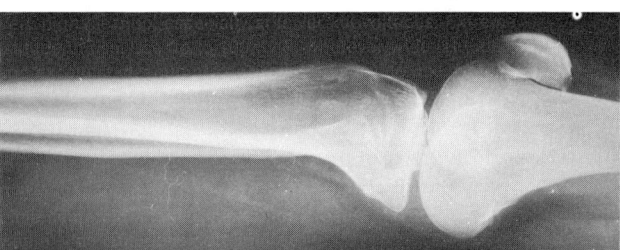

Figures 8.31, 8.32, and 8.33. Examples of long-scale contrast

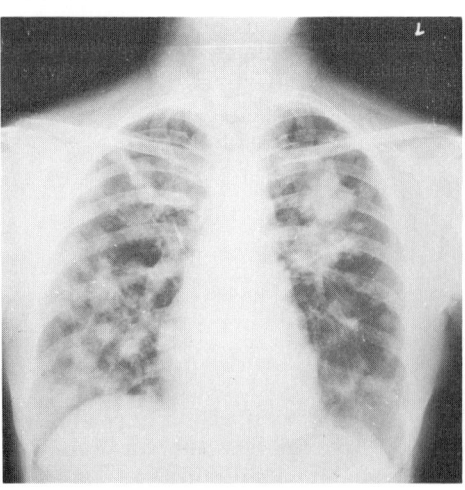
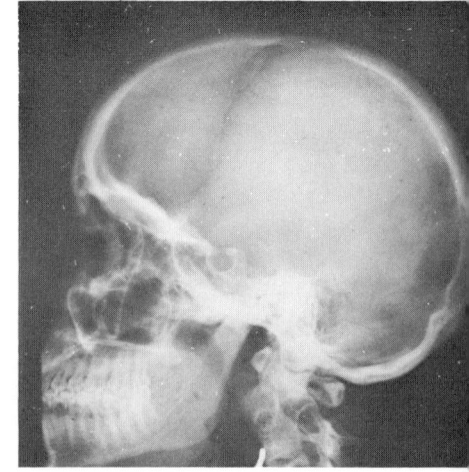

Essentials of the Radiograph

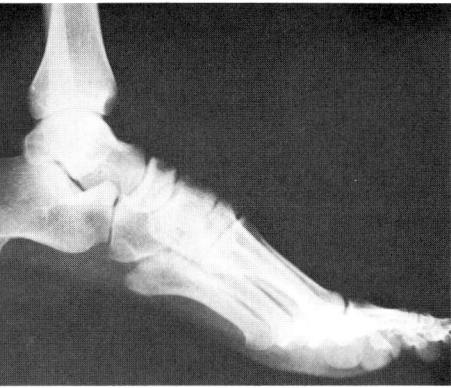

Figure 8.34. Radiograph of the lateral ankle and foot, made with regular film and screens.

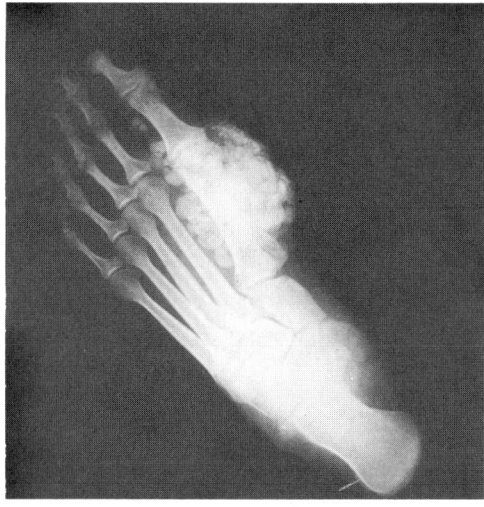

Figure 8.35. Anteroposterior view of the entire foot, made with non-screen film.

constants and thus standardized. Still other factors affecting contrast are processing (automatic vs. manual), temperature of the developer, screens (Figures 8.34 to 8.36), focus-film distance, cones, grids, pathology, compression, opacity of the part, respiration, Ma.S., secondary radiation fog, filters, old chemicals, white light or any form of radiation.

Developer contrast (manual processing)

Two types of developers are in common use. The regular type is a sodium carbonate developer that produces long-scale contrast in the radiographic

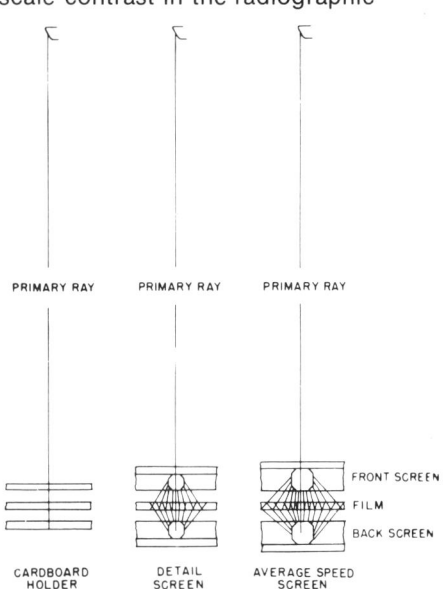

Figure 8.36. The effect of screens on detail. Though overall contrast is heightened by screens, some detail is lost, depending on the size of the crystals of calcium tungstate.

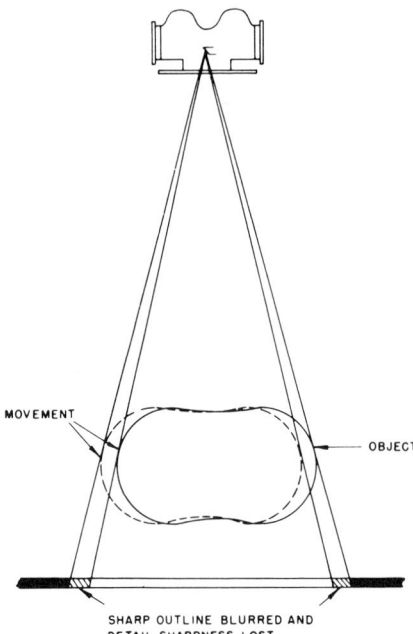

Figure 8.37. The effect of motion on detail.

image. The other is one containing a more active alkali, sodium hydroxide, which produces greater contrast in the image than that produced by regular developer. Since the type of contrast produced by the developer can be changed in some measure by the *time* and *temperature* of development, the maximum radiographic contrast from either type of development will be obtained only when *full* development is employed.

Film contrast

Screen-type film has an inherent higher contrast when exposed with screens than when the same film is exposed by direct radiation (cardboard holders) at the same kilovoltage.

Direct exposure films (non-screen) have a thick emulsion, and provide a higher contrast than the screen-type film when *direct exposures* are employed for both, using the same kilovoltage. At the *same* kilovoltage, non-screen film is about *three* times as fast as screen-type film under the same conditions.

DETAIL

Detail can be considered a visual quality that depends, first, upon *sharpness* and, secondly, upon *radiographic contrast*.

When structures are sharp and clearly delineated, and when the density differences between these structures (contrast) are sufficient for the eye to distinguish one from another easily, the radiograph is said to have good detail. Sharpness of detail is often referred to as *definition*.

The size of the x-ray tube focal spot has a great effect on detail; however,

Essentials of the Radiograph

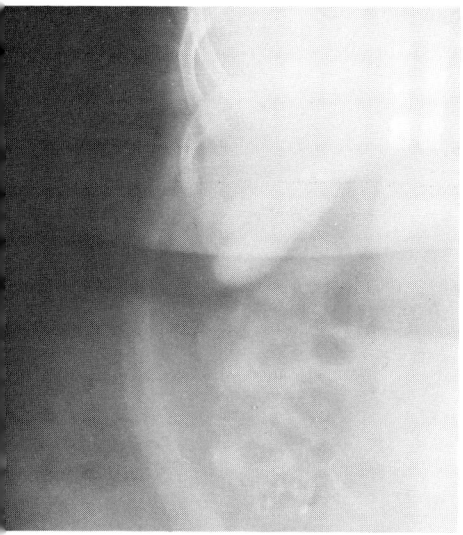 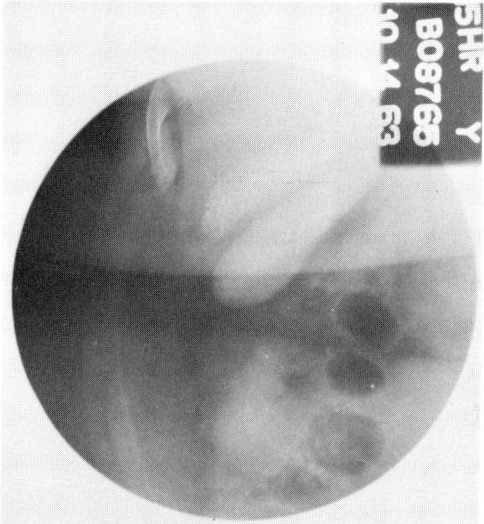

Figure 8.38. Radiograph of gallbladder in a patient weighing 270 pounds. Taken with a large port of entry.

Figure 8.39. Radiograph with a small port of entry—a cylinder cone—taken of the patient of Figure 8.38.

with present-day rotating-anode tubes this size is no longer of critical importance.

When an image is projected from a pinpoint light source, the borders of the image are sharp, but if the light source is a larger surface, such as a large focal spot of an x-ray tube, the image is ill-defined at the *outer edge* because of *penumbra* formation. To reduce the penumbra the focal-spot size must be small, and the object-film distance as close as possible. The focus-film distance should be as long as possible (see Figure 8.40).

Generally the smaller the size of the focal spot, the sharper the detail. Close subject-film contact, non-movement of the part, film, or tube during exposure, and good screen contact are essential for good detail.

The use of screens results in a loss of detail; however, it is impractical to use cardboard holders and regular film or non-screen film on heavy parts in order to obtain better detail.

Detail is dependent primarily upon:

a. Size of effective focal-spot
b. Focus-film distance
c. Object-film distance
d. Immobilization of the part (Figure 8.37)
e. Size of port of entry of primary beam (Figures 8.38 and 8.39)
f. Speed of screens
g. Screen-film contact

Other factors affecting detail are overexposure or underexposure with Ma.S. or Kv.P., filters, respiration, fog, stereo shift, grid "cut-off," Bucky, pathology, and compression.

DISTORTION

The smaller the source of radiation and the nearer the object to the film, the sharper and more accurate the image.

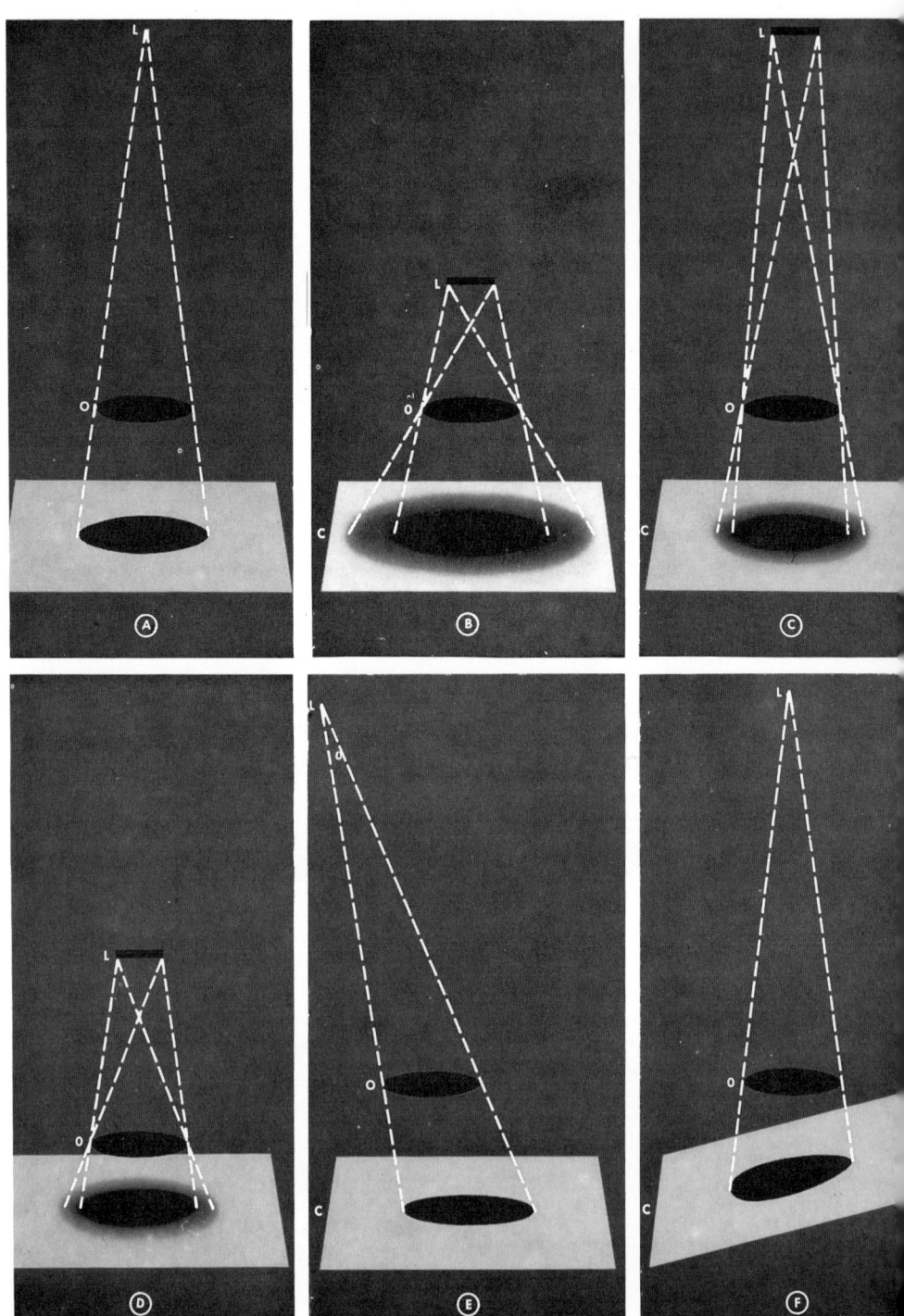

Figure 8.40. Geometric principles: the effects of changing the relative positions of source, object, and card. [Courtesy, Eastman Kodak Company.]

Essentials of the Radiograph

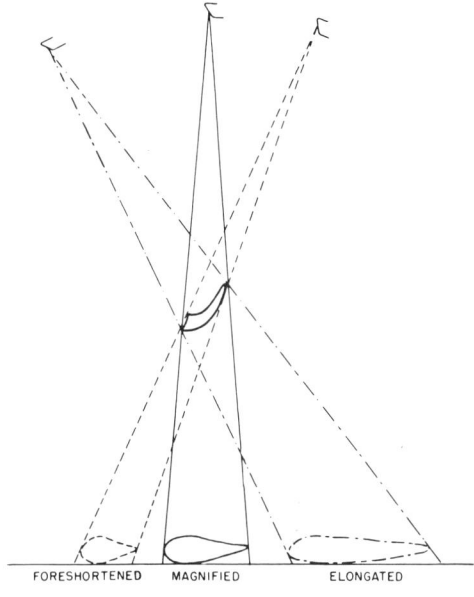

Figure 8.41. Types of distortion caused by inaccuracies in aligning the tube, the object, and the film.

Geometric principles

X-rays and gamma rays obey the common laws of light—their shadow formation may be explained in a simple manner in terms of light. The analogy between light and x-rays or gamma rays is not perfect, but the same geometric laws of shadow formation hold for both radiations.

Suppose as in Figure 8.40 that there is light from a point (L) falling on a white card (C), and an opaque object (O) is interposed between the light source and the card. A shadow of the object will be formed on the surface of the card.

This shadow cast by the object will naturally show some *enlargement* because the object is *not in contact* with the card; the *degree of enlargement* will vary according to the relative distances of the object from the card and from the light source. *The form of the shadow* also may differ according to the angle which the object makes with the incident light rays. Deviations from the *true shape* of the object as exhibited in its shadow image are called *distortion* (Figure 8.41).

The degree of sharpness of any shadow depends upon the size of the source of light and upon the position of the object between the light and the card—whether nearer to or farther from one or the other. The shadows cast when the source of light is not a small area are not perfectly sharp because each point in the source of light casts its own shadow of the object; all these overlapping shadows, since they are slightly displaced from each other, produce an ill-defined image. Figures 8.40A–F show the effects of changing the relative positions of source, object, and card. The following conditions must be fulfilled to produce a sharp, true shadow of the object.

1. The source of light should be small. Compare Figures A and C.

FORMULATING X-RAY TECHNIQUES

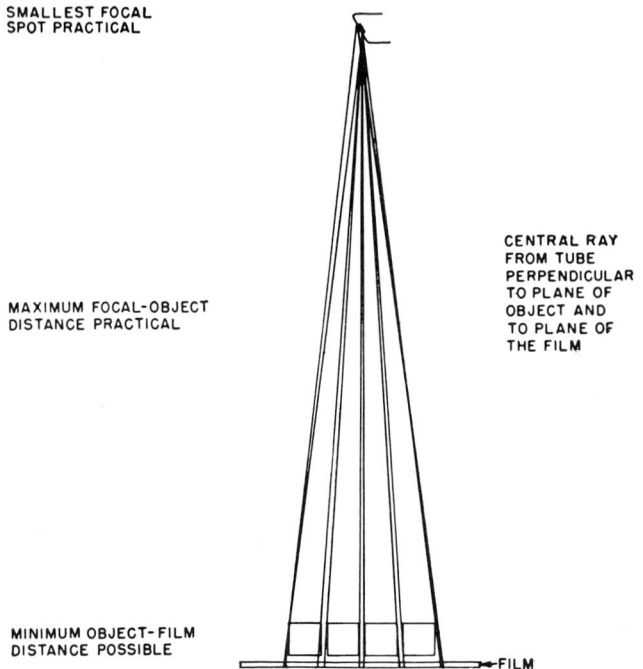

THE CENTRAL RAY DIRECTED THRU THE CENTER OF THE PART AND TO THE CENTER OF THE FILM

Figure 8.42. The best positioning of source, object, and film.

2. The source of light should be as far from the object as practicable. Compare Figures B and C, and see Figure 8.42.
3. The recording surface should be as close to the object as possible. Compare Figures B and D.
4. The light rays should be directed perpendicularly to the recording surface. See Figures A and E.

KILOVOLTAGE

Of all the four primary factors in the production of a radiograph (milliamperage, time, kilovoltage, and distance) kilovoltage has the greatest effect upon the radiographic image. Kilovoltage *influences the quality of the radiation, determines the contrast in the image, and influences exposure latitude, radiographic density, and secondary radiation fog.*

According to a long-established view, a good radiograph is the net result of favorable conditions with respect to two basic physical factors: *contrast* and *definition*. No one can say that *definition* is more important than *contrast,* or vice versa. In a radiograph with insufficient contrast, brightnesses over the areas are too nearly the same for satisfactory discrimination, while with poor definition, areas of one density merge into another so gradually that the diffuse image cannot be interpreted.

Early radiographic techniques employed the use of higher kilovoltages

Essentials of the Radiograph

Table 8.1 REVIEW OF THE RADIOGRAPHIC QUALITIES

Controlling factors			
Density	Contrast	Detail	Distortion
1. Ma.S. 2. Kv.P.	1. Kv.P. 2. Ma.S.	1. Motion 2. Focal spot 3. Focus-film distance 4. Object-film distance	1. Focus-film distance 2. Object-film distance 3. Tube alignment

Factors directly affecting		Factors indirectly affecting	
Density	Contrast	Density	Contrast
1. Thickness of part 2. Opacity 3. Pathology 4. Compression 5. Respiration 6. Focus-film distance	1. Bucky 2. Cones 3. Screens 4. Cardboard holders 5. Filters 6. Film	1. Bucky 2. Cones 3. Screens 4. Cardboard 5. Filter 6. Films	1. Thickness of part 2. Opacity 3. Pathology 4. Compression 5. Respiration 6. Focus-film distance

Factors affecting both density and contrast
1. Processing 2. Radiographic efficiency of equipment

because with low-current equipment, penetration was of paramount importance. With the development of equipment with higher milliamperage and faster film and screens, radiographic technique swung to the use of lower kilovoltages, higher milliamperage, and high film contrast. Now the trend is back to the use of higher kilovoltages, and low milliampere-second values, which permit lower patient dosage with the production of better diagnostic images. Notable among the contributors to the standard approach to this technique was the late Arthur W. Fuchs. The use of higher kilovoltages in radiography caused the factors of *secondary radiation fog, cones,* and a *higher ratio grid* to assume great importance.

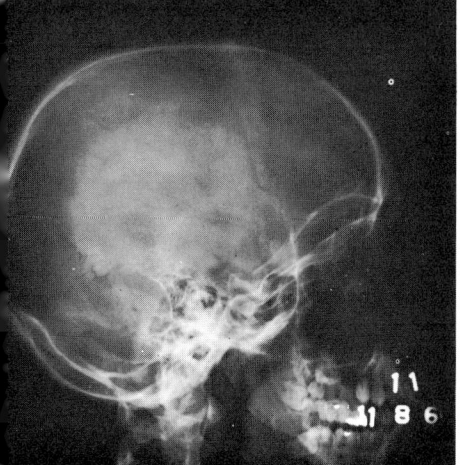

Figure 8.43. An overexposed radiograph due to essive Kv.P.

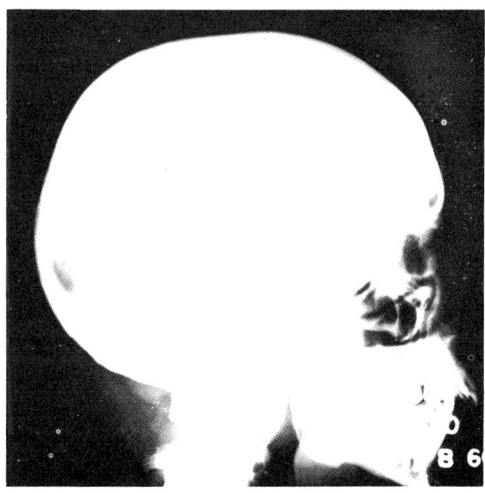

Figure 8.44. Underexposure due to inadequate Kv.P.

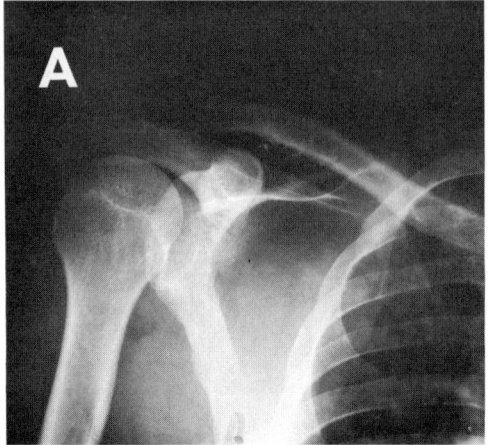
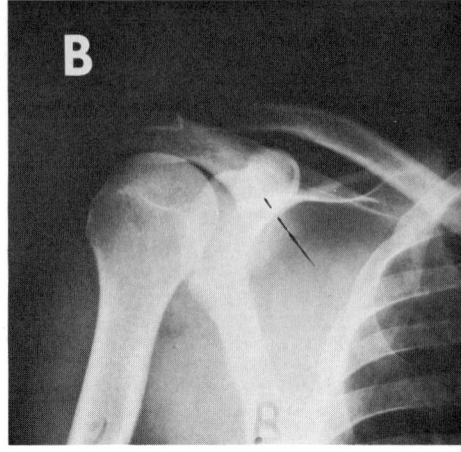
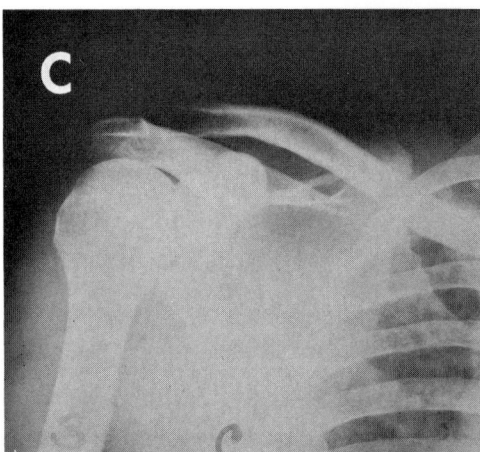

Figure 8.45. Anteroposterior view of the shoulder. A overexposure; corrected in B by reducing the Kv.P by 10. In C, insufficient Kv.P. results in underexposure

Overexposure with kilovoltage

An overexposed radiograph is gray and flat. The contrast and detail of the image are obscured. Under normal conditions, a reduction of 10 to 15 Kv.P. will improve the radiographic quality appreciably (Figure 8.43).

Underexposure with kilovoltage

A radiograph underexposed because of inadequate kilovoltage, because of the lack of penetration, is characterized by a *chalky appearance* and *insufficient contrast* (Figure 8.44). An increase of 10 to 15 Kv.P. will improve the radiographic quality; however, a slight adjustment in milliampere-seconds may be necessary to provide the optimum film quality.

Insufficient kilovoltage

It is not practical to use excessive milliampere-second values when using a kilovoltage that is inadequate to penetrate the part. High Ma.S. values and low Kv.P. increase the radiation dosage to the patient (see Figures 8.5–8.11 and 8.12–8.16).

Essentials of the Radiograph

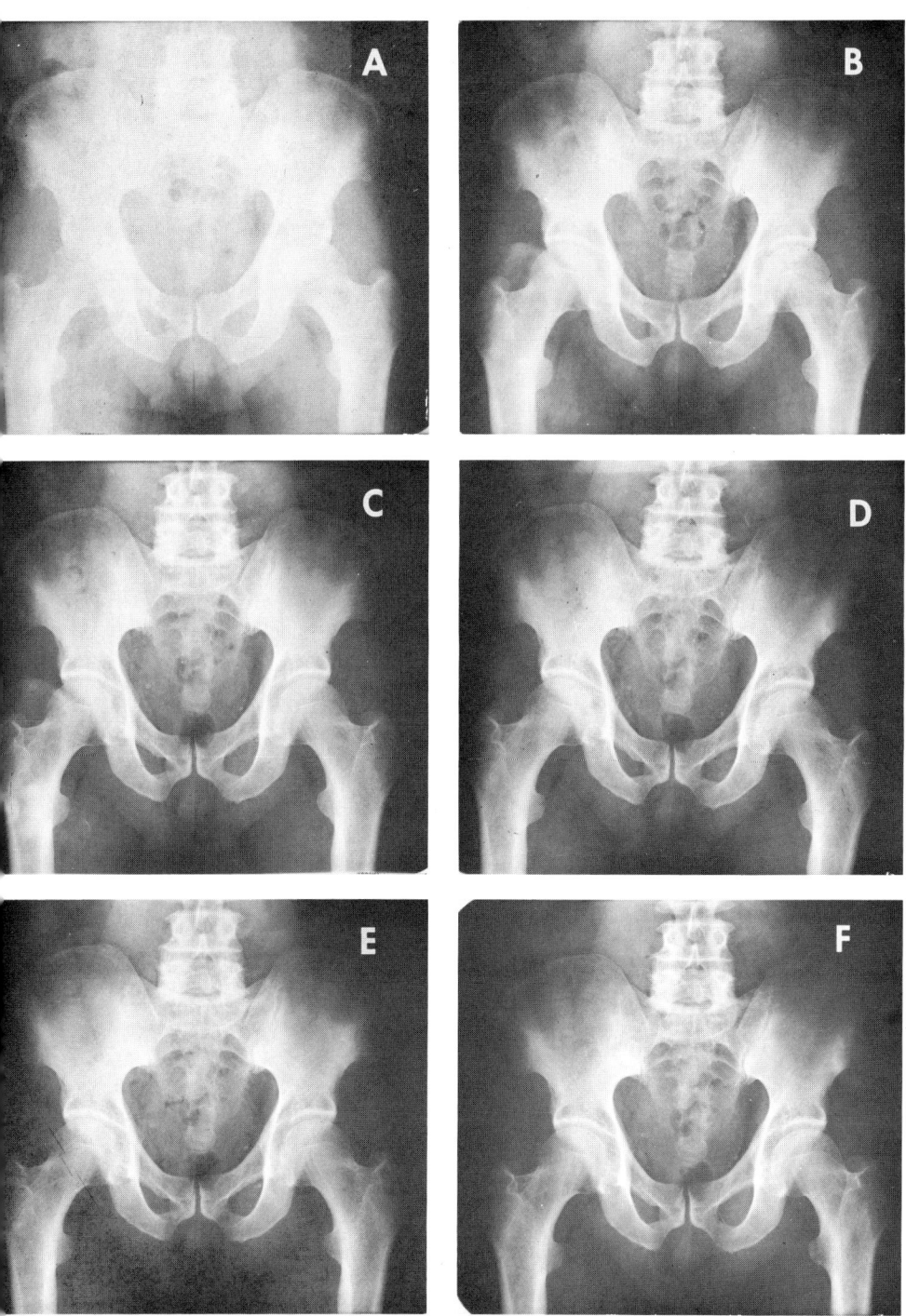

Figure 8.46. These six anteroposterior views of a pelvis show a broad exposure latitude: A — 20 Ma.S.; B — 30 Ma.S.; C — 40 Ma.S.; D — 50 Ma.S.; E — 60 Ma.S.; F — 70 Ma.S.

FORMULATING X-RAY TECHNIQUES

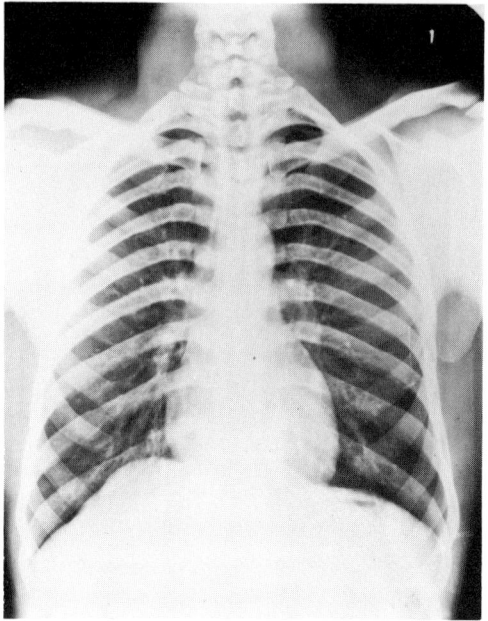

Figure 8.47. Posteroanterior view of the chest at 50 Kv.P. and 5 Ma.S.

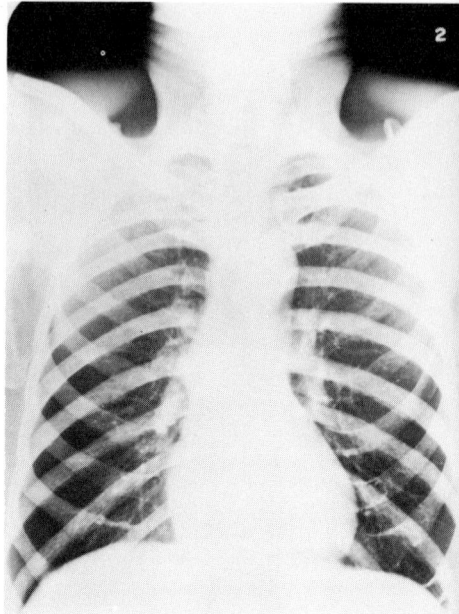

Figure 8.48. Chest at 50 Kv.P. and 10 Ma.S.

Kilovoltage and contrast

When secondary radiation and Ma.S. are controlled, kilovoltage becomes the factor of radiographic contrast. With contrast, we have detail in the image; in fact, detail in the image is dependent upon radiographic contrast (Figure 8.45).

General differences in tone value may be divided into two arbitrary scales of contrast. As radiographic contrast increases, the brightness in tone value between adjacent densities becomes greater or more abrupt. The densities that represent the thinner portions of the part increase and may become opaque. This increase may be carried to excess so that the densities which represent the thick parts become very low, to the extent of not recording detail at all. Visibility of detail in those areas is diminished and *short scale* or "high" *contrast* results. As radiographic contrast decreases, the brightness differences in tone value between densities become less; consequently, a greater number of tones are visualized over the entire image. The transition between tones is gradual since only small density differences occur. This type is known as *long scale* or "low" *contrast*.

Kilovoltage and latitude

Exposure latitude is the range between maximum exposure and minimum exposure that can be used to produce a diagnostically acceptable radiograph. Exposure latitude varies with the kilovoltage applied and whether or not screens or direct exposures are employed. With long-scale contrast technique, from higher or fixed kilovoltage, exposure latitude becomes wide, and wide errors in Ma.S. may be tolerated (Figure 8.46A–F). With

Essentials of the Radiograph

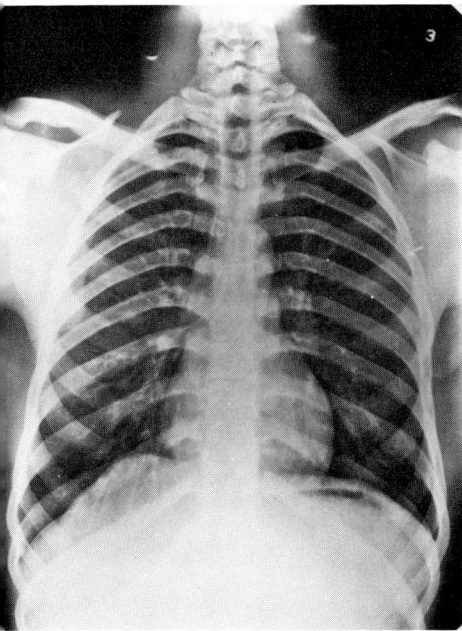

Figure 8.49. Chest at 50 Kv.P. and 20 Ma.S. Figures 8.47–49 show a narrow exposure latitude.

lower kilovoltages, short-scale contrast is produced, the exposure latitude becomes narrow, and errors in exposure become more critical (Figures 8.47 to 8.49).

The only limit to the kilovoltage that can be used in radiography is the limitation imposed by contrast. The limiting voltage is the one at which the contrast scale has become so *long* that diagnosis becomes doubtful. The limitations of contrast have been recognized by all who have investigated the use of higher voltages for diagnosis. Investigation of the grids of various ratios was the starting point for such work since the *grid,* thus far, is the best means of reducing scattered radiation. (Figures 8.50 and 8.51).

Notable among the investigators of the grid and secondary radiation are Wilsey, Trout, Groves, Slauson, Kelley, Seemann and Splettstasser. The results of Trout and Kelley proved that the 16-to-1 grid gave a considerably higher degree of contrast at any voltage than did the 8-to-1 grid. The contrast was reduced as the voltage was increased, but by using the 16-to-1 grid it was possible to use a higher voltage and to retain a degree of contrast equal to that provided by the 8-to-1 grid at a lower kilovoltage. See Figure 8.52C.

One of the real gains was the reduction of the exposure to the patient as the kilovoltage was increased. The patient dosage can be still further reduced by the use of filters.

The reduction of scattered radiation with a grid requires that additional exposure be made to obtain a satisfactory radiographic image. This may be accomplished by raising the milliampere-seconds or kilovoltage; yet so rapid is the increase in penetration with increasing kilovoltage, and so effective is the removal of scattered radiation in increasing subject contrast, that one

FORMULATING X-RAY TECHNIQUES

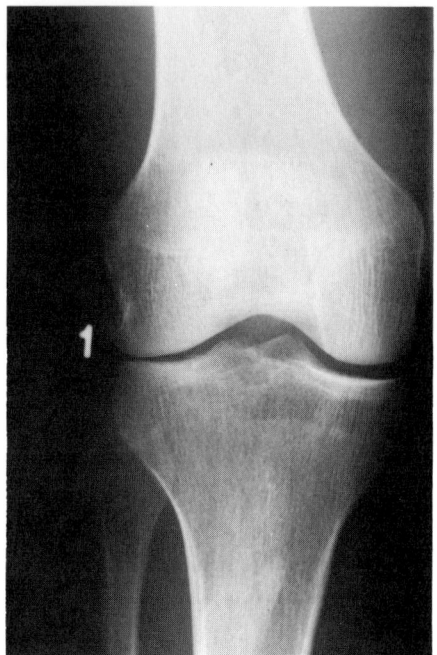

Figure 8.50. Radiograph of knee, taken without a grid.

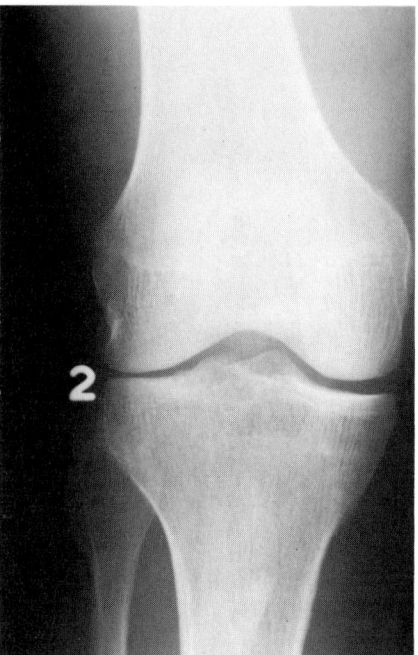

Figure 8.51. Radiograph of knee, taken with a grid, plus 20 Kv.P.

may *actually attain higher contrast at high kilovoltage with a grid than at low kilovoltage without a grid* (see in Chapter 10, Figures 10.30C and 10.32).

With small amounts of scattered radiation, an 8-to-1 grid is almost as useful as a 16-to-1 grid. A 16-to-1 grid absorbs appreciably more primary radiation than the 8-to-1 grid. The small gain in subject contrast in changing from an 8-to-1 to a 16-to-1 grid technique might not be worth while for average thicknesses, because of the increased exposure required to make up for the higher absorption. The 16-to-1 grid should be used only when it offers a significant advantage by increasing the subject contrast (see Figure 8.52C).

There has been for years among technologists a commonly held fallacy that all radiographs made with high kilovoltage are necessarily gray and flat. It is possible to produce films of as good quality with high kilovoltage as with low kilovoltage. Radiographs made at various kilovoltage values, but with suitable compensation in milliampere seconds, should be indistinguishable from each other in quality, except that one should be able to visualize an increased range of densities with high kilovoltage.

Figure 8.53 shows two exposures of the toes made on non-screen film. The anteroposterior projection was exposed at 50 Kv.P. and 25 Ma.S.; the lateral at 100 Kv.P., 10 Ma.S. Note the long range of densities from the skin to the phalanx and metatarsals. Figure 8.54 shows two exposures of the os calcis made on the same non-screen film, one exposure at 50 Kv.P., 60 Ma.S., and one exposure at 120 Kv.P. and 15 Ma.S. It will be noted that these exposures are comparable.

Essentials of the Radiograph

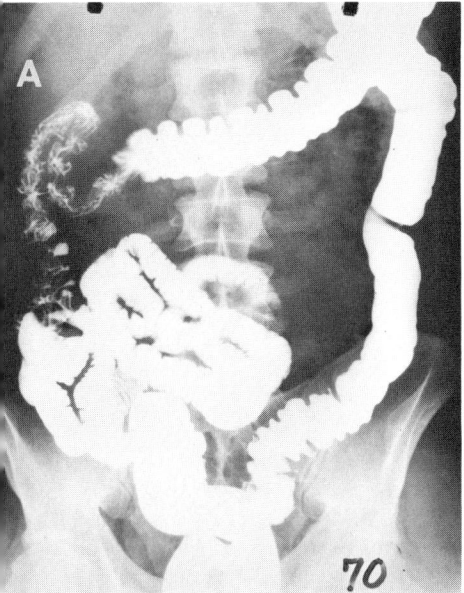
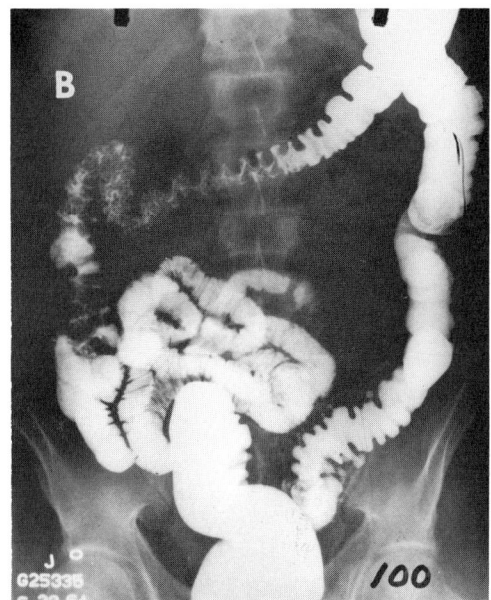
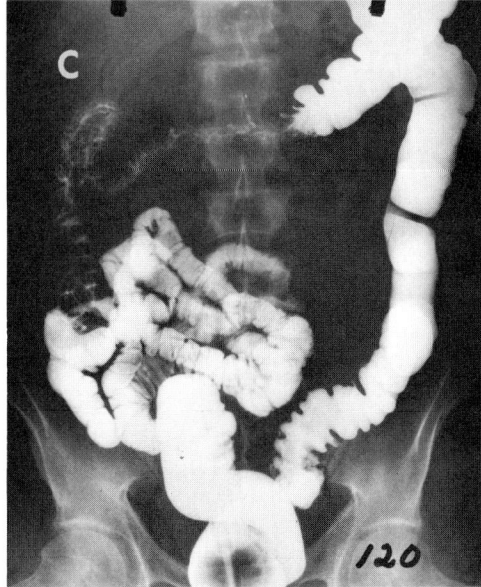

Figure 8.52. The effect of grids. Radiographs of a colon: A, at 70 Kv.P. and 60 Ma.S.; B, at 100 Kv.P. and Ma.S.; and C at 120 Kv.P. and 50 Ma.S. A and B are made with an 8-to-1 grid; C with a 16-to-1 grid. Note the detail recorded in B and C that is missing in A.

Kilovoltage and contrast studies

As a general rule, Kv.P. should not exceed 75 in performing iodinated contrast studies. This may be modified slightly by the use of different screens, grids, film and three-phase generators. The reasons for this level of Kv.P. in these studies are the following:

(1) As Kv.P. increases, film contrast decreases.
(2) The linear attenuation coefficient for fat and water (muscle) remains

FORMULATING X-RAY TECHNIQUES

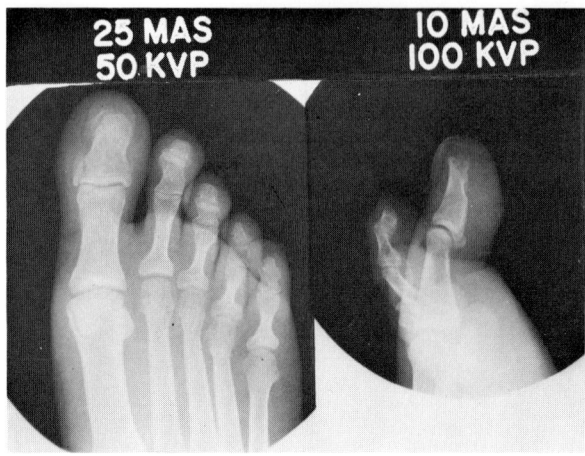

Figure 8.53. Two views of phalanges with exposures at different kilovoltages and compensations in Ma.S.: non-screen film.

about the same as Kv.P. increases.

(3) As Kv.P. increases, the linear attenuation coefficient for metals (i.e., iodinated contrast media, bone, barium sulfate suspensions) markedly decreases.

(4) In using iodinated contrast media, we try to maintain the maximum difference in linear attenuation coefficients between contrast media and soft tissues so as to better visualize the contrast media.

(5) Ideally, one should use about 65 Kv.P. for iodinated, related contrast studies; but in actual practice the Ma.S. may be too long, so one would settle for about 70–75 Kv.P., as the x-ray generators permit. In many incidents, the patient could be moved to rooms with larger generators rather than increasing the Kv.P.

Under normal conditions one would not want to use a high Kv.P. which would give a rather long scale of contrast and perhaps blend out cholesterol stones in gallbladder studies.

Kilovoltage: a review

Since kilovoltage plays such an important role in radiography, it might be

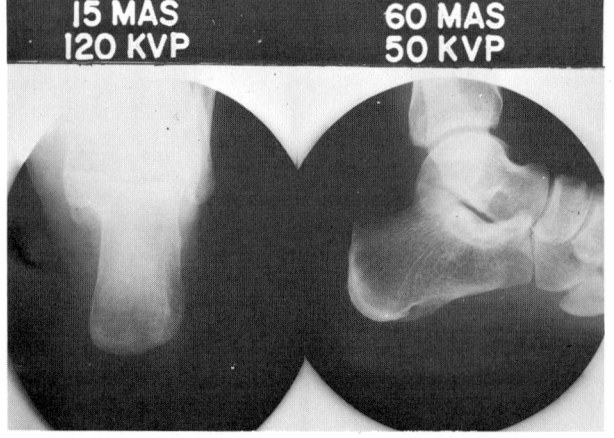

Figure 8.54. Two views of os calcis: exposures made at high and low kilovoltages with compensation in Ma.S.: non-screen film.

Essentials of the Radiograph

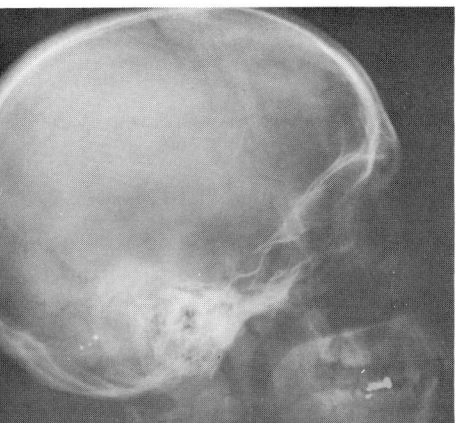

Figure 8.55. Secondary radiation fog.

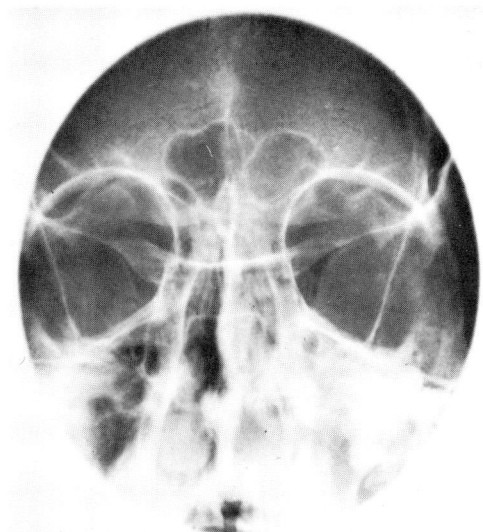

Figure 8.56. In this view, a cylinder cone has been used to reduce secondary radiation fog.

well to review the influence of kilovoltage on radiographic exposure.

When all other factors are constant, *density changes with Kv.P.; Kv.P. governs the quality of radiation; Kv.P. governs penetration; Kv.P. influences the amount of secondary radiation fog; Kv.P. regulates exposure latitude; Kv.P. controls contrast:* low Kv.P. produces short-scale contrast, high Kv.P. produces long-scale contrast.

The use of the higher kilovoltages (above the usual variable kilovoltage techniques) provides greater exposure efficiency in routine radiography because details in all tissue are recorded as translucent densities. Soft-tissue detail is often better than that produced by lower kilovoltage. See Figures 8.53, radiograph of the toe at 100 Kv.P., and 8.54.

The radiation dose to the patient is reduced as the kilovoltage increases and the milliampere-seconds decreases because the body absorbs less radiation than at lower kilovoltages.

A fixed or higher kilovoltage technique will produce more uniformity in routine radiography than a relatively low, variable kilovoltage technique, since the *latitude* and penetration at the higher kilovoltage permit more uniform results.

SECONDARY RADIATION FOG

Secondary radiation fog is a supplement density and obscures image details. Fog is characterized by a dull gray appearance and the absence of contrast and detail (see Figure 8.55).

The amount of secondary radiation fog depends upon *tissue thickness* and *density* of the *subject* matter, as well as the kilovoltage employed.

Secondary radiation fog may be controlled by the proper use of exposure factors, strict coning of the part radiographed, and the use of grids, with a grid ratio appropriate for the thickness and density of the part. It is suggested that the sections on cones, diaphragms, and grids be reviewed in order to

FORMULATING X-RAY TECHNIQUES

become more familiar with the control of secondary radiation fog. Figure 8.56 shows the effect of a cylinder cone in improving contrast by restricting the area in which secondary radiation fog is generated. See Figures 8.38 and 8.39, radiography of the gallbladder.

MILLIAMPERE SECONDS

Milliampere seconds is simply the milliamperage (Ma.) multiplied by the time of exposure in seconds (s.), the product being Ma.S.

It is most important for the technologist to become familiar with Ma.S., since proper control of this factor gives him an opportunity to fit the exposure to the problem at hand.

It is suggested that the reader refer to Table 7.9 in order to become familiar with the most common Ma.S. values used in radiography. The Ma.-time relation formula on page 102 should be reviewed until one is able to work this formula from memory.

Table 8.2 SUMMARY OF THE RADIOGRAPH AND IMAGE FORMATION

PHOTOGRAPHIC ASPECTS	GEOMETRIC ASPECTS

I. Radiographic density
    Controlled by:
        Ma.S.
        Focus-film distance
        Heel effect
    Influenced by:
        Kv.P.
        Fog
        Processing
	I. Image sharpness (definition)
	    Affected by:
	        Focal-spot size
	        Object-film distance
	        Focus-film distance
	        Motion
	        Screen-crystal size
	        Film-screen contact

II. Radiographic contrast
    Controlled by:
        Kilovoltage
    Influenced by:
        Filters
        Fog (all forms)
        Development
        Tissue contrast
        Type of film
        Pathology
	II. Image size (magnification)
	    Influenced by:
	        Focus-film distance
	        Object-film distance

III. Secondary radiation fog
    Affected by:
        Size of area irradiated
        Compression
        Cones
        Diaphragms
        Grids
        Kv.P.
	III. Image shape (distortion)
	    Influenced by:
	        Alignment of tube to film
	        Alignment of part to film
	        Object-film distance

Essentials of the Radiograph

REVIEW: DENSITY VERSUS CONTRAST

If an x-ray film is placed in the direct path of an x-ray exposure, without there being an object placed on the film and subsequently processed, the result is a film covered with about the same amount of black metallic silver at every point over its entire surface. This deposit of black metallic silver on the radiograph is known as *radiographic density*. If we were to place an object on the film and make another exposure and process the film, the image of the object would be rendered not as one density but as two or more densities. The mere fact that there are two or more densities that can be seen and compared indicates the presence of *radiographic contrast*.

To provide satisfactory radiographic contrast, each density should permit the transmission of a certain amount of light from a standard radiographic illuminator. The light value of each density is called a *tone*. Since each tone in a radiograph is a radiographic representation of some detail within the object radiographed, obviously we cannot afford to have areas in the radiographic image that are devoid of them, nor should the density be so great that it ceases to have tone value. Such areas are ordinarily useless for diagnosis.

There are two types of radiographic contrast. Where only a few tones are present and the transition between the densities is abrupt or great, we have a radiograph with *short-scale contrast*. Such radiographs are usually made with low kilovoltage. *Long-scale contrast* is evident in a radiograph by a large number of tones of varying density over the entire image. These tones differ from one another by only small amounts of density, and the transition between tones is very gradual. Radiographs possessing long-scale contrast are usually considered to have good diagnostic quality. The higher kilovoltages produce this type of contrast and provide great exposure *latitude* as well. A disadvantage encountered in the use of the lower kilovoltages is the lack of tissue penetration that so frequently results, as well as the necessity of *strict accuracy* of exposure.

X-rays must penetrate the body tissue in order to produce an image. As the x-ray beam traverses the body part, the *intensity* of the x-ray is attenuated in proportion to the kind and thickness of the tissue; bone absorbs more radiation than muscle, muscle more than skin. It is not the primary radiation that exposes the radiographic film, but the radiation leaving the body part, known as *remnant radiation*. If the radiation applied does not penetrate the part, obviously no x-ray wavelengths leave that part to produce a radiographic image. To be effective, therefore, the *quality* of the radiation must be such that the part is penetrated — irrespective of its thickness — and the quantity of radiation must be adequate to provide a satisfactory image.

Kilovoltage or penetration regulates the *quality* of radiation — its wave length and resulting penetrating power and hence the *scale of contrast*. The Ma.S. factor should be considered the *quantity* or amount of radiation reaching the film and resulting degree of density on the finished film. When a kilovoltage has been selected as desirable for a given projection, it should be established as a constant; then any change in radiographic density that may be required becomes a function of the Ma.S. or *density factor*. By first establishing the kilovoltage as a constant, the changes in contrast are minimized as compared with techniques that employ changes in kilovoltage to regulate density and for which consequently contrast varies widely.

FORMULATING X-RAY TECHNIQUES

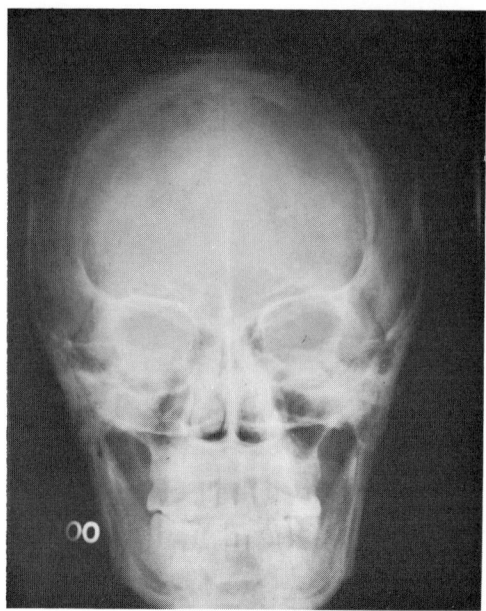
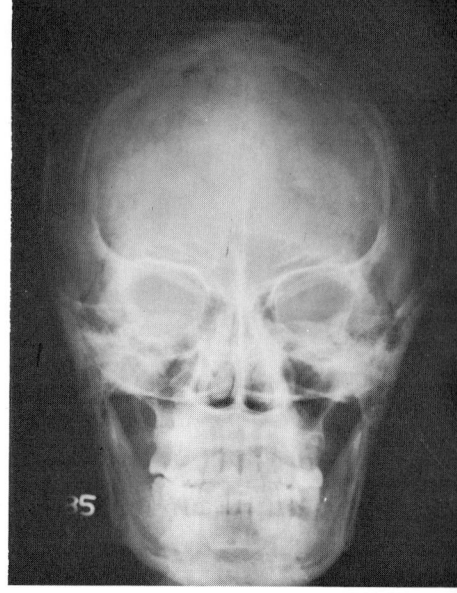

Figure 8.57. Posteroanterior view of skull at 100 Kv.P.   **Figure 8.58.** Posteroanterior view of skull at 85 Kv.P

Figure 8.45 above shows a series of radiographs demonstrating the results of (A) overexposure, (B) correct exposure, and (E) underexposure. Note opaque silver deposits in A and the absence of some silver deposits in C, indicating a loss of detail.

Assuming that a radiograph is processed by a standardized method, either manual or automatic processing, *opaque* deposits are known as *overexposures;* areas of the image possessing little deposited silver are almost totally transparent and are known as *highlights* or *underexposure.* Under the standard conditions of illumination, highlights possessing little silver, and therefore little detail, are diagnostically useless in modern radiography. Areas of overexposure may also be considered diagnostically useless, since the opaque silver deposits obscure image details when the radiograph is viewed on the standard radiographic illuminator.

In the visualization of radiographic *detail,* it is the *tone* relationship between one *density* and another that enables image details to become visible (Figures 8.57 to 8.60). This constitutes *radiographic contrast.* Radiographic contrast is a result of the difference in translucency between the various radiographic densities that compose the image. Generally speaking, visualization of details depends upon the degree of contrast and sharpness with which they are rendered (Figure 8.61).

The scale of contrast in a radiographic image is determined by the number and the tone value of the various densities. Radiographic contrast may vary widely or within some acceptable *average* range depending upon the nature of the part being radiographed. A good radiograph is one that shows a correct balance of densities over the entire contrast scale. The contrast should be such that, with the exposure techniques normally used, good differentiation is shown between tissue detail portrayed over the whole area of interest,

Essentials of the Radiograph

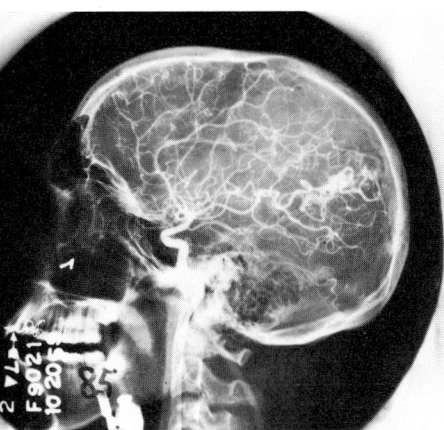

Figure 8.59. Lateral view of skull with opaque medium at 85 Kv.P.

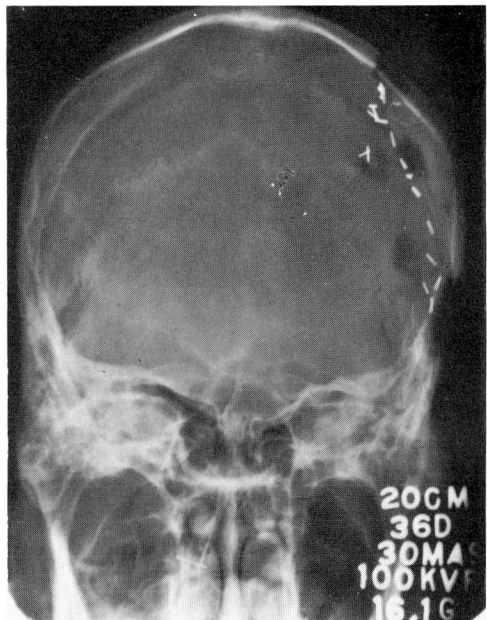

Figure 8.60. Postoperative view of skull at 100 Kv.P.

without loss of detail in the *lighter* or *darker* areas of the radiographic image.

From the foregoing we may conclude the following:

Radiographic density is the deposit of *black metallic silver* on the radiographic film that results as it has been exposed and processed. Details of the part examined are rendered as radiographic densities of varying degrees of concentration.

Radiographic detail comprises all silver deposits on a radiographic film, that is, the aggregate composing the radiographic image.

Tone value — how clearly we see the structure — of any radiographic density is influenced by the degree of silver concentration in the deposit. Tone value is considered to be the degree of light transmission or brightness value of the various densities when they are viewed as an aggregate and as an image on a standard x-ray illuminator.

Radiographic contrast is that characteristic of the image that provides sufficient differentiation between translucent radiographic densities to reveal all possible anatomical details when viewed on a standard x-ray illuminator. Contrast cannot exist unless *two or more* radiographic densities are present. Contrast precipitates the visualization of all important tissue structures irrespective of their type. Kilovoltage is the exposure factor that *regulates radiographic contrast;* hence the visibility of details. There are two general types of contrast—

> Short-scale contrast, wherein the range of image densities is *short and small* in number, and each density exhibits a large *tonal difference* from its neighbor. This type of contrast is considered to be impractical in modern medical radiography.
>
> Long-scale contrast, wherein the range of image densities is wide and

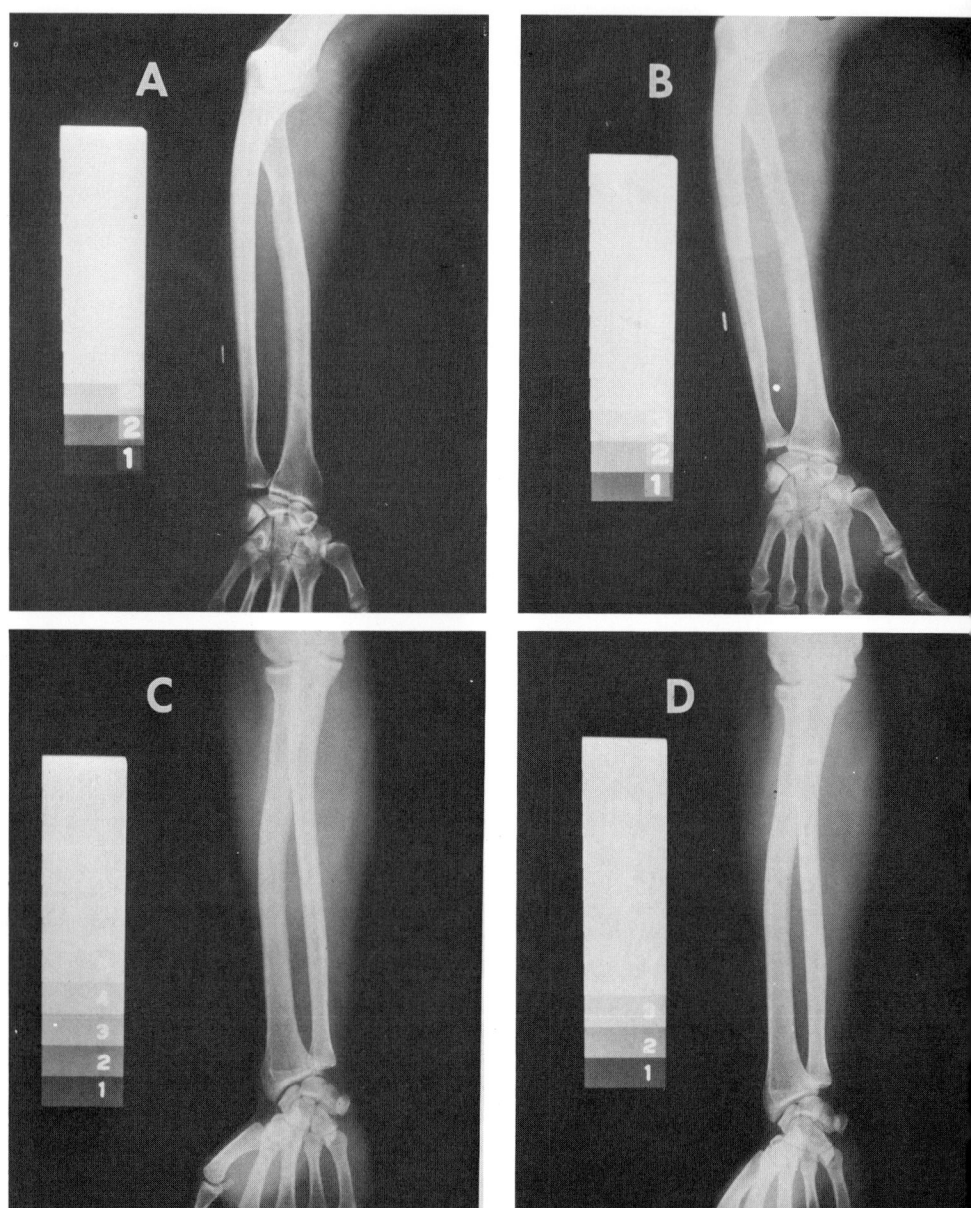

Figure 8.61. Comparison of results. The view in A was taken at 50 Kv.P. and 100 Ma.S. with regular film and a cardboard holder. B was taken at 60 Kv.P. and 70 Ma.S., also with regular film and a cardboard holder. Note the increase in overall detail. Views C and D were taken with regular film and screens—C at 60 Kv.P. and 2.5 Ma.S., and D at Kv.P. and 10 Ma.S.

great in number and each density exhibits only relatively *small tonal difference* from its adjacent structure. This scale of contrast is considered ideal for modern medical radiography.

Essentials of the Radiograph

There are times when extremely short-scale contrast *and* long-scale contrast can be used to an advantage in certain radiographic problems. Figure 11.19, for example, shows pathological destruction of the skull. Then to visualize the skin lines, a higher kilovoltage was used as depicted in Figure 11.20.

Other factors influencing contrast are properties inherent in the x-ray developer, the type of film employed, the radiographic intensifying screens when used, and the type of tissue radiographed. These all contribute to the sum total of radiographic contrast.

Penetration of the tissue is determined by the x-ray wave length, which is *directly influenced* by the kilovoltage; it is also effected by the density of the *tissue* as well as the *thickness* of the particular part.

GENERAL SUMMARY

The influence of kilovoltage and its relation to other exposure factors in altering radiographic density and contrast is summarized as follows:

(a) *Kv.P.-density relation.* When all other factors are constant, density changes with Kv.P.

(b) *Kv.P.-time relation.* With changes in Kv.P., the time of exposure must be adjusted to compensate for the density influence of Kv.P.

(c) *Kv.P.-Ma. relation.* It is impractical in routine radiography to employ this relation. The effects are the same, however, as the Kv.P.-time relation.

(d) *Kv.P.-FFD relation.* In practical radiography, the need for using this relation is extremely rare.

(e) *Kv.P.-penetration relation.* By virtue of its control of x-ray wave length (quality of radiation), Kv.P. governs the degree of x-ray penetration of body tissues.

(f) *Kv.P.-fog relation.* Kv.P. has a direct influence on the production of secondary radiation generated in the tissues; hence, Kv.P. influences the amount of secondary radiation fog produced on the radiographic image.

(g) *Kv.P.-contrast relation.* Kv.P. has a direct bearing upon the contrast scale; as Kv.P. changes, contrast changes. The lower the kilovoltage, the shorter the scale of contrast. The higher the kilovoltage, the *lower* the scale of contrast.

(h) *Kv.P.-latitude relation.* Because of its control over radiographic contrast, Kv.P. regulates exposure latitude.

The use of higher kilovoltage provides greater exposure efficiency in radiography for the following reasons.

(a) Anatomical details in all tissue thicknesses are rendered as translucent densities. The relative absorption properties between bone and flesh are reduced, making possible visualization of more structural details. Soft tissue detail is as good, if not better, than that produced by the lower kilovoltages because shorter exposures tend to reduce motion unsharpness. At lower kilovoltages, bone detail often tends to obscure details of soft tissues that lie behind the bone. Complete penetration of bone by higher kilovoltages reveals soft tissue details that are not visible at lower kilovoltages.

FORMULATING X-RAY TECHNIQUES

   (b) Greater image sharpness is obtained because shorter exposures may be employed with smaller focal spots.
   (c) The radiation dose to patients is reduced as the kilovoltage level increases because the body absorbs less radiation than at the lower kilovoltages. More radiation can, therefore, reach the film to expose it and exposures can be reduced.
   (d) Heat production in the x-ray tube is reduced because smaller energy loads can be employed, thereby increasing x-ray tube life. As the kilovoltage increases, tube efficiency increases. There is more radiation per watt of electric power consumed when using the higher kilovoltages than there is when using the lower kilovoltages. A correct exposure may therefore be produced with less heat generated in the tube.
   (e) Greater exposure latitude may be secured. As the kilovoltage increases, exposure latitude increases.
   (f) The higher kilovoltages make possible the use of many radiographic techniques that heretofore have been too difficult to perform.

The influence of Ma. and time of exposure in relation to radiographic density is summarized as follows.

   (a) **Ma.-density relation.** When all exposure factors but milliamperage are constant, radiographic density increases in direct proportion to the Ma.; hence, as time is increased, the density increases, and vice versa.
   (b) **Ma.-time relation.** When Ma. is changed, time must be proportionately changed, and vice versa.
   (c) **Ma.S.-density relation.** The Ma.S. factor is the product of Ma. and time (in seconds) and should be employed as the factor of density control.
   (d) **Time-density relation.** When all other factors but time of exposure remain constant, the radiographic density increases in direct proportion to the time; hence, as time is increased, the density increases, and vice versa.

The influence of focus-film distance and its relation to other exposure factors in altering radiographic density is summarized as follows.

   (a) **FFD-density relation.** When all factors but focus-film distance are constant, the radiographic density decreases as the FFD increases.
   (b) **Time-FFD-density relation.** The time of exposure required to produce a given radiographic density is directly proportional to the square of the FFD when all other factors are constant.
   (c) **Ma.-FFD-density relation.** The millimaperage required to produce a given radiographic density is directly proportional to the square of the FFD when all other factors are constant.
   (d) **Ma.S.-FFD relation.** The Ma.S. required to produce a given radiographic density is directly proportional to the square of the FFD when all other factors are constant.

Fog can be controlled by

   1. Limitation of the amount of tissue irradiated,

Essentials of the Radiograph

2. The use of correct exposure, and
3. The use of cones and/or grids.

Kilovoltage should be employed as the factor influencing contrast. An unrestricted beam of x-rays always causes a larger amount of secondary radiation to be emitted by the tissues than a beam confined by a cone or diaphragm. As may be expected, any method of limiting the amount of secondary radiation, produces radiographic images of better diagnostic quality. When a cone or grid is not used, kilovoltage then becomes the most important factor in the control of fog. With a knowledge of how secondary radiation fog affects the overall density of the image, and hence the quality of the radiograph, a balance of exposure factors and accessory apparatus can lead to the selection of an exposure that will be best suited to each body part examined.

(1) As kilovoltage is increased, secondary radiation fog as well as overall density increases.

(2) When secondary radiation is controlled efficiently, kilovoltage becomes the factor of radiographic contrast.

(3) When Ma.S. compensates for the density effect of the increased kilovoltage, the low level of image fog is relatively the same, irrespective of the kilovoltage.

REVIEW

When body parts of unequal thickness of tissue density are to be recorded, the following rule should be observed.

Rule. Align the long axis of the x-ray tube with the long center axis of the part and film, and direct the cathode portion of the x-ray beam toward the anatomic area of greatest tissue density thickness. It should be observed that the heel effect diminishes with an increase in the focus-film distance and with the use of small-size films, since the more uniform intensities of greatest effect are observed when the focus-film distance is relatively short, and again when a large film is employed and the body part is uneven in thickness or tissue density.

The scale of densities that determines the *contrast* and the *visibility of detail* is *directly* influenced by the x-ray *wave length,* which in turn is regulated by the factor of *kilovoltage.* This can easily be demonstrated by the student or instructor by making a radiograph of a step wedge with an exposure of *lower* kilovoltage and an exposure at a *higher* kilovoltage.

The above experiment will illustrate the fact that radiographic details of an object cannot be seen in the image unless there are discernible differences in tone value between densities, and that there must be a silver deposit on the film if a detail within the object is to be demonstrated. The experiment is typical of *short-scale* contrast technique. From a purely photographic standpoint, the result may be likened to Figure 8.63, where a large number of details in the image of Figure 8.62 are absent.

In making a similar experiment but using a shorter wave length (higher Kv.P.), we can see an entirely different result. The kilovoltage has been increased and provides radiation (wave length) that penetrates all portions

FORMULATING X-RAY TECHNIQUES

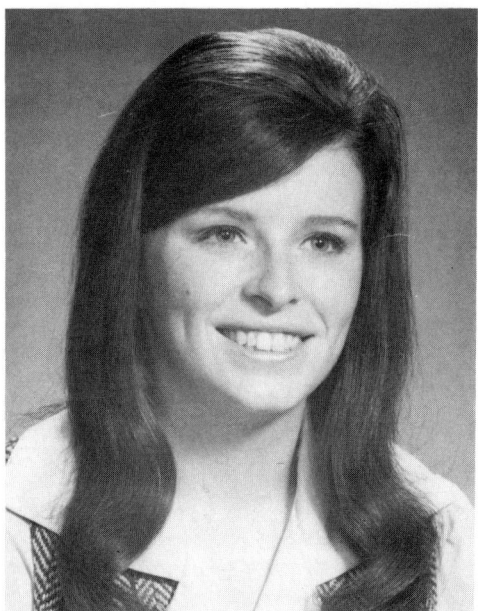

Figure 8.62. A photograph showing the characteristics of long-scale contrast.

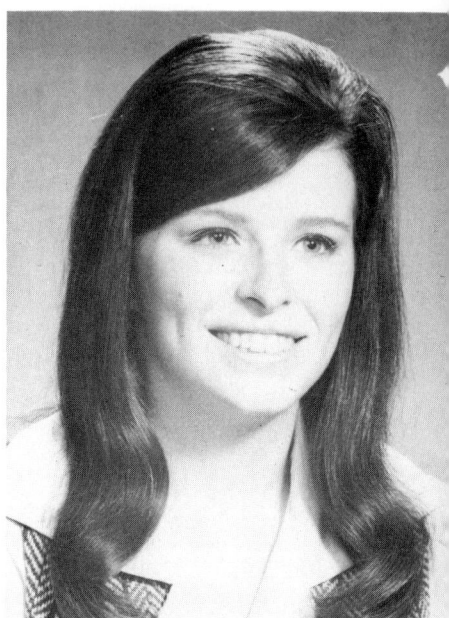

Figure 8.63. A short-scale-contrast version of Figure 8.62.

of the step wedge. The transition between tones is gradual, and each tone is distinctive. This is typical of *long-scale contrast.* From a photographic standpoint, this result may be likened to the photograph in Figure 8.62.

In the final analysis, the criterion of good diagnostic contrast is whether one sees all one expected to see.

Chapter 9. POSITIONS AND PROCEDURES; PATHOLOGY AND INJURY

It is most important from the point of view of exposure factors that the technologist know the relative differences in the composition and thicknesses of body parts. Bone is more dense to x-rays than the surrounding soft tissue. Body fluids possess about the same absorption characteristics as soft tissue. Moreover, the pathological and physiological states of the tissue are extremely important in selecting the exposure factors.

Most departments of radiology apply routine views and positions for all parts to be radiographed. If pathology is present in the routine views, the radiologic technologist, under the direction of the radiologist or physician in charge, should elaborate the technique in order to best show the pathology or to elucidate the diagnosis.

Suggested procedures are listed in Table 9.1. One should check with the radiologist or physician in charge for the position or the procedure to be used in individual departments. The information in the table is a *guide only*.

Table 9.1 ROUTINE VIEWS AND VIEWS TO SHOW PATHOLOGY

Part	Injury, pathology or diagnostic procedure	Suggested procedure
Extremities		
Hand	Routine	Posteroanterior (P.A.), and oblique
	Fracture	P.A., oblique and lateral
	Bone age (wrist)	P.A.
	Foreign body	P.A., oblique and lateral, using cardboard holders
	Pathology (tumor, etc.)	P.A., lateral and oblique
Forearm	Routine	Anteroposterior (A.P.) and lateral
Elbow	Routine	A.P. and lateral, with thumb upright
	Radial head	A.P.—hand supinated; A.P.—hand pronated
	Olecranon process	A.P.; acute flexion of elbow; A.P., lateral and oblique
Wrist	Routine	A.P., lateral and oblique
	Fracture	A.P., lateral and oblique
	Scaphoid	A.P. in ulna deviation; lateral and A.P.
	Carpal canal	Distoproximal projection
Humerus	Routine	A.P. and lateral
Foot	Routine	A.P., lateral and oblique
	Fracture	A.P., lateral and oblique
Toes	Routine or fracture	A.P., oblique and lateral

FORMULATING X-RAY TECHNIQUES

Sesamoids	Routine	Oblique metatarsophalangeal joint
Ankle		
	Bone age	Lateral
	Fracture	A.P., lateral and oblique
	Malleolus	A.P., oblique and lateral
	Tibiofibular articulation	A.P., oblique, medially, and lateral
Os calcis	Routine	Lateral and plantodorsal
Tibia-fibula	Routine	A.P. and lateral
	For veins	Lateral with a reduction of Kv.P. or Ma.S. (venogram)
Knee	Routine	A.P. and lateral
	Femoral condyles	Posterior oblique
	Intercondyloid space	A.P. knee with 60° tilt of central ray and knee flexed
Patella	Routine or fracture	P.A., lateral and axial; axial with cardboard holder
Femur	Routine	A.P. and lateral; measure part and use pelvis exposure technique
Shoulder	Routine	A.P.
	Fracture	A.P. in stereo, axial and lateral
	Subdeltoid bursa	A.P. in internal and external rotation with a reduction in Kv.P. or Ma.S.
	Coracoid process	A.P. with central ray directed 15–20° cephalad
	Glenoid fossa	A.P. with patient rotated toward affected side approximately 45°
	Acromioclavicular joint for dislocation	A.P. of both shoulders with patient in the erect position
Clavicle	Routine	P.A. shoulder
	Fracture	A.P. stereo and lateral
Scapula	Routine	A.P. and P.A. oblique
Sternum and ribs		
Sternum	Pathology	P.A., oblique and lateral, or tomography
		P.A., oblique, slow-breathing technique and close focus-film distance technique
Sternoclavicular articulation		P.A. with close focus-film distance technique
Ribs	Above diaphragm	P.A. bucky chest technique and/or grid
	Below diaphragm	A.P. abdomen or P.A. gallbladder technique
	Pathology	A.P. on 14 x 17 film transverse
Pelvis		
	Fracture	A.P. stereo
Hip	Fracture	A.P stereo and true lateral
Spine		
Atlas and axis	Routine	A.P. chewing technique or A.P. with mouth open and lateral
Cervical	Routine	A.P. and lateral and oblique
	Fracture	A.P. stereo and transverse lateral. Note: Do not move

Procedures: Pathology and Injury

		patient unless under doctor's supervision
	Intervertebral foramina	Right and left obliques; A.P. and lateral
	Tumor or disc	A.P., lateral and right and left obliques followed by myelogram studies by radiologist and neurosurgeon; flexion and extension in the lateral projection
Thoracic	Routine	A.P. and lateral; lateral using slow breathing technique
	Fracture	A.P. in stereo and lateral
	Fusion	A.P. lateral, flexion and extension
	Tumor	A.P. lateral and obliques; myelogram by radiologist and/or neurosurgeon
	Kyphosis	Lateral, A.P., employing two films: (1) A.P. with central ray directed 10° cephalad; (2) A.P. with central ray directed 10° caudad
	Scoliosis	A.P. on 14 x 17 film in upright position; include from the crest of the ilium up
Lumbar	Routine	A.P. and lateral, right and left obliques with spot film of L-5
	Disc or tumor	Same as above followed by myelogram
	Fusion	A.P., lateral and flexion and extension
	Spondylolisthesis	A.P., lateral and obliques and spot film of L-5
Sacroiliac joints	Arthritis	A.P. bilateral of entire pelvis, right and left obliques of each joint
	Separation	A.P. in stereo, right and left obliques
	Tumor	A.P. with right and left obliques
Sacrum	Routine	A.P. with central ray directed 15° cephalad
Sacral canal	Routine	P.A. in sitting position
Coccyx	Routine	A.P. with central ray directed 10° caudad, lateral spot film
Skull	Routine	A.P. stereo and lateral stereo
	Fracture	A.P. stereo, lateral stereo; brow up stereo for fluid levels
	Foramen magnum	A.P. skull with central ray directed at an angle of 45° caudad
	Base	A.P. skull with central ray directed 35° caudad, and mentovertex
	Carotid canals	Mentovertex in stereo

FORMULATING X-RAY TECHNIQUES

	Foramen ovale	Mentovertex in stereo
	Petrosae	Mentovertex, Stenvers, P.A.
	Tumor	A.P. and P.A. stereo, right and left lateral mentovertex, brow up stereo followed by air study
	Eighth nerve tumor	A.P. in stereo with central ray directed 30° caudad; O.M.L. perpendicular with tabletop, mentovertex stereo right and left Stenvers
	Labyrinth	Mentovertex stereo, right and left Stenvers, A.P. stereo with central ray directed 30° caudad
	Sella	A.P. skull with 25° caudad tilt and a true lateral
	Optic foramen	Rhese position
	Exophthalmos	Reverse Rhese position
	Inferior orbital fissure	P.A. skull with central ray directed 20° cephalad and central ray passing through the nasion
	Mastoid	Positions vary considerably; take bilateral, Law position A.P. Towne position, right and left Stenvers, Rundstrom I and II, mentovertex, Mayer position, mastoid tip projection
	Styloid (of the temporal bone)	Lateral and P.A.
	Sinuses	P.A. Caldwell, P.A. maxillary, P.A. sphenoid, true lateral
	Fluid level	Sinuses should be done in the upright projection
	Ventricular system	Cerebral pneumography
	Arterial system	Cerebral angiography
Thoracic viscera		
Trachea	Routine	A.P. and oblique, lateral; body section
	Foreign body	Right and left obliques; P.A. and lateral
Chest	Routine (lungs and heart)	P.A. and left lateral
	Heart	P.A., right oblique at 45°, left oblique at 60°, and lateral; all films should be made at a 72-in. distance
	Foreign body	P.A. chest on inspiration, P.A. chest on expiration; right and left obliques and lateral
	Diaphragm excursion	Double exposed P.A. chest without patient moving; (1) exposure on inspiration; (2) exposure on expiration; fluoroscopy
	Fluid level	P.A. lateral and decubitus
	Coin lesion	P.A. lateral and A.P. lordotic, body section

Procedures: Pathology and Injury

	Interlobar effusion	P.A. lateral and A.P. lordotic
	Heart and great vessels	Fluoroscopy, P.A. lateral and right oblique at 45°, left oblique at 60°
	Bronchial trees	Bronchography
	Aneurysm of aorta	Fluoroscopy, esophagus studies with barium and spot films, right and left oblique of chest with barium
	Mediastinal mass	Fluoroscopy; films as indicated by radiologist
	Mitral stenosis	Fluoroscopy; films as indicated by radiologist
	Hodgkin's disease	P.A. and lateral with an increase in Ma.S. or Kv.P.
	Cancer, lung	P.A. lateral, right and left obliques and P.A. lordotic
Facial bones	Routine	Waters view and lateral skull
	Fracture	Waters stereo and lateral stereo with affected side down
Facial profile		Soft-tissue technique
Nasal bones		Lateral; use cardboard holder
Zygomatic arch		Right and left for comparison; use exaggerated Waters position with chin and head extended and median plane rotated 10° right and left
Mandible	Symphysis	Inferiorsuperior projection
	Submaxillary gland	Inferiorsuperior projection with occlusal film
	Routine	Lateral and P.A.
Temporomandibular articulation		Lateral with mouth open and mouth closed, A.P. oblique body section
	Parotid and submaxillary glands	Oblique lateral projection after injection of opaque media by radiologist
Neck	Soft tissue	A.P. and lateral
	Pharynx	Lateral of neck, soft tissue with phonating "a"
Nasal pharynx		Lateral of skull with patient breathing in through the nose on inspiration only
Digestive system		
Abdomen	Routine	A.P.
	Acute	A.P., upright, lateral, and decubitus
	Abdominal aorta	Lateral of abdomen minus 6–10 Kv. or minus 30% Ma.S.; or use high-kilovoltage technique
	Tumor mass	A.P. and lateral
	Calcification	A.P. and lateral
	Fistulae and/or sinus tract	Fluoroscopy and injection of opaque media by radiologist

FORMULATING X-RAY TECHNIQUES

	Liver and spleen	A.P. abdomen, center film 6 in. higher than for routine abdomen
Gallbladder	Routine	P.A., decubitus upright and lateral; very thin patients take oblique
Biliary tract		Cholangiography; fluoroscopy by radiologist and films as indicated
Gastrointestinal tract		Fluoroscopy by radiologist and films as indicated
Stomach		Fluoroscopy by radiologist; films usually consist of P.A. obliques, serial films, and spot films
Esophagus		Fluoroscopy and films as indicated by radiologist; usually right obliques with barium and spot films
Excretory system		A.P. abdomen
Renal pelves		Urography
Urinary bladder		Cystography
Urethra		Urography
Prostate		Cystography
Female reproductive system		
Breast		Mammography; various views and exposure published by Egan and others
Fallopian tubes		Uterosalpingography
Early pregnancy		A.P. abdomen
Pelvimetry		Procedures vary considerably; Colcher-Sussmann, Thoms method, Ball method, or others

Procedures: Pathology and Injury

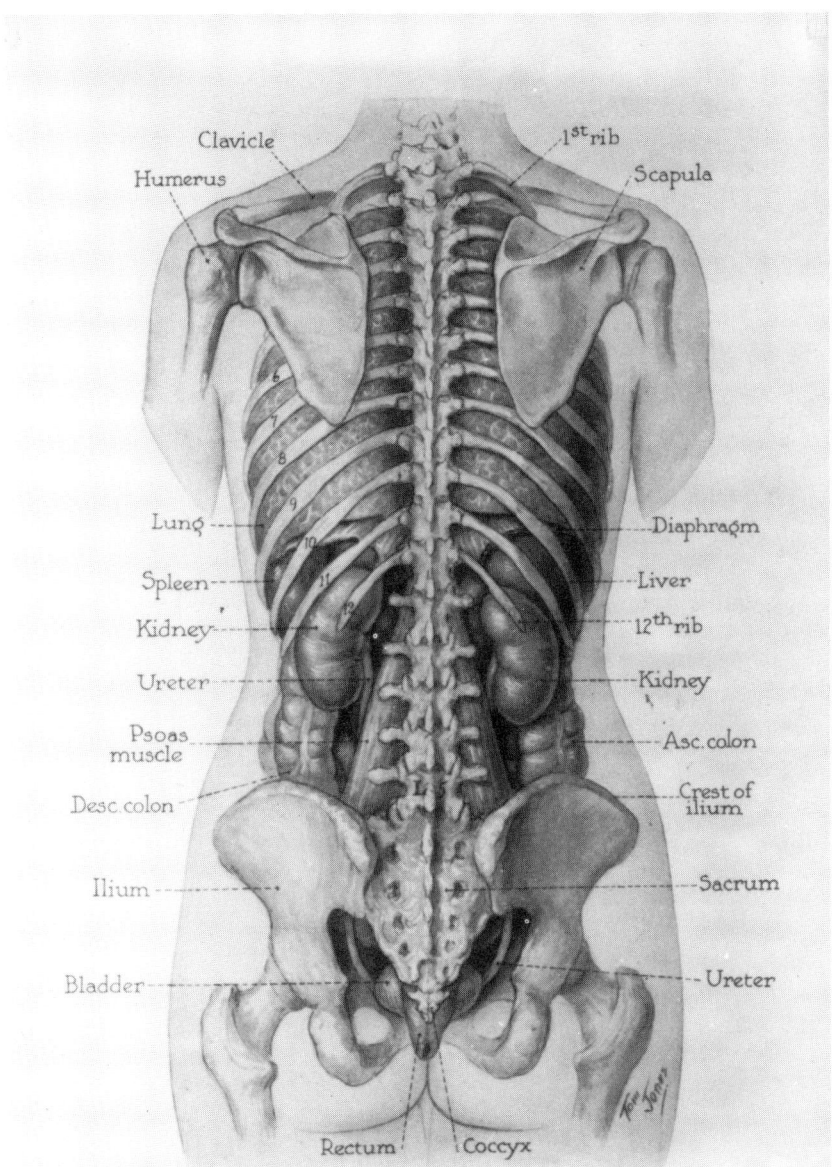

Figure 9.1. The viscera: posteroanterior view.

FORMULATING X-RAY TECHNIQUES

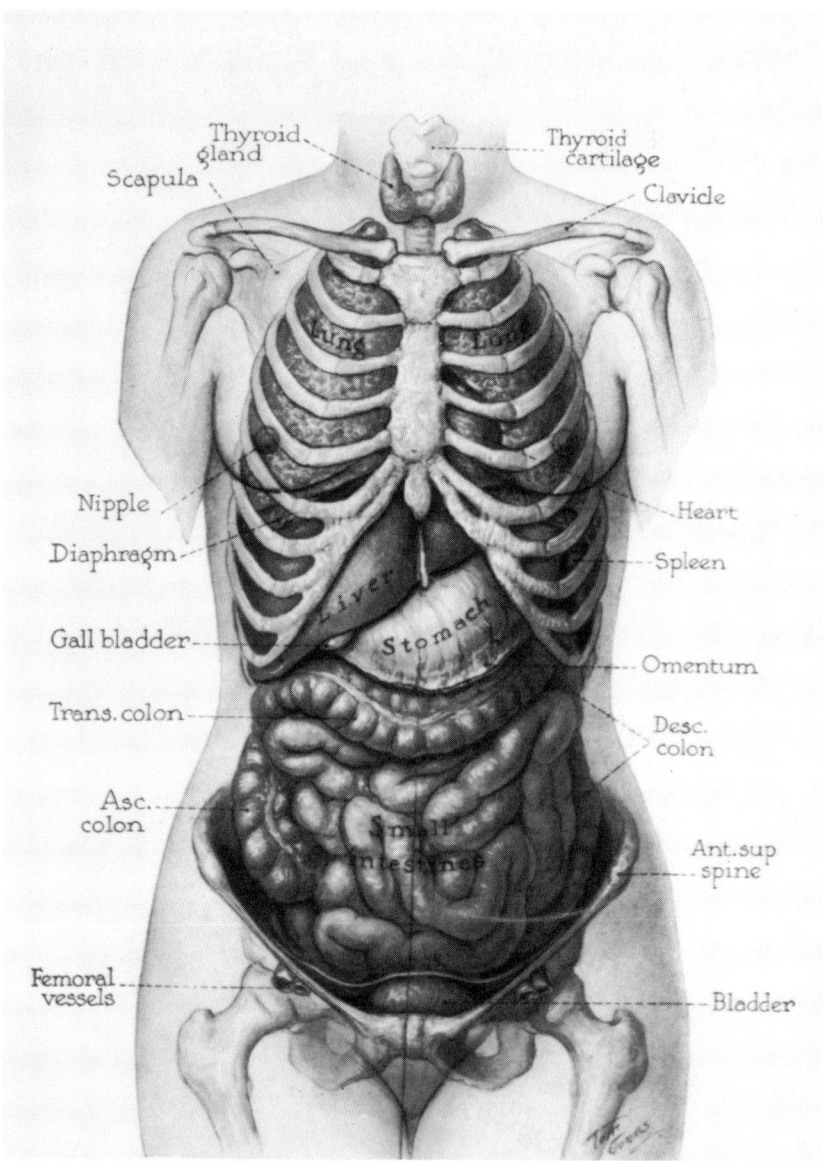

Figure 9.2. The viscera: anteroposterior view.

Procedures: Pathology and Injury

FLUID LEVEL EXPERIMENT

There are a number of clinical conditions in which the radiographic demonstration of fluid levels plays an important part in interpretation.

For very sick patients who cannot be placed in the erect position, we *usually* direct the central ray perpendicular to the film and *fail* to demonstrate fluid levels when they are present, or project them with poor detail so that the shadows cannot be identified as fluid levels.

It is a well-known fact that no matter in what position we hold a container of fluid, the fluid level will always be parallel to the floor. Therefore, if we direct the central ray parallel to the floor, no matter what the position of the container (patient), the fluid level will be demonstrated on the film as a sharp, well-defined margin.

Figure 9.3 demonstrates a bottle partially filled with a solution of water and Hypaque radiographed at an angle simulating an erect patient. The central ray is directed perpendicular to the object and film. Figure 9.4 portrays the patient in a semierect position, with the central ray directed perpendicular to the film. Figures 9.5 and 9.6 portray the patient in the semierect position, with the central ray *parallel* to the floor.

Figure 9.7 is a radiograph made of a patient in the semierect position with the central ray directed perpendicular to the patient and film. Figure 9.8 portrays the same patient radiographed in the semierect position, with the central ray directed *parallel* to the floor.

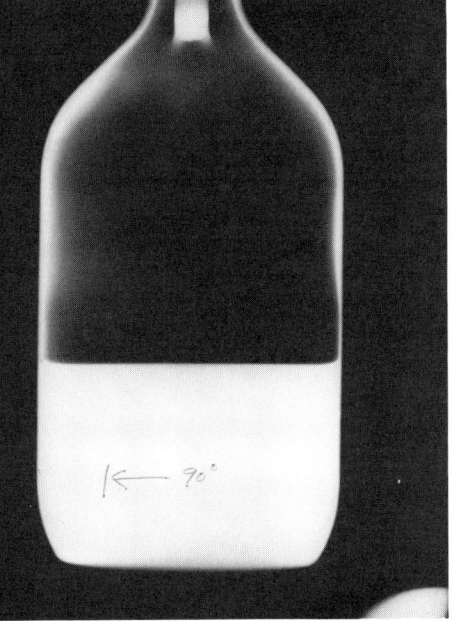

Figure 9.3. Bottle with Hypaque simulating an erect patient.

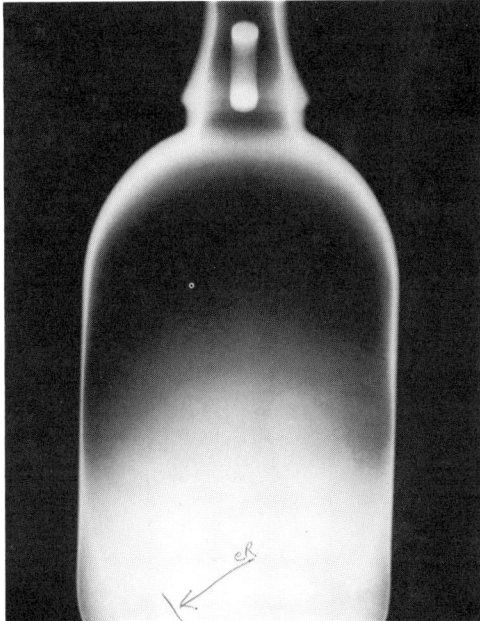

Figure 9.4. Simulation of patient in a semierect position; the central ray is directed *perpendicular* to object and film.

FORMULATING X-RAY TECHNIQUES

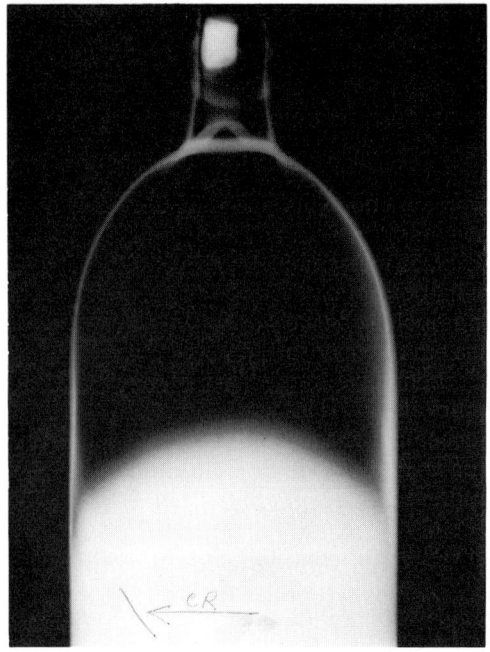

Figure 9.5. Simulation of patient in a semierect position; the central ray is directed *parallel* to the floor.

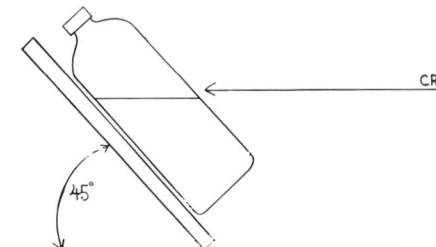

Figure 9.6. Diagram of Figure 9.5 in side view.

Figure 9.7. Radiograph of patient in the position simulated in Figure 9.4.

Figure 9.8. Radiograph of patient in the position simulated in Figures 9.5 and 9.6.

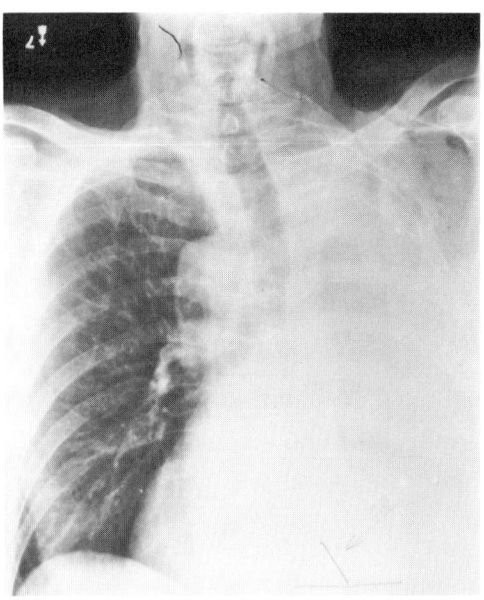
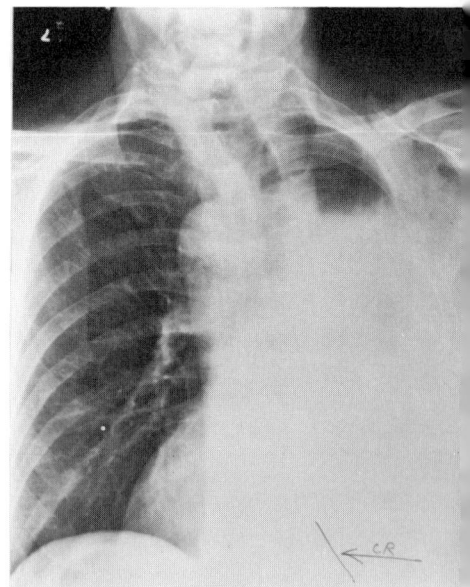

Chapter 10. FORMULATING THE TECHNIQUE CHART: VARIABLE KILOVOLTAGE METHOD

Radiography is the art of recording on a sensitive emulsion the hidden structures of the body. The permanent record which we make is called a radiograph. It is a pictorial representation of structures — a form of picture, and like all pictures, it possesses pictorial qualities, namely, *density, contrast, detail,* and *distortion.* Distortion is not thought of as a quality but is always included in this group. We speak of the qualities and we ask, how much density? A satisfactory amount. Satisfactory for whom? The *radiologist.* Contrast? Sufficient. Sufficient for what? *Sufficient to show the anatomical structure.* Detail? How much? *Maximum.* Distortion? *As little as possible.* We might also ask, what is technique? Technique is that combination of mechanical methods by which one achieves a satisfactory balance of these four factors: *density, contrast, detail,* and *distortion.*

Any technique (exposure system) is now, and always has been, subject to patient *evaluation* by the technologist.

All x-ray machines should be calibrated before one attempts to formulate a standard technique chart. Machine factors vary considerably; and in order to work for a standard production of film quality, one must know the output and characteristics of a particular machine.

The *four primary factors* involved in the production of a radiograph are *focus-film distance, milliamperage, time of exposure,* and *kilovoltage.* The focus-film distance can be measured accurately and duplicated very easily. Milliamperage can be measured accurately by the milliammeter; the timer can be tested for accuracy by the use of a spinning top or oscilloscope for exposures less than one second, and by a stop watch for exposures longer than one second.

Tube-rating chart

Before the technique chart is formulated one should refer to the tube-rating chart (Figure 10.1), since repeated exposures or even one long exposure may produce enough heat in the anode to cause serious damage. The tube-rating chart enables one to determine the combination of kilovoltage, milliamperage, and time that can be safely used for any given exposure.

Distance

The distance from the film to the tube focal-spot, known as focus-film distance, is determined to a large extent by the *ratio* and *radius* of the Potter-Bucky diaphragm or grid cassette when used (focused or parallel). The other factor influencing distance is the factor of distortion (short distance — more distortion; longer distance — less distortion).

FORMULATING X-RAY TECHNIQUES

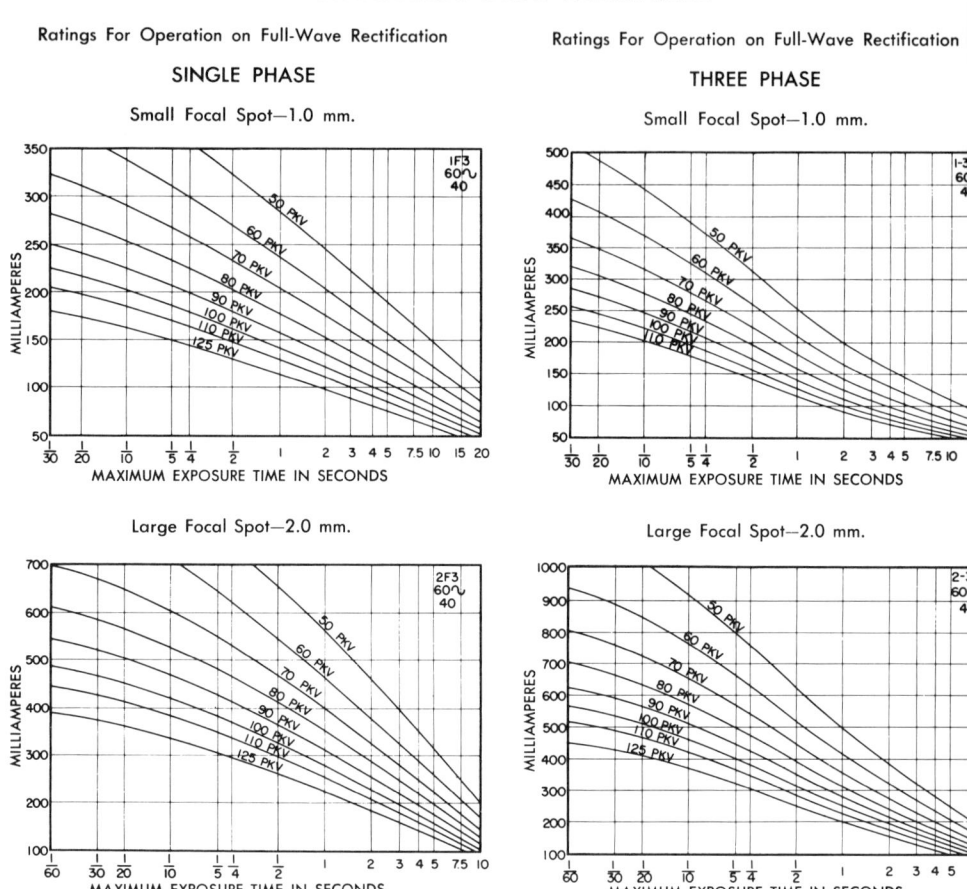

Figure 10.1. Tube-rating charts: single-phase and three-phase.

Kilovoltage

The kilovoltage should be adequate to penetrate the anatomical part. Kilovoltage governs the *quality* of the x-rays and controls contrast.

Milliamperage

The milliamperage should be high enough to produce a given density. The milliamperage governs the *quantity* or *amount* of radiation.

The time factor

The time factor refers to the length of exposure and is usually measured in fractions of a second or in seconds.

Milliampere-seconds

Milliampere-seconds (Ma.S.) is a measurement of the milliamperage and time of exposure. Example: 100 Ma. for $1/10$ of a second is 10 Ma.S.; 10 Ma. for 1 second is 10 Ma.S.; 200 Ma. for $1/20$ of a second is 10 Ma.S.

Variable Kilovoltage Method

A working knowledge of milliampere-seconds can be a great asset in *fitting the exposure to the problem.* See Table 7.9 in Chapter 7.

Cones or collimators

A cone or collimator should be used in every projection, in order to reduce secondary radiation fog.

Filters

At least 2 mm. of external aluminum filtration should be used for all exposures.

The Potter-Bucky diaphragm and grids

With few exceptions the Bucky or a grid should be used for radiography of all parts 12 cm. or more in thickness. Exceptions are the lungs, heart (except for large, heavy patients), lateral mandible, hands, wrists, ankles, legs, and sinuses.

Screens or cardboard holders

Screens should be used where speed is important and for all parts other than the so-called *small parts,* e.g., extremities and nasal bones, except in certain special techniques.

THE PATIENT PROBLEM

When the patient is ready for the radiography, the physical characteristics and region or part to be examined should be carefully observed. Any information regarding the pathology or condition of the region or regions to be examined will usually prove helpful, and the time for which the part can be held in a comfortable, steady position should be noted.

Experience will enable the radiologic technologist to judge by the physique of the patient the location of the organs, especially those of the abdomen, and particularly the gallbladder, stomach, and colon. The technologist should understand the four distinct subject types of body habitus (Figure 10.2)—hypersthenic, sthenic, asthenic, and hyposthenic; and in skull radiography (Figures 10.3 to 10.5), he should understand the three types of skulls—brachycephalic, dolichocephalic, and mesocephalic (Figure 10.6). Atypical skulls will, depending upon their shape, require more or less rotation of the head, or an increase or decrease in the angulation of the central ray. In the brachycephalic skull, which is short from front to back, broad from side to side, and shallow from vertex to base, the internal structures are higher with reference to the baseline and the long axis is more frontal in position. In the dolichocephalic skull, which is long from front to back, narrow from side to side, and deep from vertex to base, the internal structures are lower with reference to the baseline and the long axis is less frontal in position. Asymmetry of a skull should also be considered, but if the technologist will adhere to the fundamental radiographic baselines and rules of positioning, he will encounter little difficulty. Care and precision should always be used, and the use of a protractor or cardboard angles will be tremendously advantageous in producing standardized results. The mesocephalic or so-called normal skull is more or less oval in shape, being wider behind than in front. The average skull measures approximately 15 cm. in

FORMULATING X-RAY TECHNIQUES

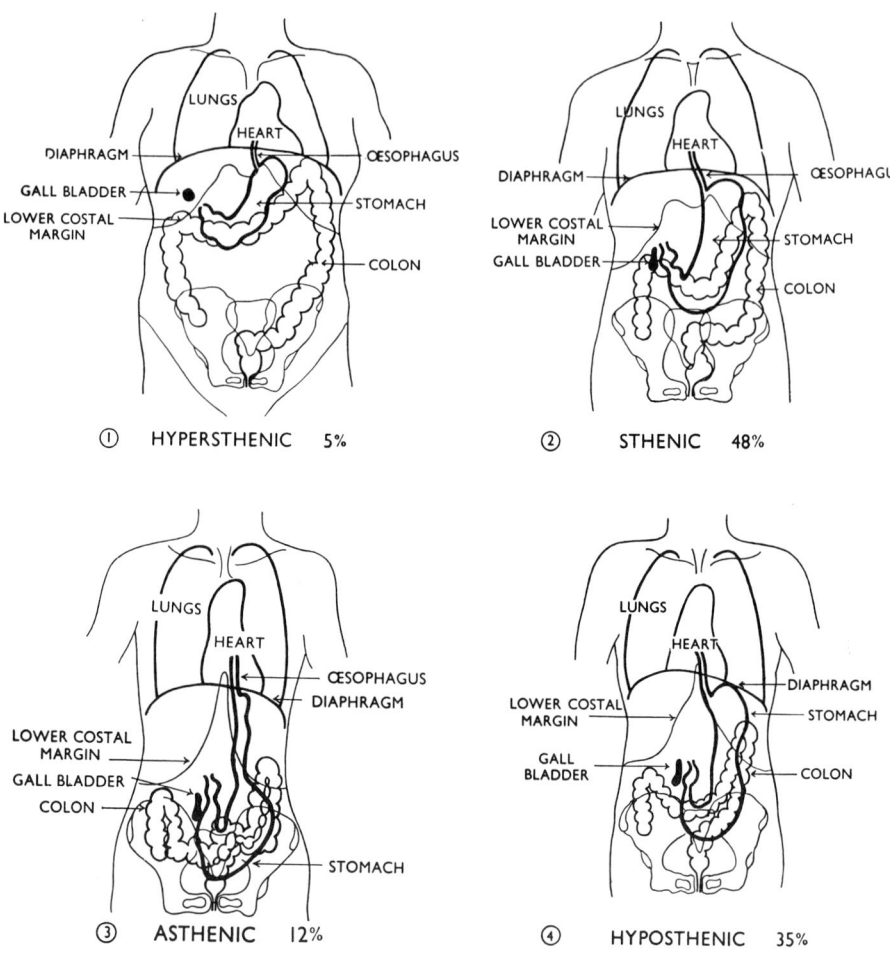

Figure 10.2. Subject types.

the lateral position, 19 cm. in the anteroposterior position, and 22 cm. in the mentovertex position. Skulls vary in size and shape with both sex and race, so that there is a variation in the position and relationship of internal parts. Internal deviations from the normal are usually indicated by the external deviations, and so can be estimated with a reasonable degree of accuracy. There is a 4-cm. difference between the lateral and anteroposterior measurements of the normally shaped skull. Any deviation from this relationship indicates a change in relationship of the internal structures which, if more than a 5° change, must be compensated for by either a change in rotation of the part or the angulation of the central ray.

THE FACTOR OF MOTION

Certain radiographic examinations—of infants and children, emergency radiography, bedside cases, and all technical procedure, if it is to be successfully utilized—must be based upon the ability of the patient to hold

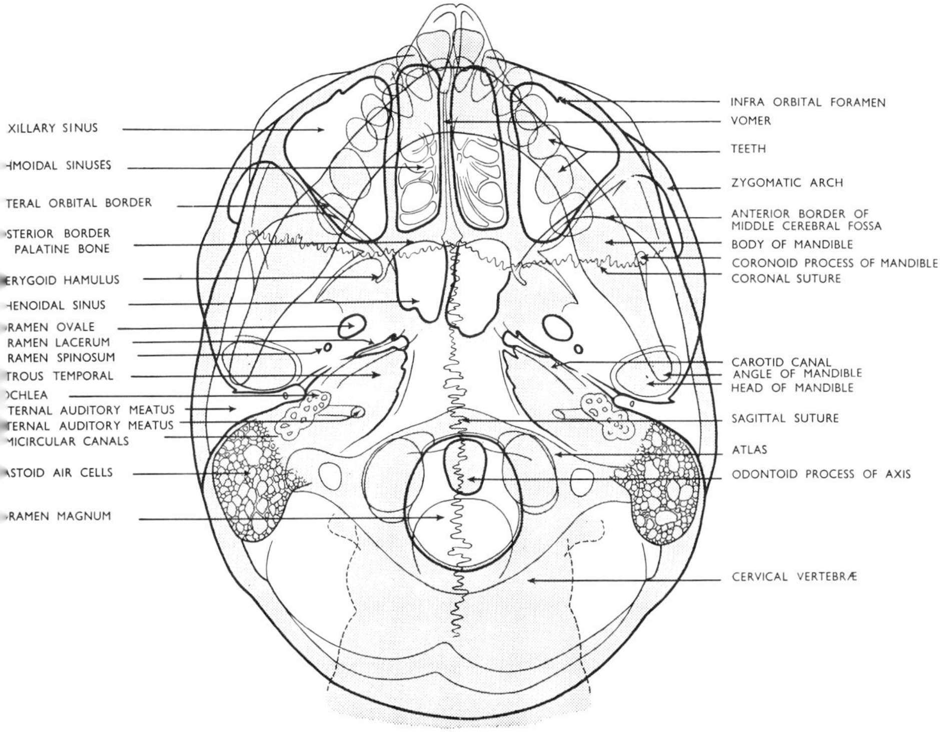

Variable Kilovoltage Method

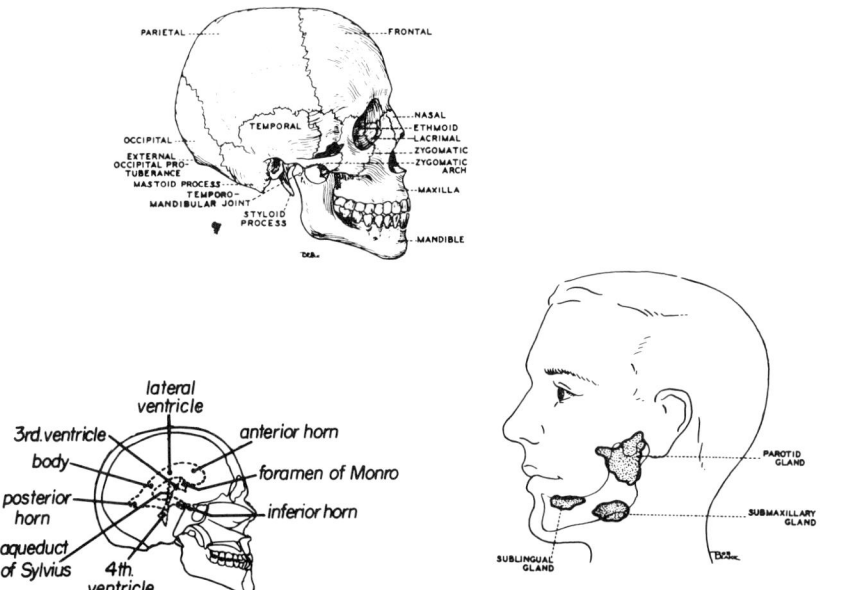

Figure 10.3. The skull.

Figure 10.4. The skull.

FORMULATING X-RAY TECHNIQUES

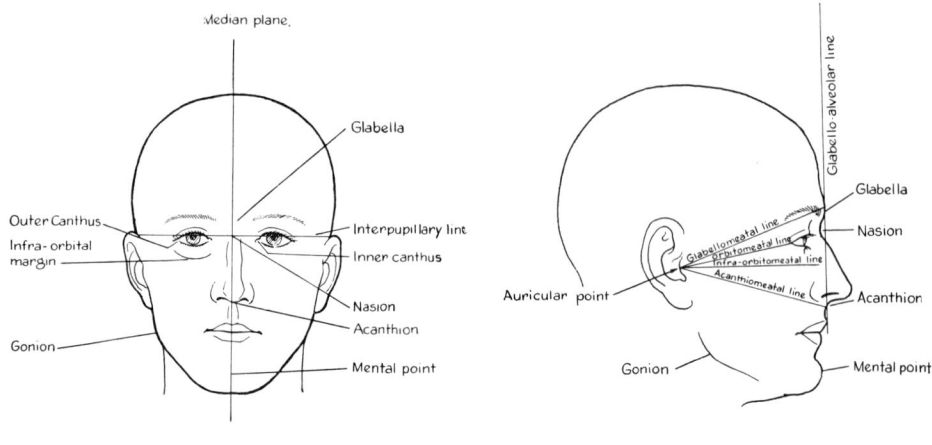

Figure 10.5. Basic localization points and planes.

still or the ability of the x-ray technologist to immobilize the patient successfully. It is of utmost importance that the x-ray technologist thoroughly understand the four prime factors in the production of a radiograph. If he is to acquire skill in his work, he must develop a keen sense of judging how long the patient or part will remain still, the ability to immobilize the part in such a way as to preclude the possibility of motion, and the ability to make the necessary changes in any of the four prime factors involved in order to attain a radiographic film of the highest quality. From the radiographic standpoint, motion may be classified into two groups: (a) physiological or involuntary and (b) accidental or voluntary. Physiological motion is ordinarily respiration, heart action, spasm, or tremor. Accidental motion refers to general body movement. Of these two forms of motion the latter may be more readily controlled. The former can be controlled by employing high milliamperages and short exposures. If high-contrast films are desired, the *time of exposure* should be as long as possible with the *kilovoltages*

Figure 10.6. The three types of skulls.

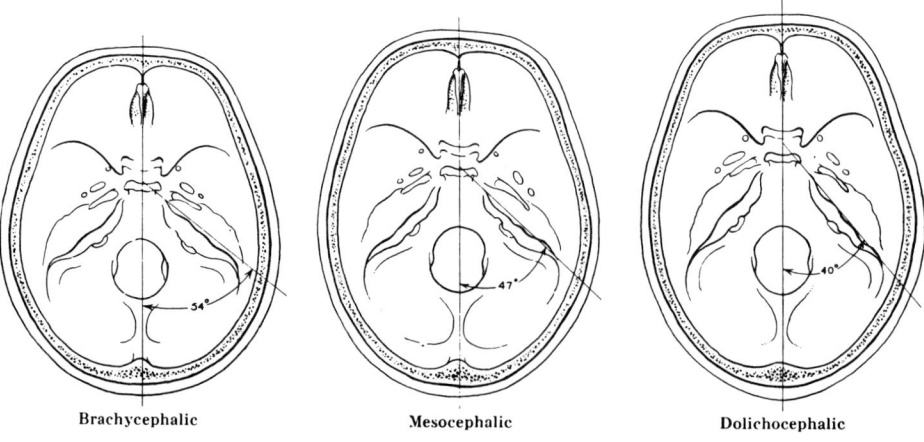

Variable Kilovoltage Method

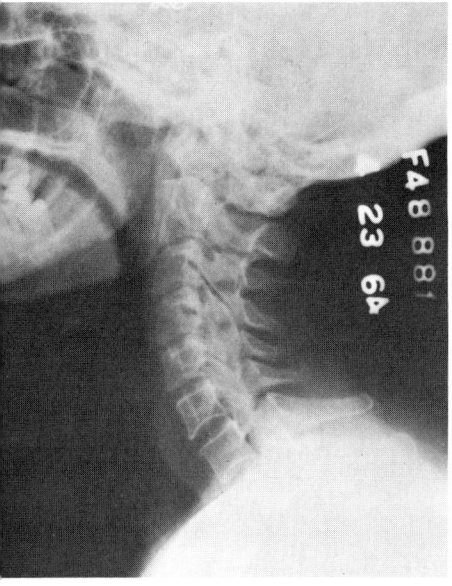

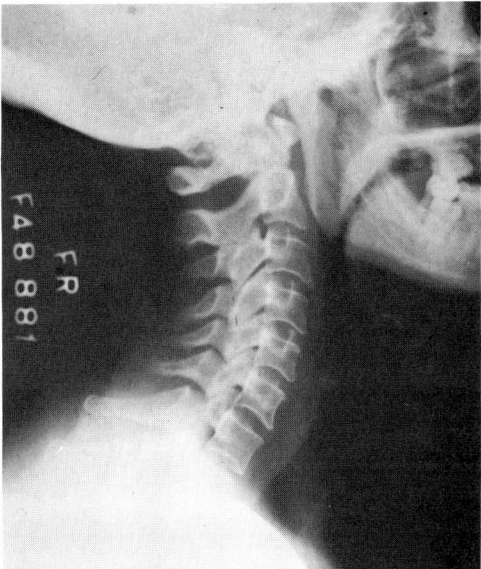

Figure 10.7. Radiograph of the cervical spine showing improper positioning of the patient and motion.

Figure 10.8. The patient of Figure 10.7 in correct position.

comparatively low. Obviously, the employment of a low penetration or Kv.P. necessitates the use of an increased amount of milliampere seconds.

In order that results of the highest quality may be obtained it is necessary to know which of the just mentioned causes of motion should be considered for each part. For example, radiography of the chest does not require that the time of exposure be based upon peristalsis, such as is found in the stomach and intestines. The three most common causes of motion in radiography of the chest are respiration, heart action, and accidental motion. Of the three, heart action ordinarily receives first consideration, since it is generally considered the most difficult to control. Were it not for the problem of motion due to the heart, obviously the time of exposure could be based either upon how long the individual can hold still, or upon the length of time the breath can be held. The normal cardiac cycle being approximately 70 beats per minute, one should try to utilize exposure factors of $1/20$ second or less.

If the region is the stomach, peristalsis and respiration—principally peristalsis—are the usual forms of motion to control. Generally speaking, exposure values for this part range from $1/30$ second to $1/2$ second.

With certain types of injuries, muscle spasms, or tremors the possibility of successful immobilization is minimal. In such cases, the time of exposure may vary considerably.

Fixed or high kilovoltage techniques can be used to an exceptional advantage in the above-mentioned group since they make use of higher than usual kilovoltage and relatively short exposure.

Positioning and measuring

Proper positioning (Figures 10.7 and 10.8) of the patient guarantees that definite anatomical structures will be projected into the active radiographic field, while proper measuring of these structures determines the necessary x-ray energies to be selected to allow the best diagnostic evaluation. *Duplicate diagnostic densities are possible only when all technologists position and measure the anatomical structure under consideration in the same manner.*

Generally speaking, the measurement in centimeter depth for any particular structure is along the line of centrally projected radiation. The part to be radiographed should always be measured by calipers. Do not simply measure to cassette or tabletop; do not make the mistake of computing the measurement of an A.P. lumbar spine by measuring depth to tabletop when the spine does not rest on the table.

Sometimes certain anatomical structures present a variable contour. In certain P.A. chest radiography, for instance, an average between the normal measurement and that of the deepest part to be projected into the active field must be considered. In other instances, like the A.P. lumbar, the measurement is indicated at a point $2\frac{1}{2}$ inches below the sternum or the lower margin to the anterior ribs, while the central ray is localized over the umbilicus. These exceptions must be carefully studied in order to guarantee satisfactory end results.

The application of compression bands may cause a considerable change in thickness of the part to be radiographed. Measurements should be made after the patient has been placed in position for the exposure.

TISSUE ABSORPTION

The x-ray-absorption characteristics of tissues are unpredictable, for it is difficult to estimate their physiologic or pathologic state even with some measure of experience. It is not practical to try to establish these variables on a precise mathematical basis. If the exposure system provides enough latitude for possible errors made in compensation, and the same body part is being considered in a given projection, a fairly close approximation may be attained. In the majority of cases, small deviations from the normal in tissue density or thickness can be ignored, but recognizable abnormal conditions of the body must be compensated for by adjustment of the variable exposure factor selected.

Classification of tissue

By classification of tissue, we refer to the relative radiolucency of different types of tissue—emaciation, superfluous flesh, muscle, and normal flesh. In bone radiography, atrophy from age, disuse, or disease must be considered. In examinations of the thorax the type of patient, age, amount and consistency of tissue, and amount of air in the lungs are determined by the structural type of the individual. Obviously, the consistent production of high-quality radiographs would be comparatively uncomplicated if all tissue had identical opacity to x-radiation. A technologist could rely on a caliper to measure the centimeter thickness of the part to be radiographed and then compensate in exposure factors according to a predetermined scale. But patients cannot be classified by thickness of part alone. Type of tissue and pathology are important factors in setting up the proper exposure techniques (Table 10.1).

Variable Kilovoltage Method

In a general way, patients may be classified as easy to penetrate, normal, or hard to penetrate. *Easy to penetrate* are the young, the aged, the underdeveloped, and those suffering destructive pathology. *Normal* are those of medium age and average development. *Hard to penetrate* are the muscular and those suffering "additive pathology" (see Table 10.1).

Table 10.1 PENETRABILITY TO X-RAYS OF PATHOLOGY OF BODY SYSTEMS

SKELETAL SYSTEM

Additive (hard to penetrate)
  Acromegaly
  Acute kyphosis
  Charcot joint
  Chronic osteomyelitis (healed)
  Exostosis
  Hydrocephalus
  Marble-bone
  Metastasis
  Osteochondroma
  Osteoma
  Paget's disease
  Proliferative arthritis
  Radiation fibrosis
  Scar-bone
  Sclerosis

Destructive (easy to penetrate)
  Active osteomyelitis
  Active tuberculosis (Beck's sarcoid)
  Aseptic necrosis
  Atrophy—disease or disuse
  Blastomycosis
  Carcinoma
  Coccidiomycosis
  Cystic conditions
  Degenerative arthritis
  Ewing's tumor (children)
  Fibrosarcoma
  Giant cell sarcoma
  Gout
  Hemangioma
  Hodgkin's disease
  Hyperparathyroidism
  Leprosy
  Metastasis
  Multiple myeloma
  Neuroblastoma
  New bone (fibrosis)
  Osteitis fibrosa cystica
  Radiation necrosis
  Senile osteoporosis
  Solitary myeloma
  Syphilis (gumma)

RESPIRATORY SYSTEM

Additive (hard to penetrate)
  Actinomycosis
  Arrested tuberculosis (calcification)
  Atelectasis
  Bronchiectasis
  Edema
  Empyema
  Encapsulated abscess
  Hydropneumothorax
  Malignancy
  Miliary tuberculosis
  Pleural effusion
  Pneumoconiosis
    Anthracosis
    Asbestosis
    Calcinosis
    Siderosis
    Silicosis
  Pneumonia
  Syphilis
  Thoracoplasty

Destructive (easy to penetrate)
  Early lung abscess
  Emphysema
  Pneumothorax
  Tuberculosis (active)

CIRCULATORY SYSTEM

Additive (hard to penetrate)
  Aortic aneurysm
  Ascites
  Cirrhosis of liver
  Enlarged heart

Destructive (easy to penetrate)
  Gout
  Leukemia

GASTROINTESTINAL SYSTEM

Destructive (easy to penetrate)
  Bowel obstruction
  Malignancy

SOFT TISSUE

Additive (hard to penetrate)
  Edema

Destructive (easy to penetrate)
  Emaciation
  Pendulous breast
  Pneumoperitoneum

FORMULATING X-RAY TECHNIQUES

To compensate for tissue differences in the small, medium, and large patient, one may use classifications of A, B, and C. A would represent the thin and emaciated patient, B the normal or medium patient, and C the large or muscular patient. For A, B, and C classifications, milliampere-seconds values are given; for example, in the lateral radiography of the three types for lumbar spine, each measuring the same thickness, A would require less milliampere seconds and C would require more milliampere seconds than the B patient. It is apparent that if the same peak kilovoltage and the same milliampere seconds were given all three patients, the A patient's radiograph would be overexposed while the C patient's would be underexposed.

Thickness of part

A variation in thickness of extremities should not cause a great deal of difficulty; it is easier to compensate for variations here than in working with the heavier parts. If the object being radiographed is an ankle swollen to the size of the average knee, then the knee technique should be used; if the individual is of such size that the normal ankle is the size of the average knee, the same thing holds true. The radiologic technologist with limited experience should spend considerable time in studying the thicknesses of the part which is being radiographed; with added experience his errors due to poor judgment of the thickness of the subject will, of course, be reduced. Variations in thicknesses and size of the pelvis, kidney, lumbar spine, etc., are much more difficult to judge even for the experienced technologist. When a lack of uniformity exists in the routine radiographs produced in the department, it is usually with the heavier parts of the body. When the subject to be taken is unusually large, there is a tendency on the part of the technologist to use too much penetration.

A film which is too light in radiographic density, but which has received full development, or a film too dark in radiographic density after full development, at once tells the radiologic technologist that the energy used has been either insufficient or too much. In either case it is relatively simple either to increase or to decrease the energy for the next radiograph. The experience gained from such a procedure will be far more valuable when the next heavy patient is to be radiographed than the experience gained from employing too much energy and improper processing.

It *must* be realized by every technologist, however, that the thickness of any body part is not an index of its physiology or its x-ray absorption qualities, and cannot be employed per se as an authoritative index of the radiographic density desired to be produced.

THE CHEST

The chest is less dense to x-rays than any other part of the body of the same thickness. The soft tissues and bones of the thoracic wall are like similar structures elsewhere, but air in the lungs reduces the average density to a marked degree.

Children and infants

The chests of adults of different thicknesses are of approximately the same radiographic density. If a given thickness of the thorax of a child, however,

Variable Kilovoltage Method

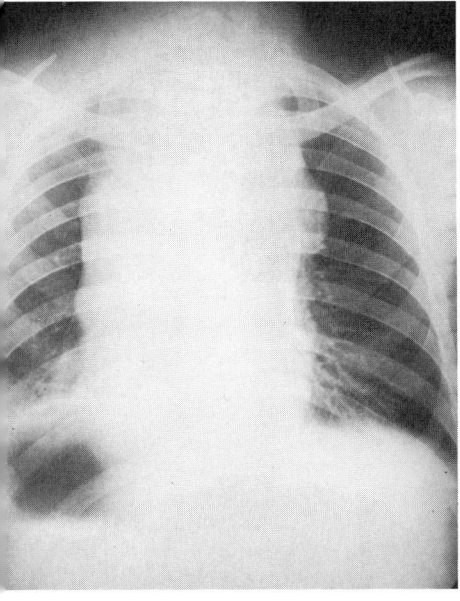

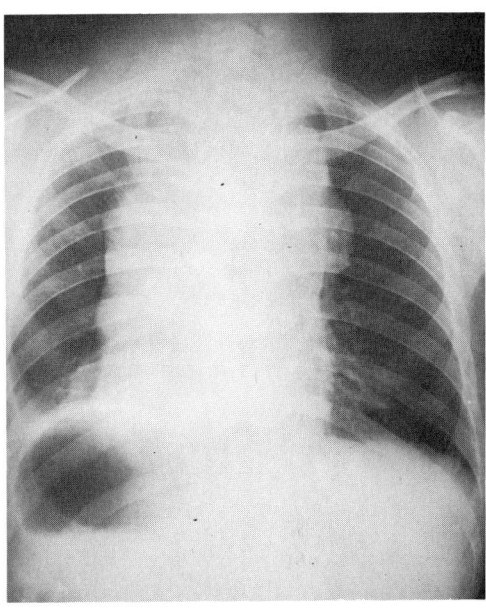

Figure 10.9. Chest with Hodgkin's disease, given normal exposure.

Figure 10.10. The chest of Figure 10.9, with the correction of an added 5 Kv.P.

is compared to a similar thickness of the thorax of an adult, the average density to x-rays of that of the child is considerably greater than that of the adult. This is most marked in infants and gradually decreases as age advances.

Figure 10.11. Chest with fluid, given normal exposure.

Figure 10.12. The chest of Figure 10.11 with the correction of an added 5 Kv.P.

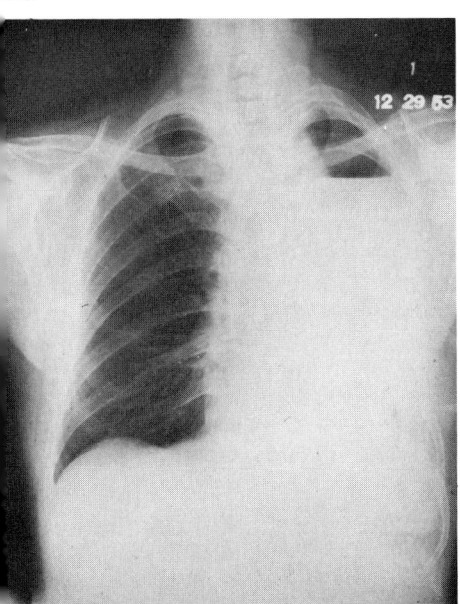

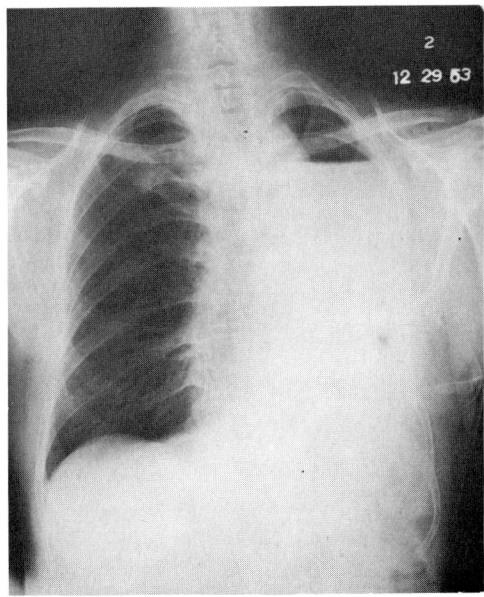

FORMULATING X-RAY TECHNIQUES

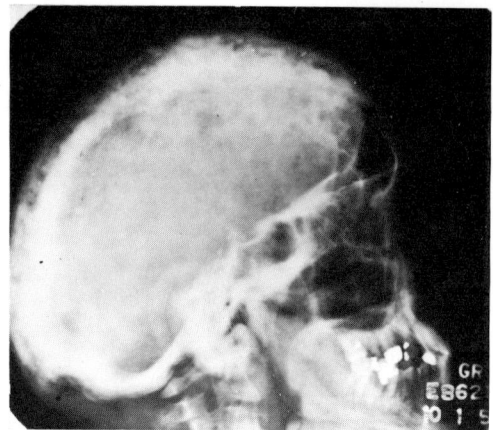

Figure 10.13. Plus 40 per cent correction factor for Paget's disease.

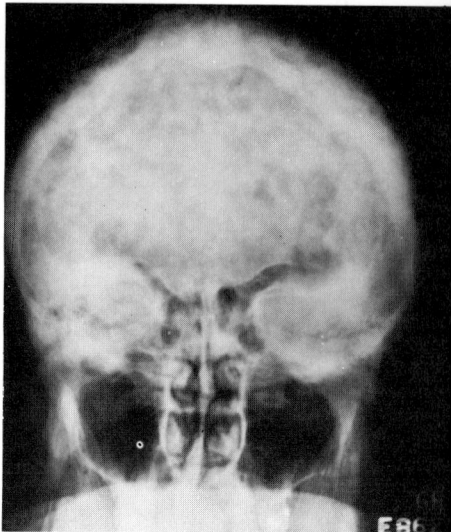

Figure 10.14. The same correction factor as for Figure 10.13.

This greater opacity makes necessary a special exposure technique for films of the chest of infants and children.

Types of thoracic cavities

Radiography of the thoracic cavity and lungs requires more attention and care than that of any other body group. Results will depend largely upon classification of patients into proper groups. There are several types of patients, and the judgment of the technologist is of great importance.

Heavy chest type. This class represents a type of individual having a heavy, dense muscular frame and normally assumes a plus percentage correction factor, depending upon tissue density. Women with very heavy frame and very large breasts should be placed in this group.

Thin chest type. Such patients are generally recognized when they are properly positioned against the cassette changer with their shoulders and arms thrown forward, because of protruding scapulae and lack of flesh. A minus percentage correction factor is necessary. (Some average patients of normal build will be found with scapulae extending beyond the normal measure.)

Very thin type. This individual is the barrel-chested type with below normal flesh, generally having good expansion, where the thoracic cavity represents practically the entire depth of the thorax. Such patients need a reduction in energy, generally through the manipulation of Ma.S. to a point considerably below that proper for a normal chest.

Pathology. The technologist should obtain specific information from the request slip with respect to suspected pathology so as to be able to apply positive percentage correction factors (Figures 10.9 to 10.20).

Variable Kilovoltage Method

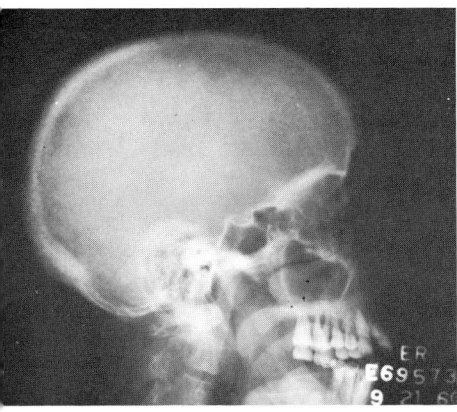

Figure 10.15. Lateral view of skull with hyperparathyroidism, with normal exposure.

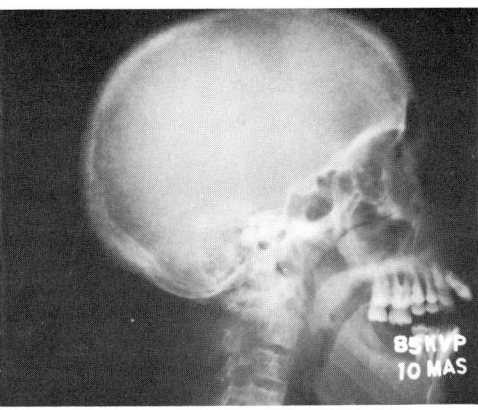

Figure 10.16. The skull of Figure 10.15, with a minus 30 per cent correction in Ma.S.

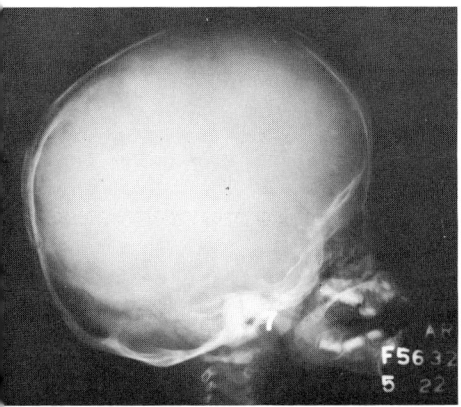

Figure 10.17. Lateral skull with hydrocephalus; plus per cent correction in Ma.S.

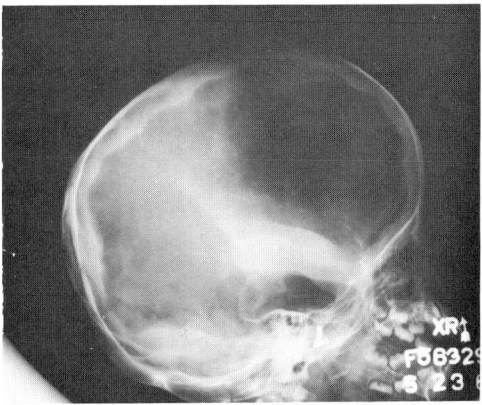

Figure 10.18. The skull of Figure 10.17 with a minus 30 per cent Ma.S. correction for hydrocephalus and an air study on the same patient.

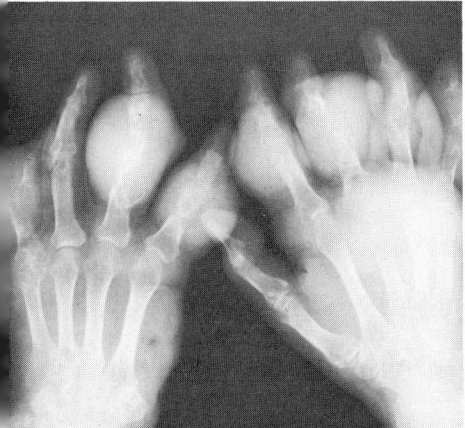

Figure 10.19. Posteroanterior view of hands, with a us 30 per cent correction in Ma.S. for gout.

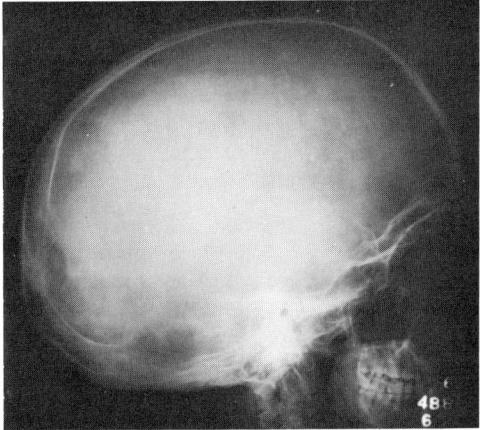

Figure 10.20. Lateral skull of a child with hydrocephalus, with a plus 30 per cent correction factor.

165

FORMULATING X-RAY TECHNIQUES

VARIABLE KILOVOLTAGE TECHNIQUE CHART—TYPE ONE

Select an individual or phantom of average size and start with any group of parts of similar density.

The lateral skull will be used as our starting point. Measure the subject in the lateral projection. On the average, this measurement will be 15 cm. *Multiply the centimeter thickness by 2 and add the figure 30 to the product.* In this manner we arrive at the figure 60, our *base kilovoltage.* In other words, a 15-cm. lateral skull would require 60 Kv.P.; a 16-cm. skull would require 62 Kv.P.; a 14-cm. skull would require 58 Kv.P.

Select the *milliampere seconds* thought to be most appropriate for this group.

Select the focus-film distance and a cone which will restrict radiation to the part.

The technical factors we will use, then, are:

Focus-film distance	36 inches
Bucky	8-to-1 ratio
Cm.	15
Kv.P.	60

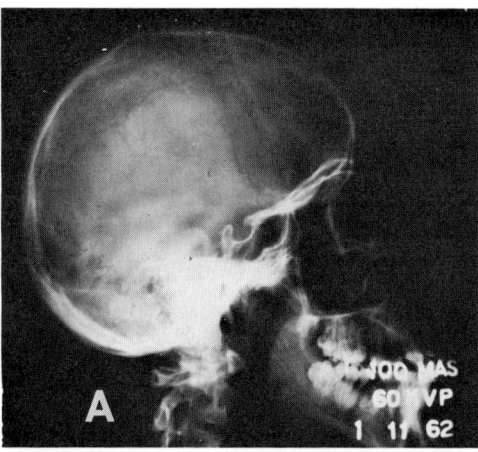
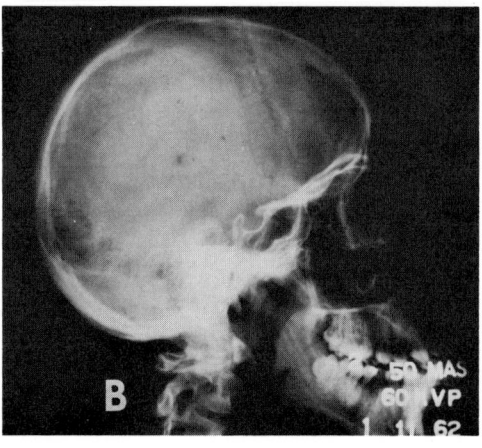
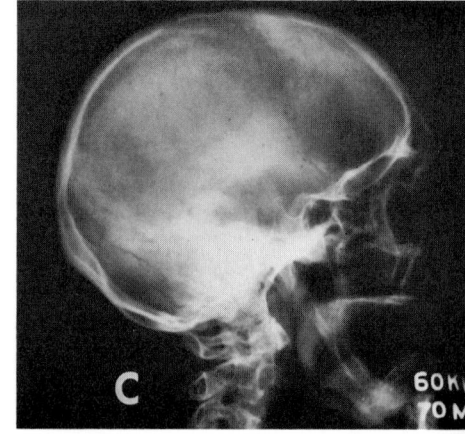

Figure 10.21. Lateral views of a skull. A, the initial film, an overexposure. In B, the Ma.S. was reduced to half to compensate, and the result is an underexposure. In C, the Ma.S. was adjusted to give a correct exposure by using the average Ma.S. for the two preceding Ma.S. values.

Variable Kilovoltage Method

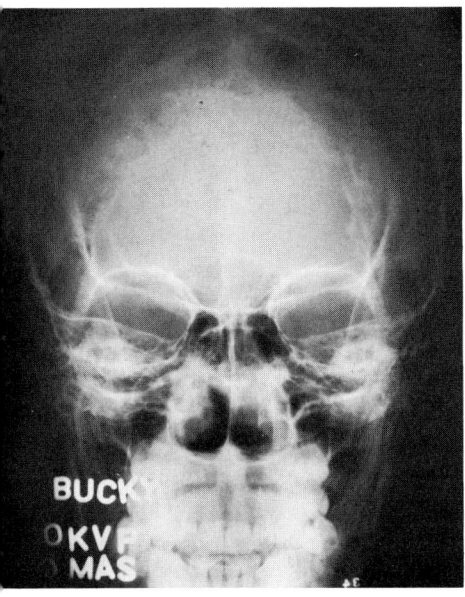

Figure 10.22. Posteroanterior view of the skull.

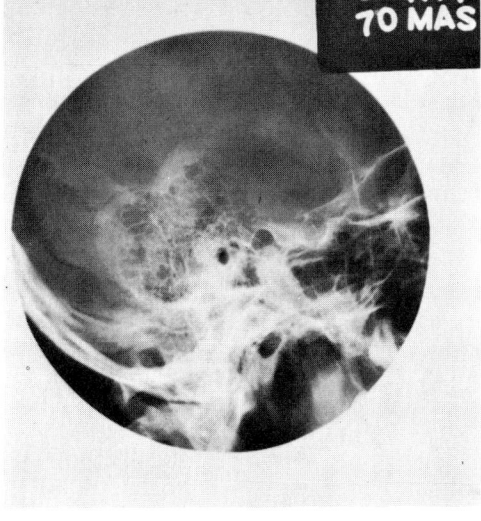

Figure 10.23. Lateral view of a mastoid, with cylinder cone at a 30-inch focus-film distance.

Ma.S. 100
Cone To Part

Place the subject in the lateral skull position and make an exposure employing the above factors. Develop the film according to *standard time-temperature* or *automatic* processing; inspect under standard illumination. If the film is overexposed (see Figure 10.21A) reduce the Ma.S. by one-half and repeat (see Figure 10.21B). If this film is underexposed, repeat, going in between 100 and 50 Ma.S. and use 70 or 75 Ma.S. (see Figure 10.21C).

If this meets our standards we now have a working technique as follows:

Region: Skull *Time:* $7/10$
Position: Lateral *Ma.S.:* 70
Cone: V-10 *Dist.:* 36
Ma.: 100 *Bucky:* Yes
Cm.: 13 14 15 16 17 18 19 20 21 22 23
Kv.: 56 58 60 62 64 66 68 70 72 74 76

These factors will hold for the entire skull group. See the following figures: 10.22, P.A. skull; 10.23, lateral view of mastoid with a cylinder cone *but* at a 30-inch focus-film distance (because of the added absorption of the cylinder cone); 10.24, Stenver's at 30 inches; 10.25, optic foramen at 30 inches; 10.26, P.A. mandible at 30 inches; 10.27, Caldwell at 30 inches, using Bucky.

Consult also Figure 10.28, a child's skull with a reduction in Ma.S. according to the age correction table, page 175, and Figure 10.29, an infant's skull, also with a reduction in the Ma.S. according to the age correction table.

The above procedure is followed throughout the entire chart for *each group* of parts of *similar density*.

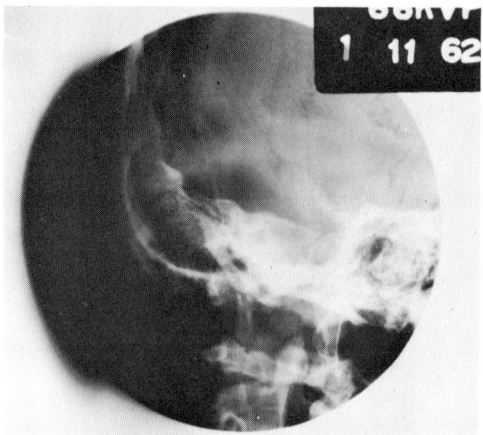

Figure 10.24. Stenvers view at 30 inches.

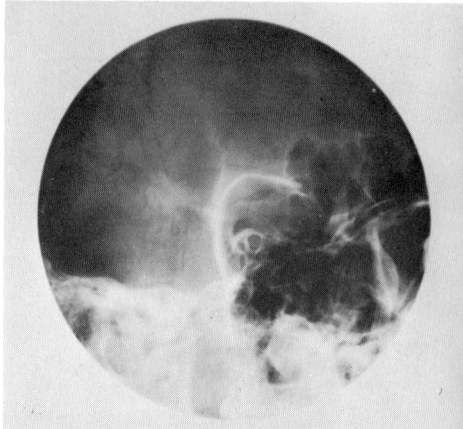

Figure 10.25. Optic foramen at 30 inches.

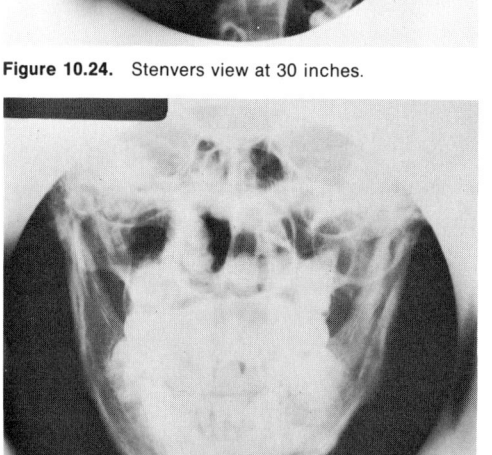

Figure 10.26. Posteroanterior view of the mandible at 30 inches.

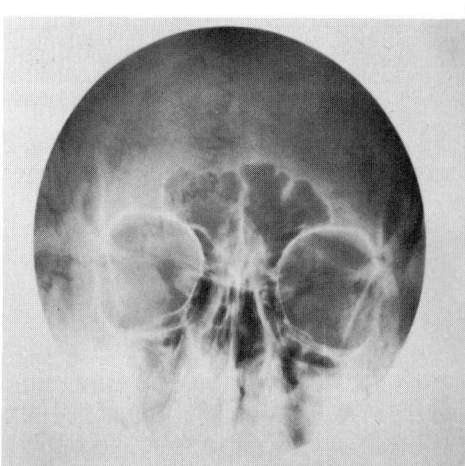

Figure 10.27. Caldwell view at 30 inches, using Bucky.

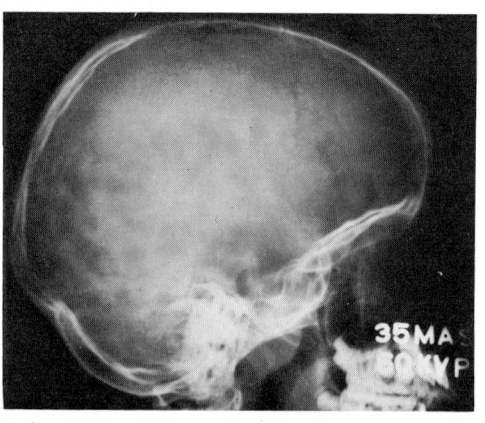

Figure 10.28. Child's skull, with reduction of Ma.S. according to the age correction table.

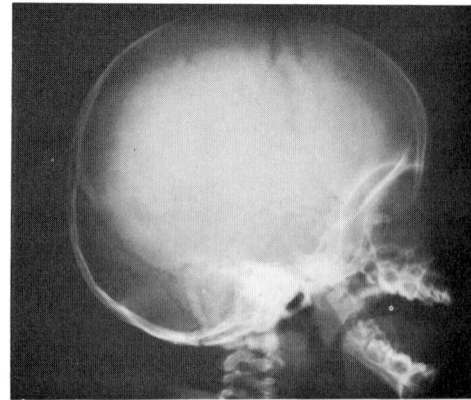

Figure 10.29. Infant's skull, with reduction in Ma.S. according to the age correction table.

Variable Kilovoltage Method

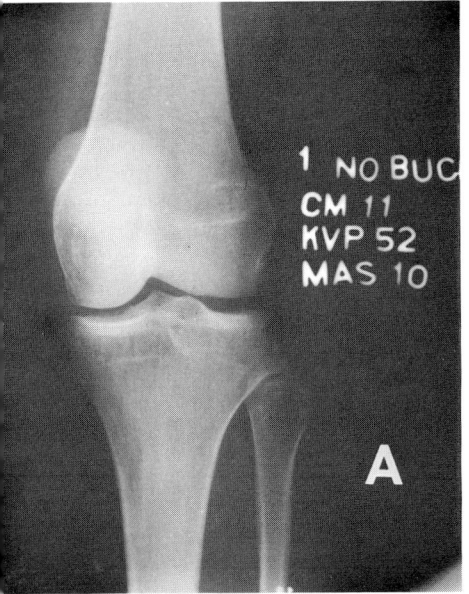
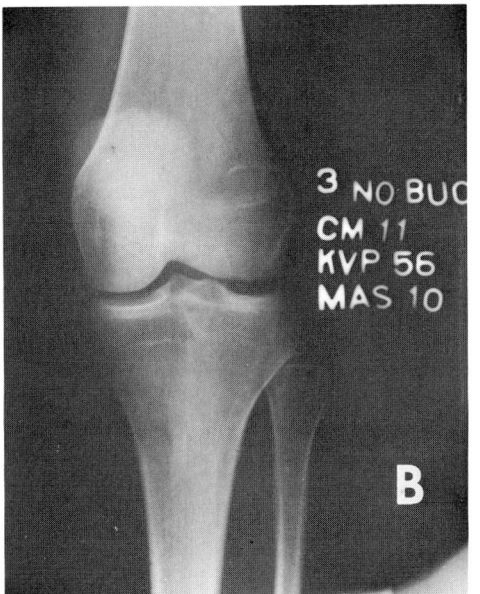
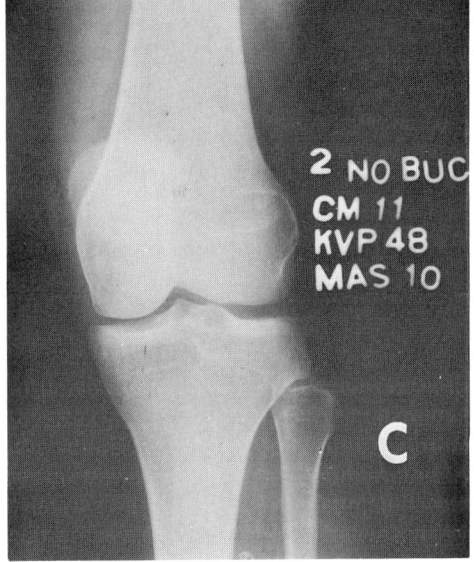

Figure 10.30. Three radiographs of the knee, all at 10 Ma.S. View A is taken at 52 Kv.P., B at 56 Kv.P., and C at 48 Kv.P.

The next step is to apply our Ma.S. correction factors for the adult patients who are above or below normal. This correction is based on a 30 per cent change in Ma.S. In other words, we would add 30 per cent to our base or normal Ma.S. for patients who are above normal, and decrease our Ma.S. by 30 per cent for patients who are below normal.

A 30 per cent change in Ma.S. will cause an increase or decrease in density. See Chapter 7, above, Figure 7.8, normal exposure; Figure 7.9, 30 per cent below normal; Figure 7.10, 30, per cent above normal.

For infants and children, with the *exception* of the *chest,* we can use the

FORMULATING X-RAY TECHNIQUES

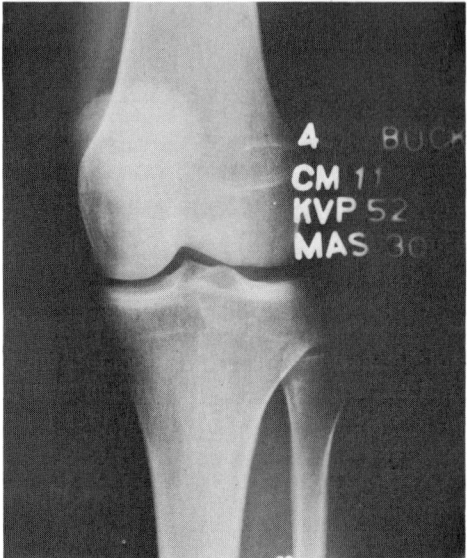

Figure 10.31. Radiograph of the knee, with Bucky, at 52 Kv.P. and 30 Ma.S.

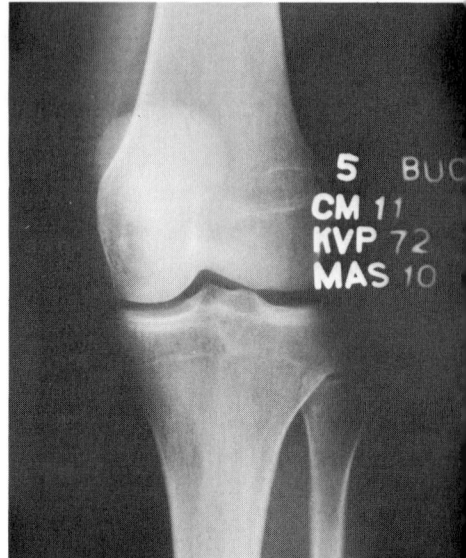

Figure 10.32. Radiograph of the knee, with Bucky at 72 Kv.P. and 10 Ma.S.

age correction table (p. 175) to obtain the correct Ma.S. and then simply measure the part and use the Kv.P. as listed under the Cm.-Kv.P. scale. A possible exception to this would be the lateral thoracic and lumbar spine.

For uncooperative patients, simply convert the Ma.S. to a higher Ma. value and a faster time. Use the time-milliamperage formula below. Example: change a 2-second exposure at 50 Ma. to $1/2$ second.

$M_1:M_2 :: T_2:T_1$
$50:x :: 1/2:2$
$1/2 x = 100$
$x = 200 =$ new Ma. for $1/2$ second

Extremity group

Let us select the knee to start this group. Select the Ma.S. you want to use. In this case we want to use 10 Ma.S. We have a choice of Ma. and time values:

100 Ma. at $1/10$ second = 10 Ma.S.
200 Ma. at $1/20$ second = 10 Ma.S.
300 Ma. at $1/30$ second = 10 Ma.S.

Since the 100-Ma. station is on the small focus, let us select 100 Ma. at $1/10$ second, a 36-inch focus-film distance and par-speed screens.

Measure the knee in the A.P. projection and add the figure 30. In this case the knee measures 11 cm.; therefore $2 \times 11 = 22$, $22 + 30 = 52$. This is our base Kv.P.

To save time, let us expose the knee at 52 Kv.P. (Figure 10.30A), another exposure at 4 Kv.P. more (Figure 10.30B), and another exposure at 4 Kv.P. less (Figure 10.30C).

All three films should be developed at standard time-temperature proc-

Variable Kilovoltage Method

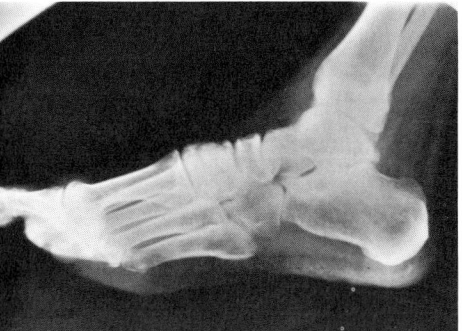

Figure 10.33A. Lateral view of foot and ankle at 5 Ma.S.

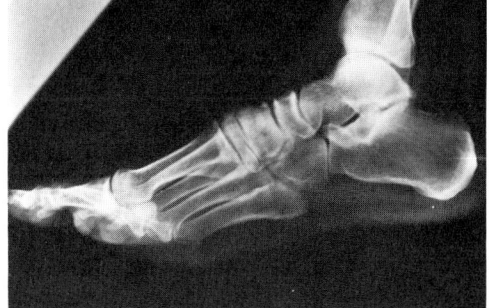

Figure 10.33B. Same view as in A. but at 10 Ma.S.

essing and then placed on the illuminator for evaluation. Suppose we select film number 1 (see Figure 10.30A). We now can insert 52 Kv.P. under 11 cm. on our scale.

If we wish to obtain more contrast and better detail we can go to a Bucky technique. We have a choice in how we make our compensation. For high contrast we can *treble* the Ma.S., which would be 30 Ma.S. All other factors remain the same (see Figure 10.31). Or if we wish to have better penetration and a reasonable amount of contrast, we *add* 20 Kv.P. and use 72 Kv.P. (see Figure 10.32). All other factors remain the same.

Extremity group: alternative method

Example: It is desired to formulate the extremity technique. Let us select the lateral foot and ankle and an Ma.S. factor that does not work out on the first exposure. To find our Kv.P. we would use 2 times the thickness of the part ($2 \times 7 = 14$) plus 30, which gives 44 Kv.P.

Cm.: 7
Kv.P.: 44
Dist.: 36 inches
Ma.: 100
Time: $1/20$
Ma.S.: 5
Cone: To film
Film: Regular
Screens: Medium
Development: Automatic
Bucky: No

Expose the part using the above factors (see Figure 10.33A). Upon inspection of the finished radiograph we find we have penetrated the part but have insufficient density. Expose a second film with an increase in Ma.S., since Ma.S. is the controlling factor for density. The second radiograph exposed at 10 Ma.S. (see Figure 10.33B) is of the desired quality. Figures 10.34A and B show the same procedure carried out with dried bones of the foot.

Cm.: 7
Kv.P.: 44
Dist.: 36 inches
Ma.: 100
Time: $1/10$ second
Ma.S.: 10
Cone: To film
Film: Regular
Screens: Medium
Development: 5 minutes at 68°
Bucky: No

By adding 2 Kv.P. per centimeter thickness to the base kilovoltage of 30, our extremity chart would be:

Ma.: 100 *Time:* $1/10$ *Distance:* 36" *Screens* *Bucky:* No. *Cone:* To Part

Cm.	2	3	4	5	6	7	8	9	10	11	12	13	14	15
Kv.	34	36	38	40	42	44	46	48	50	52	54	56	58	60

FORMULATING X-RAY TECHNIQUES

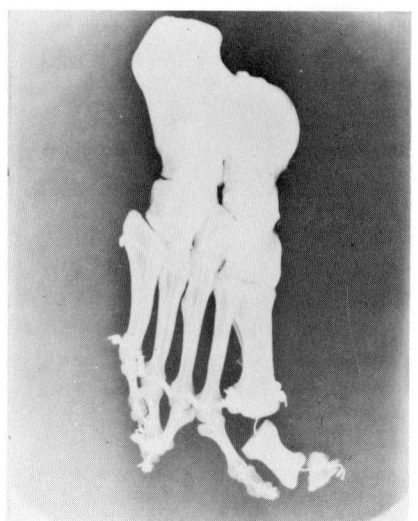 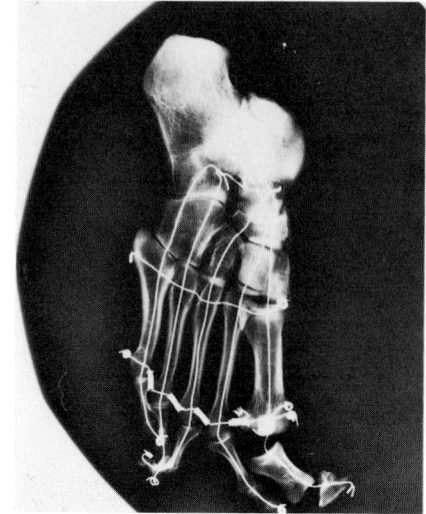

Figure 10.34. Views of bones of the foot (dried): A, at 40 Kv.P. and 1.2 Ma.S.; B, at 40 Kv.P. and 2.4 Ma.S.

To compensate for children and infants, we would use the age correction table, p. 175.

VARIABLE KILOVOLTAGE TECHNIQUE CHART—TYPE TWO

Because of the numerous variable factors in radiography it is often necessary to make two or three exposures of a part to secure the best results.

After processing the film under standard conditions, one should study the radiograph on a standard illuminator; if underexposed, the Ma.S. should be increased for the next exposure; if dense and black from overexposure, reduce the Ma.S. by one-half. If gray and flat from overpenetration, reduce the Kv.P. from 10 to 15 Kv.P.; or "chalky," increase the Kv.P. from 10 to 15 Kv.P. Further fine adjustments in Kv.P. or Ma.S. can then be made in order to give you the type of radiograph you wish.

With variable kilovoltage technique the *kilovoltage* is varied for tissue-thickness measurements of all subjects and classes which are composed of structures with *similar thickness* and *density* and are divided into groups.

1. Extremities
2. Skull
3. Sinuses
4. Trunk and pelvis
5. Lateral lumbar
6. Lateral thoracic
7. Chest
8. Gastrointestinal tract
9. Lateral cervical spine

The various parts included in each major group will vary in required Kv.P.; i.e., a shoulder and lateral skull of the same thickness will require different Kv.P. or Ma.S. In addition, patients are divided into the following classifications: A, B, and C, with B representing the normal patient, A less than normal, and C greater than normal. By using these classifications we are able to compensate for the emaciated, normal, and muscular patients as well as for atrophy and disease.

Variable Kilovoltage Method

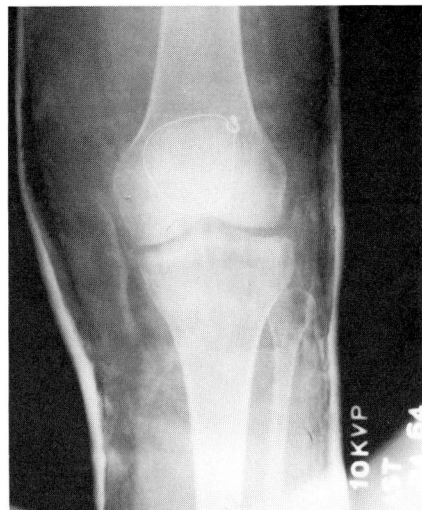

Figure 10.35. Anteroposterior view of knee with a dry cast (an added 10 Kv.P.).

By the grouping of parts, we balance the Ma.S. and Kv.P. The next step is to select the type of technique which will produce the quality of film desired by the radiologist. If the selection is made for high contrast (short-scale), the Kv.P. is low and the Ma.S. high. If the choice is for a radiograph with wide latitude and long-scale contrast, the Kv.P. will be higher and the Ma.S. lower.

There is a balance between Ma.S. and Kv.P. which must stay within reasonable limits. If the Ma.S. for a heavy part (lateral skull) is employed with a small part (knee) and the Kv.P. reduced to avoid total blackening of the film, high contrast results. Conversely, if one uses an exposure (Ma.S.) suitable for a small part on a heavy part and increases the Kv.P., extreme flatness results and the scale of contrast is too long.

Effective Kv.P.

Effective Kv.P. refers principally to the lowest possible Kv.P. with which a part can be penetrated. This minimum penetrability has almost as many variations as there are different types of machines and tubes. That is to say, some machines or tubes are *more effective* at a given Kv.P. than others; so it is impractical to set up a Ma.S. and Kv.P. balance and regard it as standard the world over.

Direct exposure

This particular type of technique is restricted in application to the small parts of the body and further restricted by the thickness of the parts themselves. This limitation can be explained by the fact that a normal amount of contrast and detail is necessary for bone radiography and beyond a certain thickness of tissue, this is a hopeless task with *direct exposure,* i.e., cardboard holder with non-screen or regular film.

There are times when one will encounter conditions which make cardboard exposures impractical. These instances are usually:

FORMULATING X-RAY TECHNIQUES

A. Necessity for increased contrast or parts thicker than 12 centimeters.
B. Necessity for increased contrast of thick muscular parts.
C. Presence of a plaster cast.
D. Necessity for increased speed of exposure.
E. Type of processing to be employed.

When these or comparable conditions present themselves, it is advisable to use screens. When screens are used, one must compensate for the increased speed by deducting Ma.S. For the proper reduction in Ma.S., one must know the *speed ratio* between screens and direct exposure. This will depend, of course, on the kind of screens being used. For example the ratio for par-speed screens to direct exposure (employing non-screen film) is 5 to 1; therefore if we have been using 50 Ma.S. for non-screen work, we would use 10 Ma.S. with screens, all other factors remaining the same. If we were using screens and 10 Ma.S. and went to non-screen film, we would use 50 Ma.S., all other factors remaining the same except *processing*. Non-screen film can be processed *only by* manual processing; it is *not to be used* with automatic processing.

Plaster cast

Convert to screens and add 10 Kv.P. for a dry cast and 15 Kv.P. for a wet cast (Figure 10.35).

RADIOGRAPHIC GUIDE: VARIABLE KILOVOLTAGE TECHNIQUE

It might seem rather difficult to follow charts with stated factors since it is commonly known that all machines will vary to a certain extent. It must be understood that the purpose of any chart in this book is to serve as a guide so that when one part has been satisfactorily adapted to existing conditions, all other parts of the same group will require the same corrections.

Variable Kilovoltage Method

Cone	Videx
C-Cone	Cylinder
Film	Regular
Screens	Medium
Bucky	8-to-1
Tube	Rotating Anode
Development	Automatic

Age Correction Factor

Age	Factor, × adult Ma.S.
Birth to 3 months	.2
3 months to 2 years	.3
2 years to 5 years	.4
5 years to 7 years	.5
7 years to 12 years	.6

Example: If adult Ma.S. is 80, then the correct Ma.S. for a 3-year-old child is 80 × .4 = 32 Ma.S.

Region	Position	Cone	Ma.	Time	Ma.S.	Distance	Bucky
Skull	Lateral	V-10	100	$7/10$	70	36	yes
	A.P.-P.A.	V-8	100	1	100	36	yes
	Vertex	V-8	100	1	100	36	yes
	Petrous-A.P.	C	100	$1 1/4$	125	36	yes
	Optic	C	100	$8/10$	80	33	yes
	Stenvers	C	100	$8/10$	80	33	yes
	Mastoid-Lat.	C	100	$7/10$	70	30	yes
	Waters	V-8	100	1	100	36	yes
	Mandible-P.A.	C	100	1	100	33	yes

Ma.S.
A – minus 30%
B – normal
C – plus 30%

Cm.	10	11	12	13	14	15	16	17	18	19	20	21	22	23	24
K.V.	50	52	54	56	58	60	62	64	66	68	70	72	74	76	78

Region	Position	Cone	Ma.	Time	Ma.S.	Distance	Bucky
Facial bones	Mandible-Lat.	C	100	$1/10$	10	33	no
	Nasal-Lat.	C	100	$1/20$	5	30	no
	T.M.J. A.P.	C	100	$1/10$	10	30	no
	Maxilla P.A.	C	100	$2/5$	40	33	no
	Zygomatic	C	100	$1/10$	10	33	no

Cm.	3	4	5	6	7	8	9	10	11	12
K.V.	34	36	38	40	42	44	46	48	50	52

Region	Position	Cone	Ma.	Time	Ma.S.	Distance	Bucky
Sinuses	Lateral	C	100	$1/10$	10	30	no
	Frontal	C	100	$2/5$	40	33	no
	Maxillary	C	100	$2/5$	40	33	no
	Sphenoid	C	100	$2/5$	40	33	no
	Lateral	C	100	$3/10$	30	33	yes
	P.A.	C	100	$1 1/4$	125	33	yes

Cm.	10	11	12	13	14	15	16	17	18	19	20	21	22	23	24
K.V.	48	50	52	54	56	58	60	62	64	66	68	70	72	74	76

Ma.S.
A – minus 30%
B – normal
C – plus 30%

Region	Position	Cone	Ma.	Time	Ma.S.	Distance	Bucky
Shoulder	A.P.	V-8	100	$1/4$	25	36	yes
Scapula	A.P. & Lat.	V-10	100	$1/4$	25	36	yes
Humerus	A.P. & Lat.	V-10	100	$1/5$	20	36	yes

Cm.	8	9	10	11	12	13	14	15	16	17	18
K.V.	54	56	58	60	62	64	66	68	70	72	74

FORMULATING X-RAY TECHNIQUES

Region	Position	Cone	Ma.	Time	Ma.S.	Distance	Bucky
Cervical	A.P.	V-8	100	1	100	36	yes
Cervical	Spot-C-1	C	100	1	100	30	yes
Dorsal	A.P.	V-14	100	1	100	36	yes
Lumbar	A.P.	V-11	100	1	100	36	yes
Lumbar	Obl.	V-8	100	1	100	36	yes
Pelvis	A.P.	V-14	100	1	100	36	yes
K.U.B.	A.P.	V-14	100	1	100	36	yes
Gallbladder	P.A.	C	100	1	100	36	yes

Ma.S.
A — minus 30%
B — normal
C — plus 30%

Cm.	11	12	13	14	15	16	17	18	19	20	21	22	23	24	25
K.V.	52	54	56	58	60	62	64	66	68	70	72	74	76	78	80

Region	Position	Cone	Ma.	Time	Ma.S.	Distance	Bucky
Extremities	All	To part	100	$1/_{10}$	10	36	no
Extremities	All	To part	100	$1/_2$	50	36	non-screen
Extremities	All	To part	100	$3/_{10}$	30	36	Bucky

Cm.	2	3	4	5	6	7	8	9	10	11	12	13	14
K.V.	34	36	38	40	42	44	46	48	50	52	54	56	58

Ma.S.
A — minus 30%
B — normal
C — plus 30%

Stomach and Colon
P.A. — Oblique — Lateral Ma: 200 Distance: 36 Bucky: yes

Cm.:	15	16	17		C.M.:	18	19	20	21	22
K.V.:	86	88	90		K.V.:	82	84	86	88	90
Time:	$1/_{10}$				Time:	$1/_5$				
Cm.:	23	24	25	26	27	C.M.:	28	29	30	31
K.V.:	82	84	86	88	90	K.V.:	86	88	90	92
Time:	$2/_5$					Time:	$1/_2$			

Region	Position	Cone	Ma.	Time	Ma.S.	Distance	Bucky
Chest	P.A.	V-14	300	$1/_{30}$	10	72	no
	Oblique	V-14	300	$1/_{15}$	20	72	no
	Lateral	V-14	300	$1/_{15}$	20	72	no

Cm.	15	16	17	18	19	20	21	22	23	24	25	26	27	28	29
K.V.	62	64	66	68	70	72	74	76	78	80	82	84	86	88	90

Special Lateral Exposure

Ma.S.
A — minus 30%
B — normal
C — plus 30%

Region	Position	Cone	Ma.	Time	Ma.S.	Distance	Bucky
	Lateral	V-8	300	$1/_{15}$	20	72	no
Cervical	Oblique	V-8	300	$1/_{15}$	20	72	no

Cm.	8	9	10	11	12	13	14	15	16
K.V.	68	70	72	74	76	78	80	82	84

Ma.S.
A — minus 30%
B — normal
C — plus 30%

Region	Position	Cone	Ma.	Time	Ma.S.	Distance	Bucky
Lumbar	Lateral	V-11	50	4	200	36	yes
L-5	Lateral	C	50	7	350	33	yes
Pelvimetry	Lateral	V-14	50	5	250	36	yes

Cm.	21	22	23	24	25	26	27	28	29	30	31	32	33	34
K.V.	72	74	76	78	80	82	84	86	88	90	92	94	96	98

Variable Kilovoltage Method

A – minus 30%
B – normal
C – plus 30%

Cm.	21	22	23	24	25	26	27	28	29	30	31	32	33	34
K.V.	48	50	52	54	56	58	60	62	64	66	68	70	72	74

Thoracic	Lateral	V-14	25	6	150	36	yes

RADIOGRAPHIC GUIDE – VARIABLE Kv.P.

Region	Position	Cone	Ma.	Time	Ma.S.	Dist.	B.	Film	Cm.	Kv.P.
Skull	Lateral	10	100	$7/10$	70	36	√	$10/12$	2	34
	P.A.	8	100	1	100	36	√	$8/10$	3	36
	A.P.	8	100	1	100	36	√	$8/10$	4	38
	Mentovertex	8	100	1	100	36	√	$8/10$	5	40
	Occipital	8	100	1	100	36	√	$8/10$	6	42
	Stenvers	C	100	$8/10$	80	30	√	$8/10$	7	44
	Petrous	C	100	$1 1/4$	125	36	√	$8/10$	8	46
	Mastoid	C	100	$7/10$	70	30	√	$8/10$	9	48
	Waters	8	100	1	100	36	√	$8/10$	10	50
	Optic	C	100	$8/10$	80	30	√	$8/10$	11	52
	Mandible, Lat.	C	100	$1/10$	10	30	No	$8/10$	12	54
	Nasal Bones	C	100	$1/20$	5	30	No	$8/10$	13	56
Spine	Cervical, A.P.	8	50	2	100	36	√	$8/10$	14	58
	Cervical, Lat.	8	300	$2/15$	40	72	No	$8/10$	15	60
	Cervical, Obl.	8	300	$2/15$	40	72	No	$8/10$	16	62
	Dorsal, A.P.	7	100	1	100	36	√	$7/17$	17	64
	Dorsal, Obl.	11	100	1	100	36	√	$11/14$	18	66
xxx	Dorsal, Lat.			see below					19	68
	Lumbar, A.P.	11	100	1	100	36	√	$11/14$	20	70
	Lumbar, Obl.	8	100	1	100	36	√	$8/10$	21	72
	Lumbar, Lat.	11	100	2	200	36	√	$11/14$	22	74
	Lumbar, Spot-L-5	C	50	5	250	30	√	$8/10$	23	76
	Pelvis, A.P.	14	100	1	100	36	√	$14/17$	24	78
Shoulder	A.P.	8	100	$1/2$	50	36	√	$8/10$	25	80
	Axial	8	100	$1/10$	10	36	No	$8/10$	26	82
Sternum	P.A. Obl.	11	100	1	100	36	√	$11/14$	27	84
	Lateral								28	86
Gallbladder	P.A.	8	100	$4/5$	80	36	√	$8/10$	29	88
	Decubitus	8	100	$4/5$	80	36	√	$8/10$	30	90
	Upright	8	100	$4/5$	80	36	√	$8/10$	31	92

FORMULATING X-RAY TECHNIQUES

Region	Position	Cone	Ma.	Time	Ma.S.	Dist.	B.	Film	Cm.	Kv.P.
Abdomen	A.P.	14	100	$4/5$	80	36	√	$14/17$	32	94
	Decubitus	14	100	$4/5$	80	36	√	$14/17$	33	96
K. U. B.	Upright	14	100	1	100	36	√	$14/17$	34	98
	Lateral	14	100	1	100	36	√	$14/17$		
Extremities	Screen	8	100	$1/10$	10	36	No	$8/10$		
	No Screen	8	200	$1/4$	50	36	No	$8/10$		
	Bucky	8	100	$3/10$	30	36	No	$8/10$		
	Infant	8	100	$1/20$	5	36	No	$8/10$		

Region	Position	Cone	Ma.	Time	Ma.S.	Dist.	B.	Film
Pelvimetry	Thoms, A.P.	10	200	1	200	36	√	$10/12$
	Lateral	14	50	4	200	36	√	$14/17$
	Placenta	See below: use barium filter						
Ribs	A.D.	14	50	$1/5$	10	36	√	$14/17$
	B.D.	14	100	$3/5$	60	36	√	$14/17$

Position	Cone	Ma.	Time	Ma.S.	Dist.	Bucky
Sinuses, Lat.	C	100	$1/10$	10	30	No
Frontal	C	100	$2/5$	40	30	No
Maxillary	C	100	$2/5$	40	30	No
Sphenoid	C	100	$2/5$	40	30	No

Cm.	12	13	14	15	16	17	18	19	20	21	22	23	24
Kv.	52	54	56	58	60	62	64	66	68	70	72	74	76

	Cone	Ma.	Time	Ma.S.	Dist.
Chest, P.A.	14	300	$1/30$	10	72
Chest, Oblique	14	300	$1/15$	20	72
Chest, Lateral	14	300	$1/15$	20	72
Chest, P.A., Grid	14	Add	20	Kv.P.	72
Chest Obl., Grid	14	Add	20	Kv.P.	72
Chest Lat., Grid	14	Add	20	Kv.P.	72

Cm.	17	18	19	20	21	22	23	24	25
Kv.	60	64	64	66	68	70	72	74	76

Variable Kilovoltage Method

Cm.	26	27	28	29	30	31	32
Kv.	78	80	82	84	86	88	90

		Cone	Ma.	Dist.	Bucky	Film
Stomach	P. A., Obl.	10	200	36	√	$10/12$
Stomach	Serial	10	200	30	√	$10/12$
Stomach	Spot Film	Use	photo	timer		$8/10$

Cm.	15	16	17	18	19	20	21	22		23	24	25	26	27	28	29	30	31
Kv.	86	88	90	82	84	86	88	90		82	84	86	88	90	86	88	90	92
Time	$1/10$			$1/5$						$2/5$					$1/2$			

Note: This type chart is formulated by 2 times the part plus 30. The Ma.S. has been corrected for each group except the chest. The chest, as well as the lateral thoracic spine, has a Kv.P.–Ma.S. balance of its own.

SPECIAL EXPOSURE

Lateral Dorsal Spine

MA: 50   Time: 3 sec.   Dist.: 36"   Bucky: yes
CM: 23   24   25   26   27   28   29   30   31   32   33
KV: 52   54   56   58   60   62   64   66   68   70   72

Infant Chest
MA: 50   Time: $1/20$ Dist.: 36"   Bucky: no
CM: 8   9   10   11   12   13   14   15
KV: 44   46   48   50   52   54   56   58
Oblique: add 6 Kv.P.
Lateral: add 10 Kv.P.

Child's Chest

MA: 300   Time: $1/20$ Dist: 72"   Bucky: no
CM: 12   13   14   15   16   17   18
KV: 54   56   58   60   62   64   66
Oblique: add 6 Kv.P.
Lateral: add 10 Kv.P.

Placenta — Lateral
300 Ma.S.   36" Dist.
Small: 60 Kv.P.   Medium 65 Kv.P.
              Large: 70 Kv.P.

The Kardex type technique chart (variable kilovoltage) is shown below.

Part: Skull   Position: Lateral

Remarks:

Ma.	Time	Dist.	Bucky	Cone	Film	Screen	Cardboard
100	$7/10$	36	yes	V-10	10 × 12	par	no

Cm.	13	14	15	16	17	18
Kv.	56	58	60	62	64	66

FORMULATING X-RAY TECHNIQUES

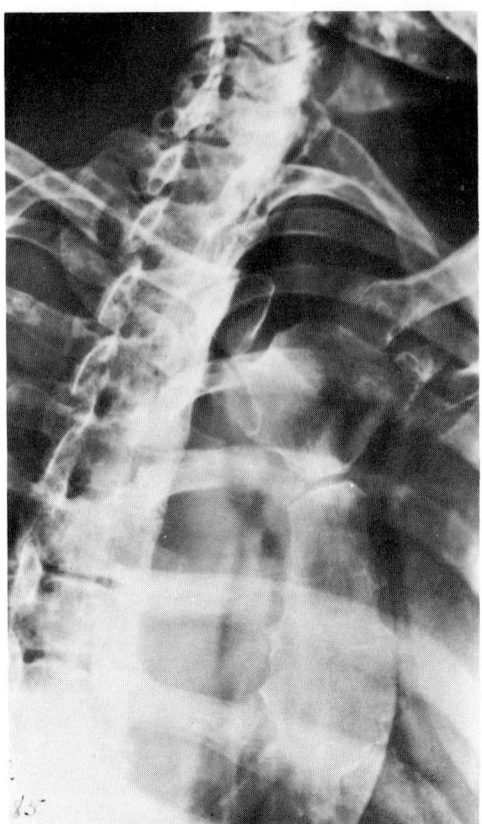

Figure 10.36. Close subject-tube distance techniqu posteroanterior view of a sternum at 50 Ma.S. and Kv.P.; distance 30 inches, cone to part, 8-to-1 gri medium screens.

CLOSE SUBJECT–FOCUS-FILM DISTANCE TECHNIQUE

Under certain conditions a short focus-film distance, i.e., focal spot 30 inches from the subject being radiographed, will be of value (Figure 10.36).

The short distance takes advantage of the wide divergence of the x-rays. The close position of the tube or focal spot causes blurring of the superimposed parts distant from the film, while the part to be radiographed, being in close contact with the film, still remains sharply outlined. This technique can be used in radiography of the sternum in the P.A. oblique position, the temporomandibular joint, and differentiation of gallstones and kidney stones.

EXPOSURE NOMOGRAMS FOR POLAROID TLX FILMS

Directions for use: Figures 10.37 and 10.38 are nomograms based on original experimentation done at the Duke University Medical Center and at the Polaroid Corporation. These nomograms may be used with any medium-speed film.

Take a clear plastic ruler and place it across the column headed KV at the point that represents the kilovoltage you are now using for routine radiography. Connect this point with the point in the third column (headed Wet

Variable Kilovoltage Method

10.37. Nomogram relating Polaroid TLX exposures to techniques developed for regular film and *high-speed screens*.

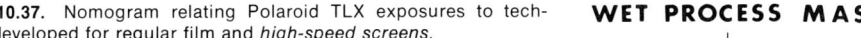

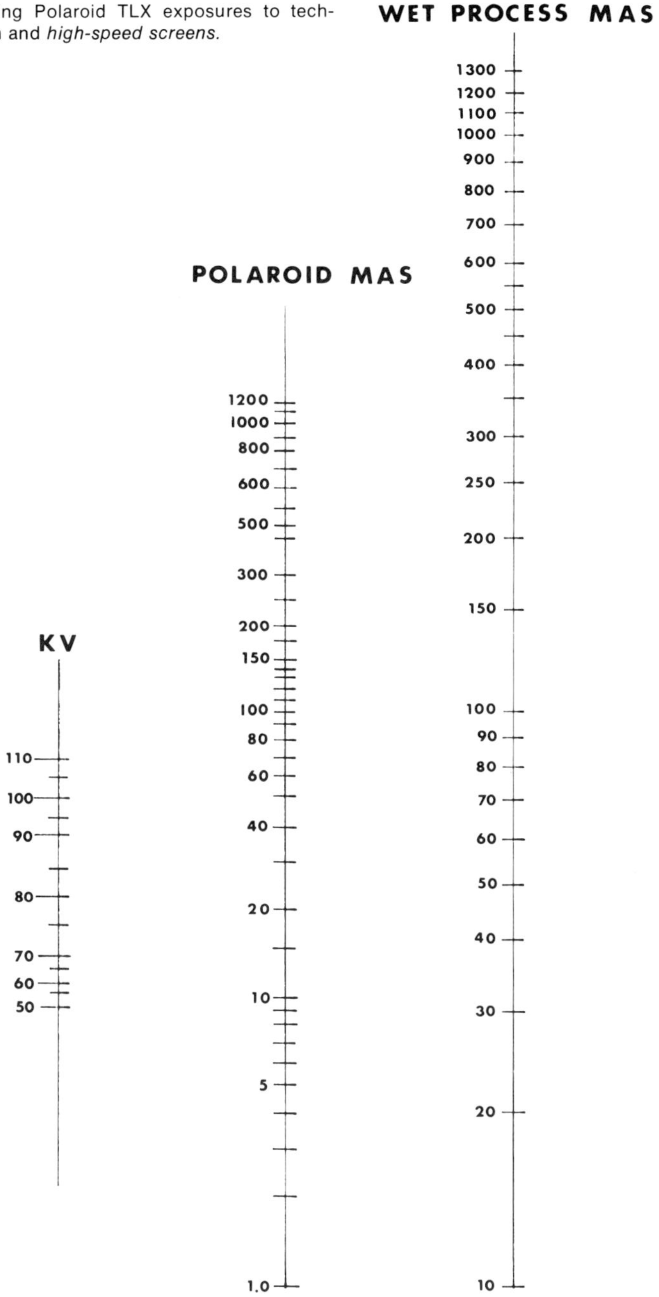

Process MAS) representing the Ma.S. you are now using. The point where the ruler crosses the second column represents the new Ma.S. to be used with Polaroid TLX film.

Example: With regular film and high-speed screens a technique calls for 60 Kv.P. and 100 Ma.S. Following the above directions we would use 30 to 33 Ma.S. with Polaroid TLX film.

FORMULATING X-RAY TECHNIQUES

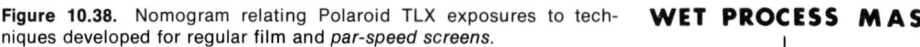

Figure 10.38. Nomogram relating Polaroid TLX exposures to techniques developed for regular film and *par-speed screens*.

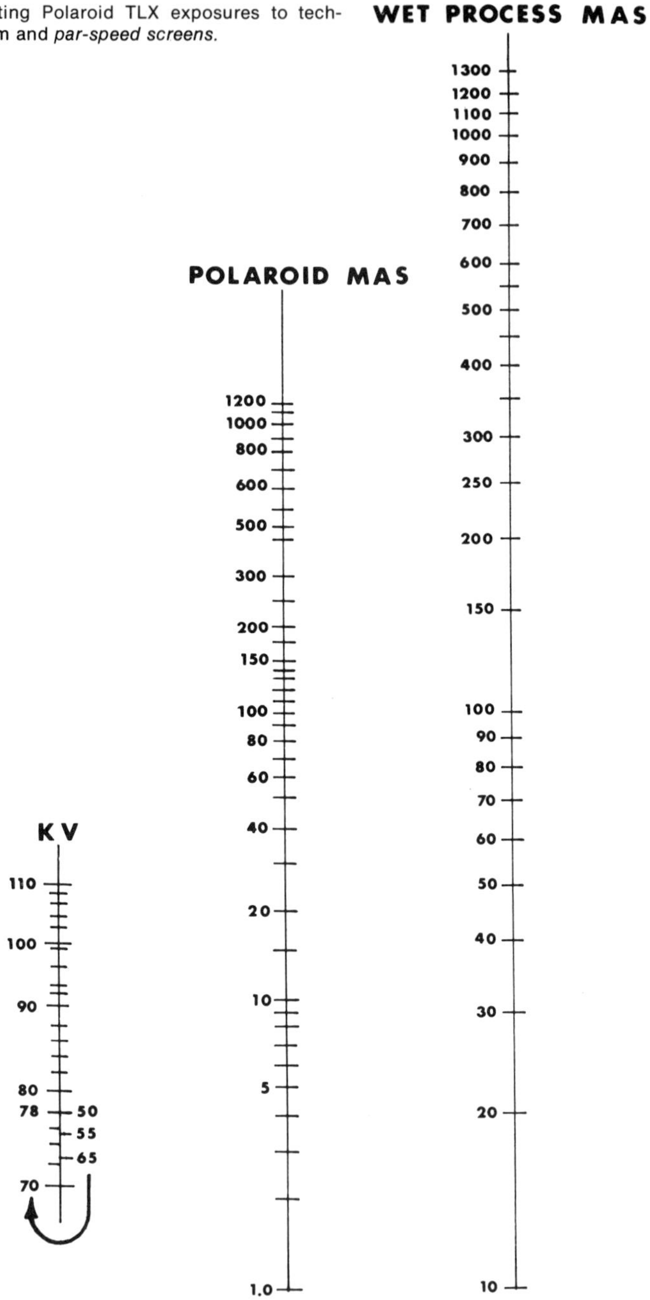

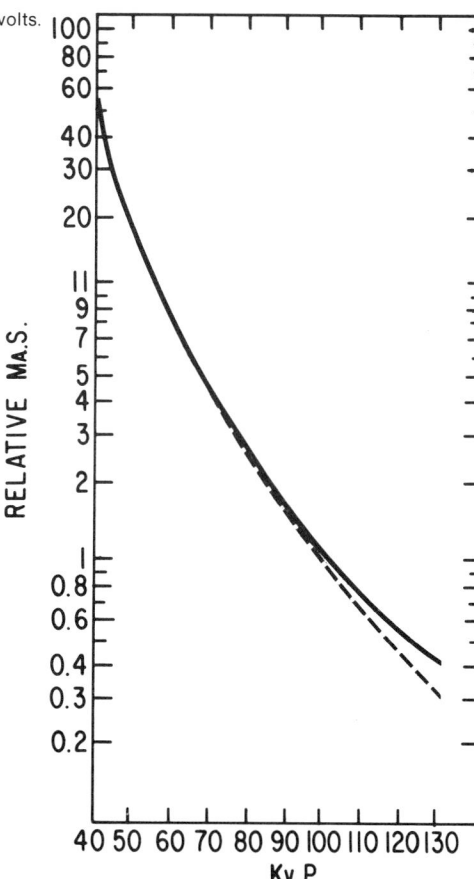

Figure 10.39. Conversion curve of density vs. kilovolts.

TECHNIQUE CONVERSION TO HIGHER VOLTAGE RANGE

The graph of Figure 10.39 shows a conversion curve based on visual densities obtained of radiographs throughout the range of 40–130 kilovolts. With the conversion curve, it is possible to determine the change in milliampere seconds for any desired kilovoltage, or the change in kilovoltage for any given change in milliampere seconds. Conversion would be made, of course, from any radiograph which produced the satisfactory degree of density in the normal voltage range. There are two curves on the chart — one with a solid line and one with a dotted line. The solid line represents constant density throughout the voltage range. However, a slight decrease in density can be tolerated if penetration is adequate with a considerable gain in radiographic contrast; this is represented by the dotted line.

Equation

$$\frac{\text{Relative Ma.S. at new Kv.P.}}{\text{Relative Ma.S. at old Kv.P.}} = \frac{\text{new Ma.S.}}{\text{old Ma.S.}}$$

Problem 1: Suppose a lateral skull radiograph is made using the following factors: 20 Ma.S. and 70 Kv.P. It is desired to change to 5 Ma.S. Find the new Kv.P.

FORMULATING X-RAY TECHNIQUES

Step 1: Determine the relative Ma.S. at starting Kv.P. This, on the graph, is 4.5.

Step 2: The relative value (4.5) is inserted into the equation so that the equation now reads

$$\frac{\text{Relative Ma.S. at new Kv.P.}}{4.5} = \frac{\text{new Ma.S.}}{\text{old Ma.S.}}$$

Step 3: The stated Ma.S. factors in the problem are inserted into the equation and x is used for the unknown, so that our equation now reads

$$\frac{x}{4.5} = \frac{5}{20}$$

Step 4: The problem is solved (ratio and proportion):

$$20x = 22.5$$

$$x = 1.125 = \text{relative Ma.S. at new Kv.P.}$$

Step 5: This new relative Ma.S. value (1.125) is located on the curve and the new Kv.P. will be found directly below, on the longitudinal axis of the graph, which is in this example, 100 Kv.P.

Problem 2: Suppose we have a technique using the factors 200 Ma.S. and 70 Kv.P.; we wish to use 110 Kv.P. What would the new Ma.S. factor be?

Step 1: Using the equation that precedes Problem 1 and the conversion curve, the relative Ma.S. at the new Kv.P. will be 0.8, so the formula will read

$$\frac{0.8}{\text{Relative Ma.S. at old Kv.P.}} = \frac{\text{new Ma.S.}}{\text{old Ma.S.}}$$

Step 2: Relying on the conversion curve, the relative Ma.S. at old Kv.P. will be 4.5, so the equation now reads

$$\frac{0.8}{4.5} = \frac{\text{new Ma.S.}}{\text{old Ma.S.}}$$

Step 3: The stated Ma.S. value of 200 is now inserted into the equation:

$$\frac{0.8}{4.5} = \frac{\text{new Ma.S.}}{200}$$

Step 4: x is inserted to replace new Ma.S., and the equation is solved:

$$\frac{0.8}{4.5} = \frac{x}{200}$$

$$5.5x = 160$$

$$x = 35.5, \text{ the new Ma.S.}$$

CHARTING RADIOGRAPHIC EXPOSURE

It may be desirable to formulate an exposure chart by charting exposure on a graph and then transferring the desired technique to a permanent place in the control stand. Usually it is best to have *one variable factor* and keep the others constant. Either the voltage or the time of exposure (Ma.S.) is most often varied.

As an illustration, suppose a chart is to be made for the lateral lumbar-sacral spine. We should first refer to the capacity of the x-ray unit and also the tube rating chart.

Let us select the following factors:

Focus-film distance: 36 inches
Screens: par speed

Variable Kilovoltage Method

Milliamperage: 100
Cone: to part
Processing: standardized
Kv.P.: 85

For the chart, take a sheet of graph paper. Mark along the left margin the exposure time in seconds. At the bottom of the chart, mark the thicknesses of the patient in centimeters. When the first patient is radiographed, measure the thickness of the lumbar spine in the lateral position, select the exposure time *thought* to be most appropriate to the thickness, and make a dot on the chart at the intersection of the exposure time and thickness. Process the film under standard processing procedure, study the film for detail and contrast with the illuminator which is to be used for interpretation. If the radiograph thus produced is found to be satisfactory, the dot may be checked; if found to be overexposed, the dot may be replaced by a plus sign; if underexposed, by a minus sign.

This procedure should be followed until several entries are made on the chart. Some of these will indicate underexposures and some overexposures, but most of them will show correct exposures along a curved line upward, the exposure increasing with an increase in part thickness.

This method may be employed for special procedures or for any technique when charting exposures in which one factor, either the time or voltage, is varied according to the centimeter thickness of the part being radiographed.

Chapter 11. THE EVOLUTION OF RADIOGRAPHIC TECHNIQUE

The early radiograph lacked density and contrast, in some measure because of the low-power equipment and photographic plates available and in some measure because of the lack of knowledge of x-radiation. Regardless of the length of exposure, some aftertreatment of the radiograph was often necessary to obtain a satisfactory image from the plates (Figure 11.1). It was soon realized that there must be some systematic basis for exposure instead of the "hunch method" of trial and error.

As early as 1898 Rollins stated some of the desirable requirements for the production of a radiograph: "The wavelength depends on the potential [Kv.P.] and degree of exhaustion in the tube; a low potential and vacuum giving waves of such length as to make strong contrast between bones and soft tissue in the human body; a high vacuum and potential giving less contrast because the shorter waves generated passed through the bones. To see through greater thickness and yet have marked contrast, increasing the amperage is recommended, *thus keeping the wavelength unchanged.* If more detail is desired in the bones, we must develop waves of shorter length; and when this is done by increasing the potential, the bones can be made bright because the light is less scattered."

Figure 11.1. Radiograph of the chest made on a glass plate.

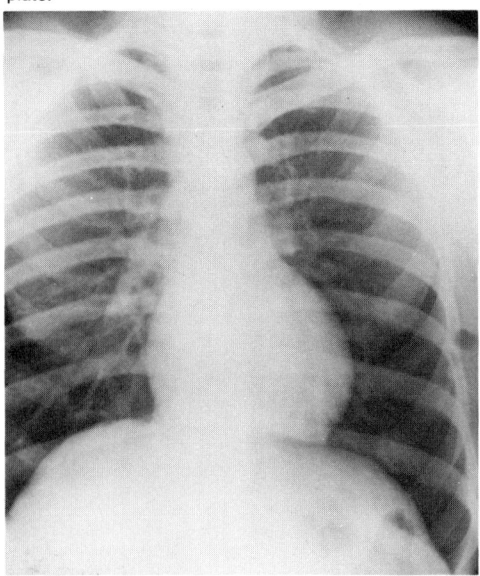

Figure 11.2. Round opening versus square opening

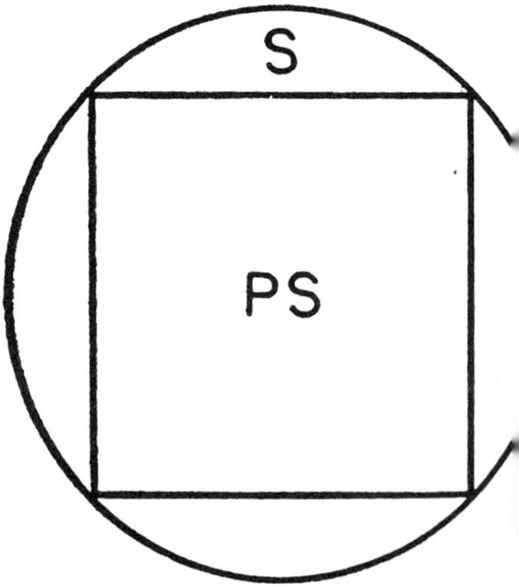

Evolution of Technique

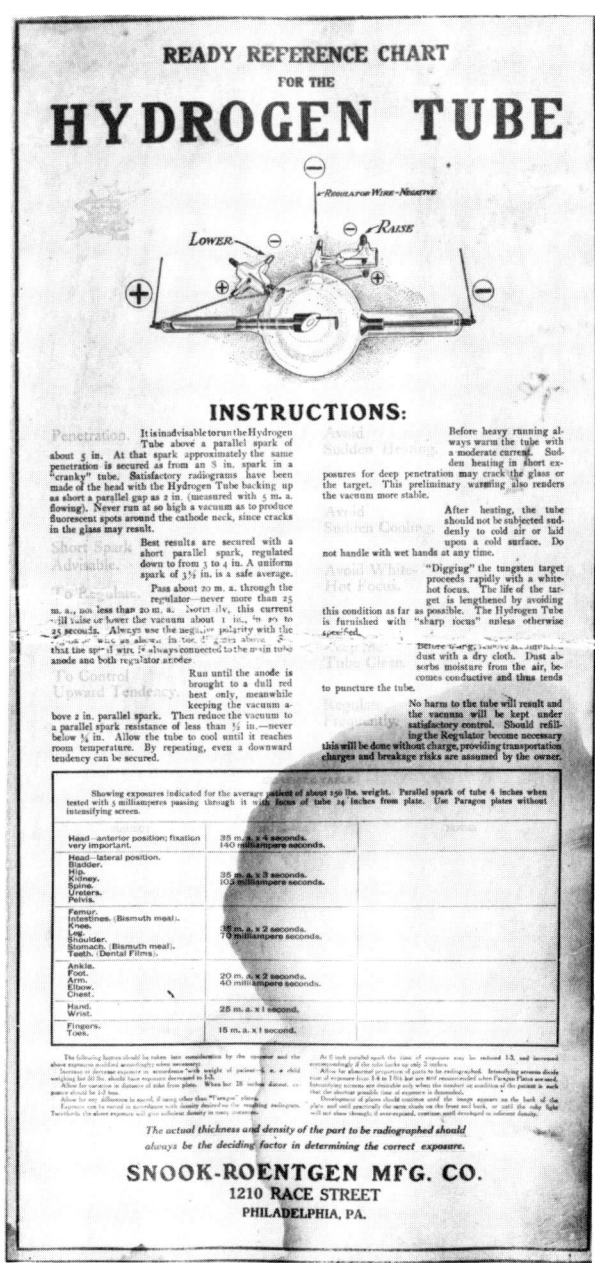

Figure 11.3. An early exposure chart.

Some five years later, in the *Electrical Review* of 4 April 1903, an article on "The Form of the Opening in the Diaphragm Plate of the X-Light Tube Box and a Means of Adjusting the Size of the Beam of X-Light" made the following statement: "The opening in the diaphragm plate of the X-light tube box should be rectangular for diagnostic and photographic work because this is the form of the fluorescent screen and photographic plate. If we use a

FORMULATING X-RAY TECHNIQUES
X-RAY PHYSICS

Part.	Time sec.	Part.	Time sec.
Head, A-P	12	Hip joint	5-7
Head, Lat.	6	Pelvis	5-7
Neck	3	Knee	2
Shoulder	3-1/2	Ankle	1-1/2
Elbow	1-1/2	Lumbar spine	5-6
Wrist	1	Teeth (slow film)	4
Kidney	3-5	Teeth (fast film)	1-1/2
Bladder	3-5	Chest (at 28")	2-1/2-4

Note: For parts above average thickness, increases time considerably more than in proportion to increase of thickness.

Note: All exposures on 5" gap, 40 M.A. 20" distance except chest which is at 28".

Figure 11.4. Technique table based on Shearer's formula (1917).

round opening, the section of the cone of X-light escaping from the tube box is a circle (Figure 11.2). It is evident that the only part of the illumination which will be useful will be that included in the rectangular area of the largest plate or screen. All the X-light [radiation] which strikes the patient outside the rectangular area is objectionable, for it is unwise to expose a patient unnecessarily; besides, the excessive illumination fogs the plate."

By 1905, x-ray plate and equipment manufacturers were supplying exposure charts for use with their manufactured products (Figure 11.3). The trend to a more standardized exposure system began to show promise. In 1916 Professor John S. Shearer of Cornell University published a formula that provided a reasonably accurate means for compensating variations in factor change for a limited voltage range by changing any one of the four exposure factors. His formula, known as the photographic effect, was stated thus:

$$\text{Photographic effect} = \frac{\text{Ma.} \times \text{Kv.P.}^2 \times \text{time}}{\text{distance}^2}$$

Professor Shearer's formula led to the publication of a technique table (Figure 11.4) that was successfully employed with military units during World War I (1917–18). All factors except time were established as constants.

In 1925 Jerman advocated keeping the kilovoltage constant and varying the time of exposure, using as a basis a 150-pound normal person. In other charts which followed his 1925 publications (1926–27), he recommended varying the kilovoltage according to the centimeter thickness of the part (now known as the variable kilovoltage technique). The choice of technique depended upon what type of tube was used, a universal broad-focus Coolidge

RADIOGRAPHIC TECHNIQUE CHART

COMPUTED FOR USE WITH SUPER-SPEED DUPLITIZED FILMS

AVERAGE PATIENT 150 LBS. - - - - - - - - - - USE 1/4 MORE TIME PER 25 POUND INCREASE
SIZE OF FILM - - - - - - - - - - - - - - - - - USE SMALLEST SIZE FOR AREA DESIRED
SIZE OF CONE - - - - - - - - - - - - - - - USE SIZE APERTURE TO INCLUDE AREA DESIRED
INTENSIFYING SCREENS - - - USE SCREENS WHEN A SHORT EXPOSURE TIME IS ADVANTAGEOUS
POTTER-BUCKY DIAPHRAGM - - - USE FOR EXPOSURE OF HEAVY PARTS TO INCREASE DETAIL

PART	VIEW	PEAK KILOVOLTS	EQUIVALENT POINT GAP	M. A.	FOCAL DISTANCE	SECONDS EXPOSURE TIME: WITHOUT SCREENS AVERAGE	WITHOUT SCREENS CORRECTED	WITH DOUBLE SCREENS AVERAGE	WITH DOUBLE SCREENS CORRECTED	BUCKY DOUBLE SCREENS AVERAGE	BUCKY DOUBLE SCREENS CORRECTED
ANKLE	LATERAL	70	4″	10	25″	3		⅜			
ANKLE	A. P.	70	4″	10	25″	4		½			
CHEST	P. A.	80	4⅞″	30	30″	1¾		¼			
COCCYX	A. P.	80	4⅞″	20	25″	12		1½		4-6	
COLON	P. A.	80	4⅞″	30	25″	7		1		3	
ELBOW		70	4″	10	25″	6½		¾			
FERMUR	LAT. OR A. P.	80	4⅞″	20	25″	6		¾			
FIBULA AND TIBIA	LAT. OR A. P.	70	4″	10	25″	5¼		⅝			
FINGERS		50	2¾″	10	25″	2½					
FOOT		70	4″	10	25″	4		½			
GALL BLADDER	P. A.	80	4⅞″	30	25″			1¼		3¾	
HAND		70	4″	10	25″	3					
HEAD	P.A. OR A. P.	80	4⅞″	20	25″	15		2		6-8	
HEAD	LATERAL	80	4⅞″	20	25″	7¾		1		3-4	
HEART	P. A.	90	5¾″	30	7 FEET			3			
HIP	A. P.	80	4⅞″	20	25″	12		1½		4-6	
INTESTINES	P. A.	80	4⅞″	30	25″			1		3	
KIDNEY	A. P.	80	4⅞″	30	25″			1¼		3¾	
KNEE	LAT. OR P. A.	80	4⅞″	10	25″	5¼		⅝		2	
PELVIS	A. P.	80	4⅞″	20	25″	12		1½		4-6	
SHOULDER	A. P. OR P. A.	80	4⅞″	10	25″	6¼		¾		2¼	
SPINE											
CERVICAL	A. P.	80	4⅞″	20	25″	4		½		1½	
CERVICAL	LATERAL	80	4⅞″	20	25″	4		½		1½	
DORSAL	A. P.	80	4⅞″	20	25″	6½		¾		2½	
DORSAL	LATERAL	80	4⅞″	20	25″	8½		1¼		3¾	
LUMBAR	A. P.	80	4⅞″	20	25″	12		1½		4-6	
LUMBAR	LATERAL	90	5¾″	20	25″	24		4		15-24	
STOMACH	P. A.	80	4⅞″	30	25″			1		3	
TEETH		70	4″	10	15″	1½-3					
TIBIA AND FIBULA	LAT. OR A. P.	70	4″	10	25″	5¼		⅝			
TOES		50	2¾″	10	25″	2¼					
WRIST		70	4″	10	25″	3¼					

RAPID TECHNIQUES

CHESTS

FOCAL FILM DISTANCE 40 INCHES DOUBLE INTENSIFYING SCREENS

INCHES DEPTH OF CHEST	VIEW	PEAK KILOVOLTS	EQUIVALENT POINT GAP	M. A.	FOCAL DISTANCE	EXPOSURE TIME
6	P. A.	60	3⅜	80	40″	[illegible] SEC.
7	P. A.	70	4	80	40″	[illegible] SEC.
8	P. A.	80	4⅞	80	40″	[illegible] SEC.
9	P. A.	90	5¾	80	40″	[illegible] SEC.
10	P. A.	100	6⅝	80	40″	[illegible] SEC.
11	P. A.	110	7½	80	40″	[illegible] SEC.

NOTE

THE KELEKET OVERLOAD RELAY AND CIRCUIT BREAKER MAY BE USED FOR THE [illegible] SEC. TECHNIQUE. (USE RELAY SET AT EASIEST TRIPPING POINT.)

STOMACHS

FOCAL FILM DISTANCE 25 INCHES DOUBLE INTENSIFYING SCREENS

USE SAME TECHNIQUE PER DEPTH AS INDICATED FOR CHESTS CHANGING EXPOSURE TIME TO ¼ SECOND

THE KELLEY-KOETT MFG. CO., INC.
COVINGTON, KENTUCKY, U. S. A.

Figure 11.5. The Keleket technique chart.

tube or a 5–10 radiator-type Coolidge tube. Apropos of Jerman's work, his contemporaries believed that his charts were based primarily on Shearer's photographic effect formula.

Prior to 1926 x-ray technique was more or less on a trial-and-error basis until a technique satisfactory to the radiologist was formulated. The use of the Potter-Bucky diaphragm or grid was just beginning, and most radiography was done without grids. In 1928, the Keleket X-Ray Company published a "new" type of technique chart (Figure 11.5). Early in the 1930's the General Electric X-Ray Company published a conversion chart to be used in maintaining radiographic density by altering either the milliampere seconds, kilovoltage, or focus-film distance, whichever was preferred (Figure 11.6).

FORMULATING X-RAY TECHNIQUES

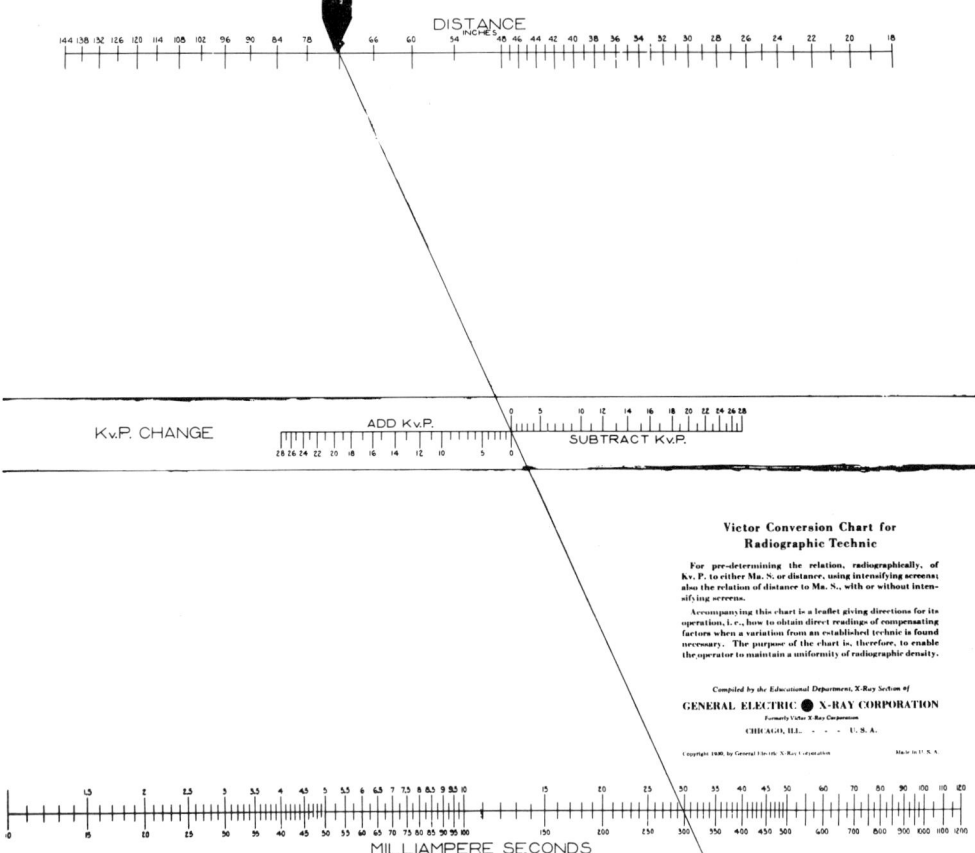

Figure 11.6. General Electric conversion chart.

During the 1930's Keleket's technical expert W. W. Mowry did much to bring about a practical approach to radiographic technique when he published reliable though elaborate tables of exposure based on the thickness of the various body parts. He designed a machine called a Techron with autotransformer steps of approximately 2 Kv.P. He called these steps *techrons*. He next incorporated into the apparatus a selection panel of different fields to be examined—i.e., gallbladder, lumbar spine, dorsal spine, skull, extremities, and so on. In use, the anatomical field to be examined was measured in centimeters, and 2 Kv.P. was added per centimeter of thickness to the numerical value of 27, known as the base Kv.P.

In 1931 Glen W. Files of the General Electric X-Ray Company established various tables of exposure using low kilovoltage and high milliampere-second values for adults of average build, with variations for large and small patients. For infants he recommended using one-fourth the exposure time and for children one-half the exposure time.

In 1933 Dr. Darmon Rhinehart pursued the concept of adequate collimation: "It is not a good practice to use a beam of Röntgen rays that is much larger than the size of the film area being exposed." Dr. Rhinehart kept an

Evolution of Technique

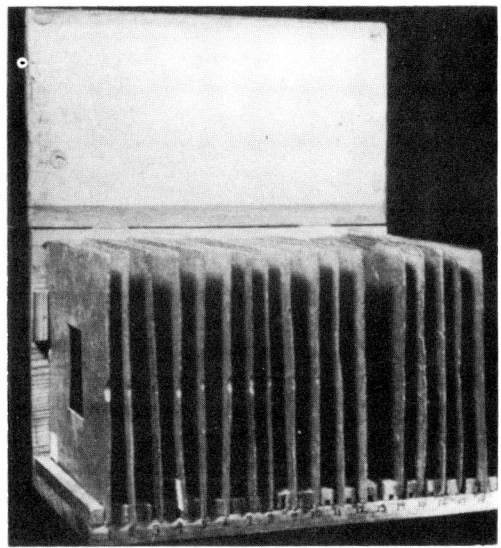

Figure 11.7. Rhinehart's square lead diaphragms.

assortment of *square* lead diaphragms in each radiographic room (Figure 11.7). A more modern version of Professor Shearer's original formula for technique was published by Fuchs and used extensively with military units during World War II in 1942–45 (Figure 11.8).

In 1945 the development of the collimator and the Videx cone took the guesswork out of localizing and centering the part to the film. Scattered radiation was controlled, producing better radiographic contrast; and there was a reduction of radiation to the patient. The collimator *exactly* outlined the body area to be exposed *before* the exposure was made.

In 1950 Dr. L. R. Sante used the formula of 2 times the thickness of the part, measured in centimeters, plus the numerical value of 25, for his base kilovoltage. His book and technique guides were a great asset to technologist and radiologist alike.

Bierman and Boldingh in 1950 proved that kilovolt potential and milliampere seconds could be related by the expression

$$\text{Exposure} = \text{Ma.S.} \times \text{Kv.P.}^5$$

A method of putting this formula to use was published by van Dijk. In 1955 Wynroe published the rule: To reduce the milliampere seconds by one-half, add 15 per cent more kilovolts at any level of kilovoltage.

In late 1955 Fuchs published two tables (non-Bucky and Bucky) for use in approximating densities with milliampere seconds when using the fixed or optimum kilovoltage (which he originated) for any given part. These tables were based largely on empirical values. They were later refined (1959) to include more reliable absorption data, and the values were adjusted to assimilate the results of more extensive experiments. These data were used in the construction of a circular slide rule, the Kodak Kv.P.–Ma.S. Computer, March 1959 (Figure 11.9).

During 1958–59 Cahoon and then Warren independently published a per

FORMULATING X-RAY TECHNIQUES

TECHNIC FOR SELF-RECTIFIED APPARATUS

REGION		AVERAGE THICKNESS (ADULT) CMS.			BASIC MA.S.	OPTIMUM KV.P.	DIST-ANCE
		AP	PA	LAT.			
THUMB - FINGER		1.5 - 4			45 F	50	
HAND		3 - 5					
			7-10		120 F		
WRIST				5-8			
		3 - 6			45 F		
FOREARM		6 - 9			75 F	60	30″
			7-10		105 F		
ELBOW		6-9			120 F		
			7-10				
ARM		7-10			5 S		
			7-10		3.75 S		
SHOULDER CLAVICLE		12-16			15 S		
			13-17				
FOOT		6 - 9			52.5 F		
				6-9			
ANKLE				6-9	90 F	65	
		7-10			105 F		
LEG		9-12			5 S	60	
				8-11	3.75 S		
KNEE		10 - 14			5 S	65	
				9-13	3.75 S		
THIGH		14-17			30 SG	75	
				13-16	22.5 SG		
HIP		17-21			60 SG		
CERVICAL VERTEBRAE	C1-7			10-13	15 S	85	60″
	C1-3	12-15			60 SG	65	
	C4-7	11-14			45 SG		
THORACIC VERTEBRAE		20-24				75	
				28-32	60 SG		
LUMBAR VERTEBRAE				27-32	150 SG	85	
		18-22					
PELVIS		20-23			90 SG	70	
GALL - BLADDER			20-24				30″
G-I. TRACT		18-22			25 SG		
			18-21		30 SG		
				13-17	15 SG	85	
SKULL		16-23			37.5 SG		
PARS PETROSA (STENVERS)				INF.-SUP. 20-25	75 SG		
				POST. LAT. 15-19	22.5 S	70	
SINUSES	ALL			13-17	12 S	65	
	FRONT.	18-21			22.5 S		
	MAX.	18-22			45 S	75	30″
FACIAL BONES		18-22			30 S		
MANDIBLE			9-12		7.5 S		
Mastoid, Temp-Mand. Jt.			14-17		15 S	70	
CHEST	SMALL		- 19		1.875 S		
	AVERAGE		20-25		3.75 S		
	LARGE		26-29		7.5 S	80	
	HUGE		30 -		15 S		60″
		20-25			7.5 S		
			OBL.	27-32	30 S	85	
				24-30	18 S		

Figure 11.8. The Fuchs technique of 1942.

cent factor for reduction of exposure from the adult technique chart for infants and children.

An interesting contribution to x-ray technique was made in 1959 by Dr. W. W. Wasson. His work correlated the physiologic characteristics of body parts with motion and the use of short exposure to secure greater image sharp-

Evolution of Technique

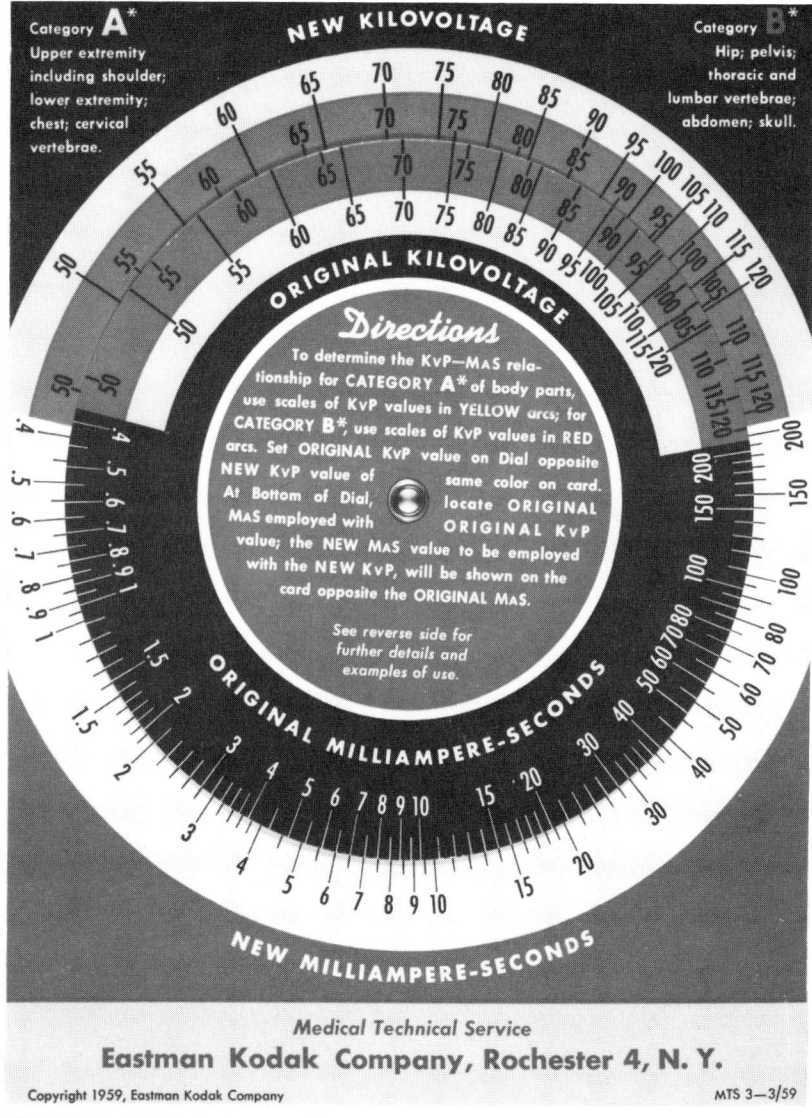

Figure 11.9. Kodak circular computer.

ness. Often during fluoroscopy of the chest Dr. Wasson noted the movements of the heart and great vessels. He saw that motions were transmitted to the bronchi and arteries and that they moved along a certain path according to the systole and diastole of the heart. With a pair of calipers he measured this path and calculated the distance that an artery and bronchus would move during systole and diastole. On the basis of the heart rate, he was then able to calculate *what the speed of exposure should be in order to stop motion.* He concluded that an x-ray exposure of the chest should be no longer than $1/10$ second. Not satisfied with $1/10$-second exposures, he attempted to reduce the exposure to $1/20$ second by modifying the construction of the timer. Dr.

FORMULATING X-RAY TECHNIQUES

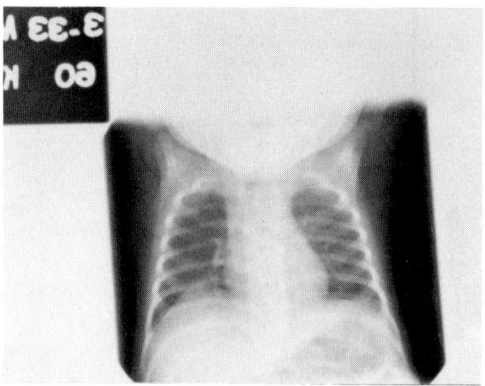

Figure 11.10. Chest of a premature infant.

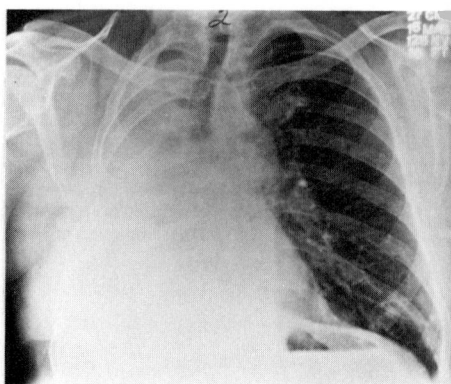

Figure 11.11. Air-gap chest radiograph at 125 Kv.P.

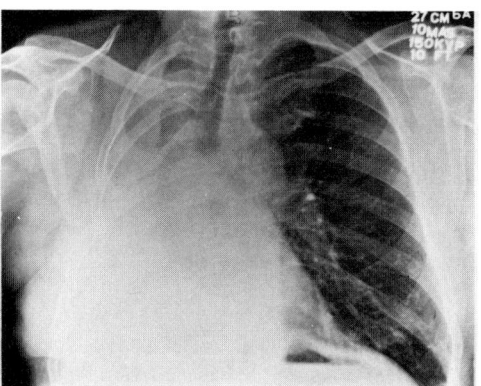

Figure 11.12. Air-gap chest radiography at 150 Kv.P.

Wasson also saw the need for sharper images which could only be obtained by the use of a fine-focus tube.

In July 1959 Mahoney made available through the Picker X-Ray Company a slide rule for Kv.P.–Ma.S. compensations. Prior to Mahoney's slide rule there had been a similar technique, described first by Hodges and later by Reed. Since that time, many slide rules for technique conversions have been placed on the market in this country, as well as in others. In 1960 Schwarz published a system for Kv.P.–Ma.S. relationships and in 1961 the Unit System of radiographic exposure technique. In 1971 the General Electric X-Ray Company published a reliable per cent factor for reduction of exposure to children and infants when using the *variable* or *fixed kilovoltage* system of exposure.

In the author's opinion, it is not possible to construct a technique chart that is precisely workable on all types and makes of apparatus, for by design they have varying degrees of efficiency. The standardization of exposure factors is predicated upon the use of apparatus that is adequately calibrated. There is no technique chart that will work precisely in every installation. There are and always will be slight variations in exposure due to screen speed, line voltage variations, and inherent machine characteristics. However, if the kilovoltages are optimum for the part, there is sufficient exposure

Evolution of Technique

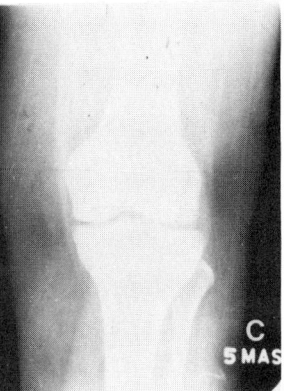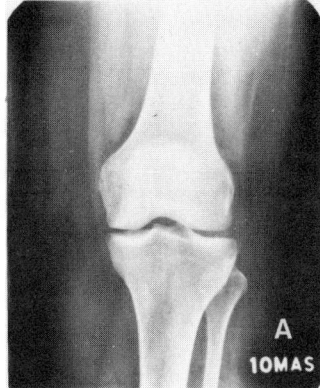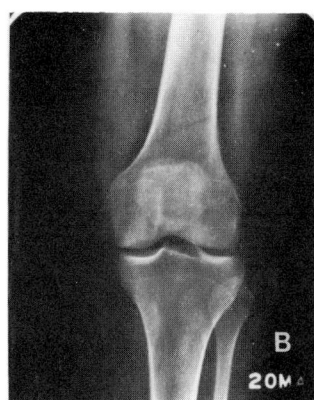

Figure 11.13. Test radiographs.

latitude to compensate for these variations. Small adjustments in milliampere-second values are to be expected.

MODERN SYSTEMS OF EXPOSURE TECHNIQUE

There are today two basic systems of radiographic exposure technique — fixed Kv.P. (Chapter 12) and variable Kv.P. (Chapter 10). The fixed kilovoltage system of technique, developed by the late Arthur W. Fuchs, employs a fixed or optimum kilovoltage for a given anatomical part. The kilovoltage selected is based upon the penetrating quality of the radiation for the average adult tissue thickness of a given part and the scale of radiographic contrast desired. All other factors are constants except the exposure time (milliampere-second factor). Ma.S. is the variable used to compensate for part thickness. If the part is smaller than normal, *one-half of a standard Ma.S. is used.* If the part is thicker than normal, twice the standard Ma.S. is used. However, refinements in the relationship between milliampere seconds and thickness should also be made for best results, especially in radiography of the thicker parts. Since the technique employs a fixed kilovoltage, the radiographic contrast remains substantially constant from one radiograph to the next. Milliampere-second compensations are made for pathological or physiological conditions that influence the x-ray-absorption characteristics of the tissues.

Contrary to some opinion, not all chest radiography need be done at 80 Kv.P. For example, in chest radiographs of premature infants made at Duke University Medical Center, a fixed kilovoltage of 60 was found to be satisfactory for this class of patients. The exposure factors were 200 Ma., $\frac{1}{60}$ second, 60 Kv.P., 40-inch focus-film distance, par-speed screens, the average thickness range 7 to 10 cm. (Figure 11.10). If a 72-inch focus-film distance should be desired, the Kv.P. or Ma.S. is adjusted. Kilovoltages of 100 and above may profitably be employed in chest radiography using stationary grids. Air-gap chest radiography at 125 to 150 Kv.P. can be successfully employed without a grid (Figures 11.11 and 11.12).

Thickness ranges with corresponding kilovoltages and starting milliampere-second values have been established and published by Fuchs for

FORMULATING X-RAY TECHNIQUES

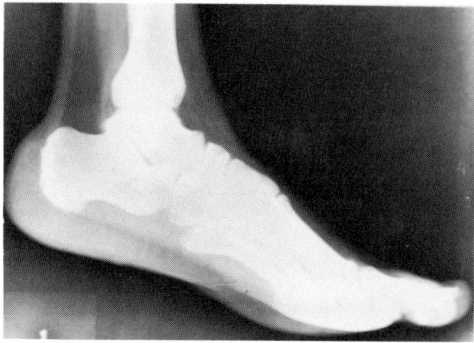

Figure 11.14. Ankle and foot in lateral projection, as example.

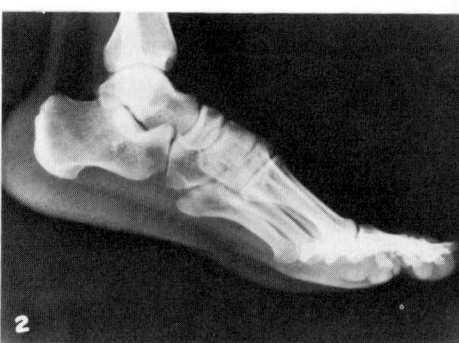

Figure 11.15. Improved version of view of Figure 11.14.

a number of parts when using the fixed kilovoltage system of exposure. To determine the milliampere-second value for a given projection, a series of three test radiographs is made. The first radiograph is made with the kilovoltage listed as optimum for the part and with a milliampere-second value *estimated* to be correct. This value of milliampere-seconds may be designated as X (Figure 11.13A). A second radiograph is made with a milliampere-second value that is twice that used for the first radiograph. This would be classified as 2X (Figure 11.13B). Then a third radiograph is made with one-

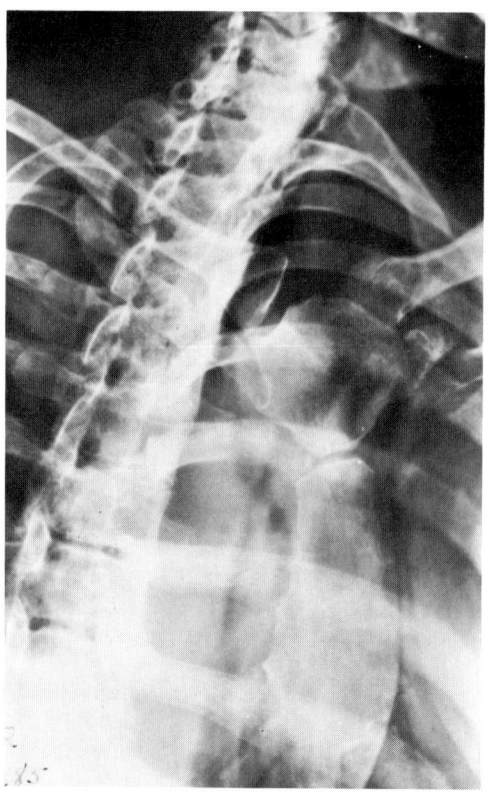

Figure 11.16. Sternum with low-voltage technique.

Evolution of Technique

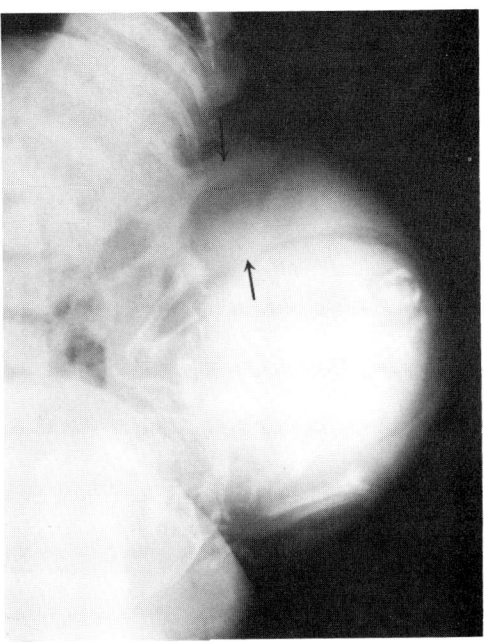

Figure 11.17. Radiograph of placenta.

half the original milliampere-seconds or $\frac{1}{2}$X (Figure 11.13C). All other factors should be constant. The three radiographs are viewed, and the appropriate density or Ma.S. for the part is then chosen.

In 1960 Cahoon developed a fixed kilovoltage technique for children and infants, as well as special procedure techniques.

The Variable Kilovoltage Exposure System requires that the focus-film distance remain constant; but the *kilovoltage* and *milliampere seconds* are varied to compensate both for thickness and for density of the part. This method has the *disadvantage* that the radiograph of any given part will vary in *contrast*, since the thinner structures will require a lower kilovoltage and the thicker structures will require a higher kilovoltage.

A complicated modification of the Variable Kilovoltage System was used by Fletcher and later by Lynch. This system required various classifications for small, medium, large, muscular, obese, and racial characteristics of the patient. Each required a different milliampere-second ratio.

To formulate a technique for variations in kilovoltage per centimeter of part thickness, a group of body parts of similar thickness is usually selected. For convenience, let us consider the ankle and foot in the lateral projection. The part is measured in centimeters. This value is multiplied by 2, and the numerical value 30 is added to the product. In this instance the part measured 7 cm., which gives a base kilovoltage of 44. Other factors are a 36-inch distance, 100 Ma. $\frac{1}{20}$ second (= 5 Ma.S.), and medium-speed screens (Figure 11.14).

Upon inspection of the finished radiograph, it is noted that the image has insufficient density and contrast. Using Ma.S. to control density, a second film is then exposed with the same factors but with twice the Ma.S., i.e, 10 Ma.S. The density and contrast are now satisfactory, so we have a technique for the extremities (Figure 11.15) based on a kilovoltage of 30 plus 2 for each centimeter of thickness, and employing an Ma.S. factor of 10.

At times, a special low-voltage technique must be worked out by trial and error. Let us suppose that in a P.A. oblique projection of the sternum we choose a short focus-film distance to utilize magnification. The film will be exposed at a 30-inch focus-film distance, 60 Kv.P., 50 Ma.S., using an 8-to-1 grid and medium- or par-speed screens. For this, 10 Ma. at 5 seconds was used to take advantage of a slow-breathing technique to eliminate lung shadows and low kilovoltage and bring out the thin density level of the sternum (Figure 11.16).

Other special cases, such as placenta radiography, lend themselves to short-scale or low-voltage high-contrast technique. Cahoon and Reeves stated in 1952: "Since publication of our 1948 paper, we have experimented extensively with the higher kilovoltages and employment of the anode-heel effect in an effort to eliminate the use of opaque plastic filters and low kilovoltage in order to reduce patient dosage in placenta radiography. Although there is no doubt that results obtained with this technique are superior to many of those published, our conclusions based on 100 comparison tests were that the radiographs made with low voltage, high milliampere-seconds and an opaque plastic filter possessed the best contrast and were superior from the standpoint of overall rendition of detail through the uterine area" (Figure 11.17). This procedure has now given way to Nuclear Medicine and Echogram techniques.

HIGHER KILOVOLTAGE RADIOGRAPHY

The only limit to the kilovoltage that can be used in radiography is that imposed by contrast. The limiting kilovoltage is the one in which contrast has been reduced to the point that density differentiation or diagnosis becomes doubtful. All who have investigated the use of higher kilovoltages for radiography realize its contrast limitation.

The immediate acceptance of any technical procedure that alters to a marked degree the appearance of the radiograph is not to be expected. Everyone recognizes the need for maximum contrast in some types of work, but there are examinations in which the increased penetration and increased exposure latitude are desirable and necessary. In Figure 11.18, the lateral radiograph of the skull at 70 Kv.P. shows pathology in the occipital region. Figure 11.19 is the same skull at 60 Kv.P., and Figure 11.20 at 100 Kv.P. Note the changes in contrast and detail in the visualization of the pathological and anatomical structures. Generally, few advocate the use of higher kilovoltages (100 Kv.P. and above) for *all* examinations; but the higher kilovoltages have been widely accepted in studies of the gastrointestinal tract and colon, the lateral view of the lumbosacral spine of obese patients, and pregnancy studies, and in various pathological studies. Langfeldt routinely uses 90 to 105 Kv.P. for demonstration of the auditory ossicles. The use of the higher kilovoltages is indicated because of better penetration of dense structures of the petrous bone and fluid, reduced exposure to the patient, and increased exposure latitude.

Although not generally a routine procedure, air-gap chest radiography may be performed with a 10-foot focus-film distance and a 6-inch object-film

Evolution of Technique

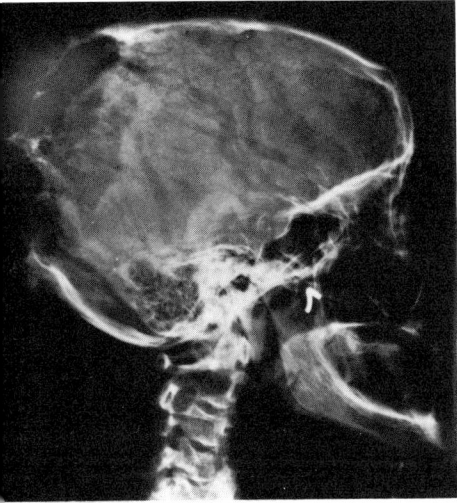

ure 11.18. Radiograph of lateral skull, with hology, at 70 Kv.P.

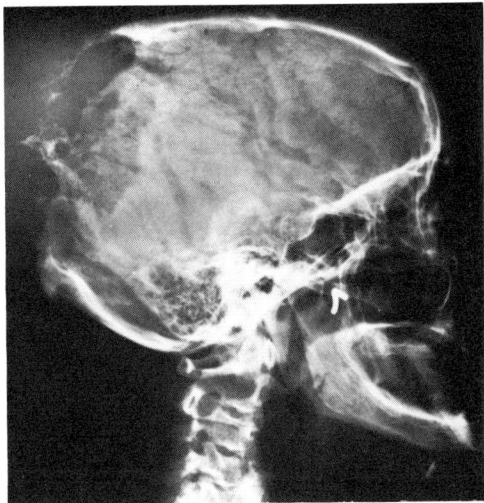

Figure 11.19. The skull of Figure 11.18, at 60 Kv.P.

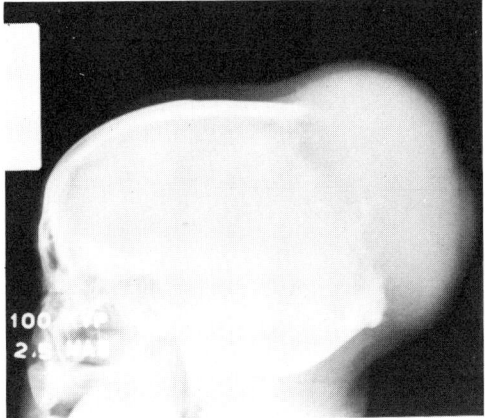

Figure 11.20. The skull of Figure 11.18, at 100 Kv.P.

distance, with 125–150 Kv.P. and without a grid (see Figure 11.11 and 11.12). A comparison of a 27-cm. chest at 80 and 125 Kv.P. is shown in Figure 11.21.

Some radiologists routinely use 150 Kv.P. for chest radiography with a 7-to-1-ratio grid. It is interesting to note that in some of the Scandinavian countries the kilovoltages have been increased to 150 Kv.P.; and the radiographic quality, according to Samuel, equals that of work done at a lower range. He has also developed exposure tables based on the circumference of the patient's chest.

We have found over a period of twenty years that the fixed kilovoltage technique is more economical in time and in the use of materials and apparatus. There is much less physical and mental strain on the part of technical personnel. Its simplicity of operation and consistency in quality of results have served to promote greater technical accuracy. It can be easily

FORMULATING X-RAY TECHNIQUES

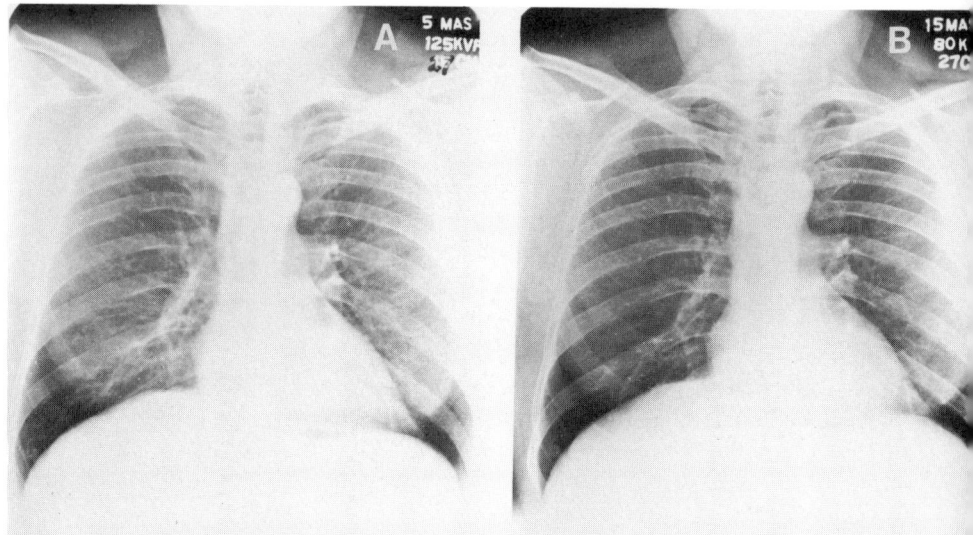

Figure 11.21. Air-gap chest radiography: A, at 125 Kv.P.; B, at 80 Kv.P.

taught, for it involves the application of only the basic radiographic exposure principles.

Radiography in the supervoltage range is of interest in selected cases because of the possibility of visualizing lesions obscured by bone, especially in the chest. Tuddenham and his associates have experimented with million-volt x-ray equipment for diagnostic purposes.

In our investigation as well as in that of others, radiographs made with the higher kilovoltages are satisfactory when the exposure factors have been correctly balanced. It is perfectly possible to produce good-quality, fog-free radiographs of the thicker parts with a higher kilovoltage. Good-quality radiographs employing different kilovoltages can be made as long as there are suitable compensations in milliampere seconds. However, the higher kilovoltages should be avoided in radiography of thin parts, e.g., the hand, or when using iodinated contrast material.

SECONDARY RADIATION

Secondary radiation is probably the greatest single hindrance to good quality in radiography. The intensity of secondary radiation is dependent on the density of the subject, the total volume of tissue irradiated, and the kilovoltage. As is well known, the most effective method of eliminating the greater part of secondary radiation is the use of *cones, collimation, grids,* or *air-gap techniques* (Chapter 4).

Absorption of secondary radiation by a grid naturally requires that additional primary radiation be used to obtain a satisfactory image. This is accomplished by raising the *kilovoltage.* For the same heat load on the focal spot, higher kilovoltage makes more useful radiation available to the film; and the radiation dosage received by the patient may be considerably lessened.

Evolution of Technique

In routine radiography, an 8-to-1-ratio grid is quite satisfactory. The higher-ratio grid absorbs appreciably more primary radiation than the 8-to-1-ratio grid. Actually, the small gain in subject contrast to be made by using a higher-ratio grid technique may not be worthwhile because of the increased exposure required to make up for the higher absorption of the grid. The higher-ratio grid should be used only when it offers a significant advantage by increase in the subject contrast, as in gastrointestinal radiography, where the use of a 12-to-1 grid has now become popular since it offers good cleanup and provides reasonable contrast latitude.

COMMON EXPOSURE SYSTEMS

Phototiming

With the exception of fluoroscopic spot-filming devices, phototiming has not generally been accepted for routine radiography. Whether this neglect is due to film speed versus photo-reaction time, cost, deficiencies in equipment, or lack of proper utilization is not known. However, the potential of phototiming, adapted to computerized techniques, indicates a future trend in this direction.

A computer-programing special-procedures unit employing vacuum cassettes has been developed, utilizing a film changer similar to the Schönander, but without the problems of variable loading to improve film sequence. Film sequence is controlled by a pre-punched IBM card inserted into a small computer. Each examination has its own sequence punched into the card. If two separate series of films need to be done on the same examination, two separate rows are punched on the card, and the computer does the rest. By employing vacuum cassettes, detail is extremely good. At the present, with serial-type radiography, the technical aspects can be synchronized: controlling the exposure, triggering the injection of contrast media, and bringing into play whatever auxiliary techniques may be desired—videotaping, cinefluorography, EKG, and so on.

With computer programing, the punch card can be used over and over again for the titled examination, assuring exact duplication of the procedure every time. With such a technique the chance of misunderstanding or human error is automatically ruled out.

One can foresee moving into the computer-programed type of technique at a rapid pace, and more will be required of the technologist.

Variable kilovoltage technique

With this type of technique the milliampere seconds remain constant and the kilovoltage changes according to the centimeter thickness of the patient. Normally one would expect the technique to increase in increments of 2 Kv.P. per centimeter thickness.

With variable kilovoltage technique the Ma.S. is sometimes typed into classes—A class, 75 Ma.S.; B class, 100 Ma.S.; and C class, 125 Ma.S. Essentially, this classifies the patient as small, medium, or large, using the milliampere-seconds most appropriate and then using the Kv.P. appropriate for the centimeter thickness.

Why are variable low-voltage techniques used today? The function of *contrast* is to enhance the *visibility of detail.* Accordingly, many radiologists

FORMULATING X-RAY TECHNIQUES

with a preference for short-scale contrast limit their technologists to techniques of the 40 and 90 Kv.P. range. In the 1920's and 1930's, low-voltage techniques were used because of equipment limitations and because devices such as 8-to-1 and 12-to-1 grids supplying adequate control of secondary and scattered radiation fog were not available. Radiologists became accustomed to interpreting films that were, *by definition,* of *high contrast.* However, most low-voltage films have areas that are not completely penetrated and thus lack silver deposits. Basically, areas lacking in silver deposits are diagnostically useless; yet because of the *pictorial quality* of low-voltage films, many subjectively feel that they are superior in radiographic quality. It is surprising to see even today that lateral lumbar spines are still radiographed at 75 Kv.P. and 600 Ma.S.

A technologist with enthusiasm and know-how can do remarkably good work with the variable kilovoltage technique, although the radiation exposure is higher than with a fixed or high Kv.P. technique and the contrast scale changes with each part thickness. No matter what radiographic exposure system he chooses, the radiologic technologist must be certain of the calibration of the radiographic equipment, since it becomes impossible to formulate standardized techniques without proper calibration of equipment.

The other problem in any department of radiology is processing. This must be standardized if one is to have consistently good diagnostic and acceptable radiographs, whether it be manual or automatic processing.

Fixed kilovoltage technique

In this technique the kilovoltage is fixed according to the part being radiographed, and the Ma.S. is varied to compensate for patient thickness. While Ma.S. controls density, the kilovoltage is fixed at a level which will penetrate the part irrespective of its size. The fixed kilovoltage system of technique has become popular since the Kv.P. controls or affects many factors—contrast, density, quality of radiation, production of secondary radiation, scattered radiation, and exposure latitudes, to name six of them. All six factors may vary with the variable kilovoltage technique, and so it becomes difficult to maintain a balanced scale of contrast, because when voltages are changed to compensate for part thickness, the contrast scale also changes.

One must bear in mind that the radiologic technologist also has a moral obligation to the patient. The radiation exposure to the patient is more likely to be greater with a variable kilovoltage technique than with a fixed or high kilovoltage technique, since tissue-absorbed dose is related to high Ma.S. values.

High kilovoltage technique

High kilovoltage refers to 100–150 Kv.P. by definition, and in some countries to 100–200 Kv.P. Various institutions in this country have already made use of the high kilovoltage technique in radiography of the chest (employing air-gap technique without grids), lateral lumbosacral spines, barium studies, and obstetrical cases. As more radiologists are influenced by the techniques used in Europe, we can expect greater utilization of the 150-Kv.P. generators now being manufactured in this country. High kilovoltage techniques permit more latitude, shorter times of exposure, sharper deatil, and fewer repeats.

Evolution of Technique

Variable kilovoltage and/or fixed kilovoltage technique charts work quite well if used properly. The *successful* application of *either* technique depends on a thorough understanding of what we have always referred to as the *four prime factors of a radiograph* — density, contrast, detail, and distortion — and the *four prime factors in the production of a radiograph* — kilovoltage, milliamperage, time, and distance.

The part to be radiographed should always be measured with a caliper, all radiographic units should be calibrated, the primary beam should be collimated precisely to the area of interest, and all films must be processed by strict time-temperature and/or rigidly controlled automatic processing.

Although a thorough knowledge of all the foregoing is available, further dividends will accrue if the film illuminators are checked regularly to see that illumination and intensity are matched. After all, one should always take pains to present one's work to the best possible advantage.

RADIATION DOSAGE

There has been much discussion in past years on the subject of exposure to radiation. As recently as 15 November 1972 a panel convened by the National Academy of Sciences concluded that federal standards for exposure to radiation must be tightened up if the United States is to avoid an increase in cancer deaths over the next thirty years. Calling the guidelines for exposure to radiation "unnecessarily high," the Academy panel strongly recommended that the federal government reexamine public exposure to x-rays, nuclear medicines, and other man-made sources of radioactivity. The discussion has occurred not only in scientific journals but also in the lay press, where many radical opinions have been expressed concerning diagnostic radiology.

According to scientific literature, the following facts can be accepted. Radiant energy can produce genetic mutations; the number of mutations increases with the amount of radiation absorbed; most mutations may be considered harmful to the human race.

It should be remembered that x-rays are not the only cause of genetic mutations; cosmic rays, various chemicals, and other things, may be factors.

At Duke University Medical Center, research has been done toward obtaining the radiation skin dosage from diagnostic procedures for the two major methods of technique: the fixed kilovoltage technique and the tissue-measurement or kilovolt-variation-per-centimeter-thickness technique. The results are similar to those of other investigators. See Appendix A.

Regardless of exposure system, Gianturco, Miller, and Neucks state: "Low-dosage techniques require some retraining of the technical staff who must understand the importance of each factor employed. Ultimately, technologists are the key to high-kilovolt, low-milliampere-second, or low-dosage radiography because the greatest reduction of exposure comes from doing the *right thing the first time.*" In many instances the tissue measurement technique gives radiation dosages as much as *three times* that of the optimum or fixed kilovoltage technique.

The proper use of filters markedly reduces the radiation dosage. In many instances the use of a filter will reduce the absorbed x-ray dose and, by reducing the scattered component, produce a better radiograph from the diagnostic standpoint.

FORMULATING X-RAY TECHNIQUES

It is the author's opinion that the lower voltage technique, employing *kilovolt* variation per centimeter, is obsolete. The future trend is toward the use of higher kilovoltage values and a more widespread knowledge regarding the radiographic function of each exposure factor.

A major equipment company for a long time associated with technical education has reversed its policy in the preparation of exposure charts. They now advocate fixed or higher kilovoltage rather than variable kilovoltage techniques.

It is the prerogative of the radiologist to specify the type of radiograph which best suits his requirements, but it is the obligation of the radiologic technologist to have a thorough understanding of exposure principles and the ability to interpret these principles so as to obtain the best diagnostic quality in radiographs.

The term "technologist" means one skilled in a specific field; and in our particular case, it is radiologic technology. Radiologic technologists are skilled in the art and science of radiographic technique and should be able to produce any type or quality radiograph at any given time.

For three-quarters of a century there has been a progressive refinement of radiographic technique to produce satisfactory radiographs and at the same time restrict radiation exposure to the patient. These refinements have led to the development and utilization of fixed or high Kv.P. technique which can substantially reduce radiation to the patient. Promising developments with phototiming and computer-controlled radiographic techniques may allow *ultimate* development of exposure techniques in the future.

Chapter 12. THE FIXED KILOVOLTAGE SYSTEM OF TECHNIQUE

Present-day radiography requires standardization of apparatus and technique in order that all operations performed may entail a minimum of time and yield results of the best quality.

The results of the beginning student in radiography, whether good or poor, are usually unintelligible to him. For that reason he must early become acquainted with the kind of radiograph that is most useful to the radiologist — one that possesses correct diagnostic quality. The student cannot acquire that knowledge except by actually making such radiographs under careful guidance. His familiarity with satisfactory radiographs, based on experience in making them, instills in him a self-confidence that is of immeasurable value in the field of radiography.

To facilitate this training, there is a simple yet exact exposure system — the fixed kilovoltage technique developed by the late Arthur W. Fuchs — which requires little applicatory effort on the part of the student and instructor. Wherever practical, the exposure factors are reduced to constants, thereby eliminating many possible sources of error. This system enables the student to quickly become acquainted with radiographs of better than average quality that are produced in the course of instruction. It precludes floundering about, seeking exposure factors for making a particular radiograph the quality of which he is often incapable of judging in the early stages of training. The fact that the fixed kilovoltage system requires the elimination of nonessentials or variables from the technical procedure accounts for the success of the technique, since it provides a clear-cut method of procedures, assures the technologist of better than average results, and is easily understood and applied by the beginner as well as the experienced radiologic technologist.

The fixed kilovoltage system does not require actual measurement of the body parts. With some experience, the technologist *learns to estimate* the thickness and is able to classify the part as *small, average,* or *large.* Since the average classification predominates, he may successfully place about 90 per cent of all patients in this category. The basic constants of kilovoltage and milliampere seconds are so few in number that they are easily memorized, and for ready reference, the factors may be placed on a small card (see Figure 11.9 in the preceding chapter).

The employment of the fixed kilovoltage technique will consistently produce radiographs of good quality with a minimum of effort. Since the method is standardized, shifting of personnel from one room to another should not interfere with the uniformity of results; each technologist trained in it should produce a radiograph of the same quality and type as his predecessor. The radiographic densities produced by this method are uniform — a point of considerable diagnostic value because any differences from the normal

FORMULATING X-RAY TECHNIQUES

density may be attributed to pathological changes within the tissues. Duplication of results is easy to obtain in follow-up cases.

The tendency in present-day radiography has been to use high milliamperages to perform work which they are not always capable of performing. It must be understood that for a given thickness of a particular body part, the wave lengths of the x-rays employed to penetrate the tissues must be adequate. Since the kilovoltage governs the *wave length* and *penetration,* all that is then necessary to secure a satisfactory image is to have a sufficient number of x-rays reach the film. The milliamperage and time control the *number* of x-rays or *intensity* of radiation, and proper adjustment of these factors will produce adequate exposure of the radiographic film. When the x-ray wave length is correct, a lesser amount of milliampere seconds is usually needed for the exposure that is habitually employed for the same purpose with lower kilovoltages. This is most important where conservation of tube life is necessary, for it is the milliampere seconds that commonly destroy tubes—not kilovoltage. Less milliampere seconds will permit a greater number of radiographs to be made over a given area before the limit of radiation safety is reached.

In determining a fixed kilovoltage system of technique a premise has been established as to the diagnostic acceptability of the image. The image should be as near 100 per cent acceptable as possible. The scale of contrast should be such that all anatomical details are readily visible. This, of course, depends upon the penetration. Each part should be adequately penetrated. Only a minimum of secondary radiation fog should be tolerated. The average density level should be such that the majority of densities are translucent when the standard type of illuminator is used.

HOW THE FIXED KILOVOLTAGES WERE DETERMINED

The determination of fixed kilovoltage for various projections involved quite a bit of preliminary experimentation, with subsequent testing.

1. A series of exposures were made of a particular part employing a given projection. The radiographs were made at various kilovoltages, usually 40 to 100, in 10-Kv.P. steps. At first, a number of values were employed, but later the kilovoltages were narrowed to three of four for trial. The Ma.S. value used with each Kv.P. was adjusted so that the average overall densities of the radiographs were approximately the same. The densities for the same anatomical area were balanced for each radiograph.

When it was determined that a given Kv.P. would be adequate, it was tried on a large number of patients using a single basic Ma.S. value. In some instances the radiographic densities were adjusted to suit the average range of tissue densities. As soon as the radiographs assumed a measure of uniformity, the Kv.P. and basic Ma.S. factors were established as constants.

2. Measurements of tissue for a given projection were carefully made. Calipers were employed and skin-to-skin measurements were made without compression of tissues. When these measurements were obtained, correlation with anthropometric data was secured so that frequency and reliability of the measurements could be assured.

The frequency of measurement to establish the average thickness ranges was established by Fuchs as shown in Table 12.1 below. The kilovoltage was

Fixed Kilovoltage System

established to suit the nature of radiography to be done—whether screen, direct exposure, or screen-grid exposures—and the greater frequencies were then tested radiographically, using the kilovoltage selected as optimum for the projection.

When measurements were encountered that were greater or less than average, some adjustment in the Ma.S. was necessary. However, the kilovoltage was to remain constant. Borderline thickness ranges were established. In some instances, compensation could be made by halving the Ma.S. with those parts measuring less than the average and doubling the Ma.S. for those parts greater than the average. This could usually be done where the per cent frequency was very high, as with the P.A. view of the hand.

As the per cent frequency of thickness became lower, refinements in the thickness divisions had to be made. Considering the basic Ma.S. as x, then the halfway point between it and $2x$ would be $1\frac{1}{2}x$. Also, with x and $\frac{1}{2}x$, the halfway point would be $\frac{3}{4}x$.

For example, if 80 Kv.P. was initially established for the chest projection (P.A.) with a basic Ma.S. of 3.3 at 72 inches using screens, then these factors were used on 82 per cent of all adult patients entering the department

Table 12.1 PROJECTION AND RANGES OF AVERAGE THICKNESS—ADULT

Region		Average thickness adult—cms.			Per cent frequency 1	Kv.P. 2
		A.P.	P.A.	Lat.		
Thumb, Fingers, Toes			1.5–4		99	
Hand		3–5			99	
				7–10	93	50
Wrist		3–6			99	
				5–8	98	
Forearm		6–8			94	
				7–9	92	
Elbow		6–8			96	
				7–9	87	
Arm	(S)	7–10			95	
				7–10	94	60
Shoulder	(S)	12–16			79	
Clavicle	(S)		13–17		82	
Foot			6–8		92	
				7–9	91	

FORMULATING X-RAY TECHNIQUES

Region		Average thickness adult—cms.			Per cent frequency 1	Kv.P. 2
		A.P.	P.A.	Lat.		
Ankle		8–10			86	
				6–9	96	
Leg	(S)	10–12			85	
				9–11	89	65
Knee	(S)	10–13			92	
				9–12	92	
Thigh	(S + PB)	14–17			77	75
				13–16	76	
Hip	(S + PB)	17–21			76	75
Cervical Vertebrae	(S) C1-3	12–14			77	65
	(S) C4-7	11–14			98	
	(S) C1-7			10–13	90	85
Thoracic Vertebrae	(S + PB)	20–24			76	75
				28–32	81	85
Lumbar Vertebrae	(S + PB)	18–22			69	70
				27–32	77	85
Pelvis	(S + PB)	19–23			78	70
Skull	(S + PB)		18–21		96	85
				14–17	88	
Sinuses (S)	Frontal		18–21		97	70
	Maxillary		18-22		88	
				13–17	96	
Mandible	(S)			10–12	82	
Chest	(S)		20–25		82	80
		Obl.		27–32	84	90
		24–30			83	85

(1) Per cent frequency of average thickness in various projections, and (2) required kilovoltages that assume complete penetration. (It is assumed that when needed average-speed screens (S) and 8 to 1 PB diaphragm (PB) are used).

Fixed Kilovoltage System

and measuring 20 to 25 centimeters. Cases measuring 25 to 29 centimeters were exposed with 2x Ma.S.; those measuring 16 to 20 were exposed with $\frac{1}{2}x$ Ma.S. These figures were later revised so that for a 21- to 24-centimeter range, x Ma.S. was used; $1\frac{1}{2}x$ Ma.S. was used for 24 to 27 centimeters; and 2x was used for 27 to 30 centimeters. For the 18 to 21 group, $\frac{3}{4}x$ was used, and $\frac{1}{2}x$ was used for the 16 to 18 group. See the graph for the chest, Figure 12.1. The same procedure was employed for all projections.

Adjustment of the kilovoltage should always be made when a *new* projection is established. Just as soon as new conditions are introduced into a standard projection, then it should be considered a new one and factors should be laid down to satisfy the requirements of that projection.

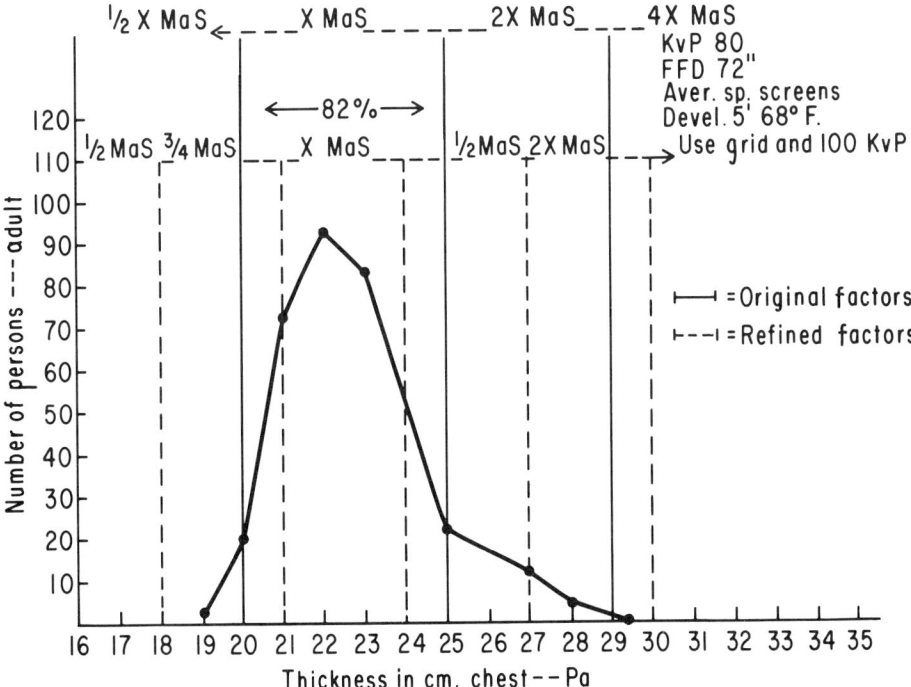

Figure 12.1. Graph for the chest.

It is not possible to construct a technique chart that is precisely workable on all types and makes of apparatus because of varying degrees of calibration efficiency. The best that can be accomplished is a compromise in which all factors but one are reduced to constants. The variable factor employed should have only one function—to influence the amount of silver deposited on the film (radiographic density).

No technique chart is a cure-all or an answer to good radiography. It is only an aid in that direction. Training in positioning, the application of suitable immobilization devices, and cones and grids (when employed), all contribute to the quality of the radiograph. Clinical experience in estimating the relative x-ray absorption characteristics of the patient as altered by disease,

FORMULATING X-RAY TECHNIQUES

trauma, or age also has a decided bearing upon the results. Adjustments for relative absorption can be approximated by using Ma.S. values in the next lower or higher thickness category.

The exposure charts in this chapter, which are designed for use with full-wave rectified equipment, list suggested exposures for various routine projections. It may be found practical to adapt these factors to the routine radiographic work required by your department. It is most important that the appropriate Ma.S. and Kv.P. values, suffixed by the same symbol, be used together. Cones of the correct size must also be employed, as well as standardized processing.

Formulating the fixed-voltage guide

Referring to Table 12.1, we find that the lateral skull will be from 14 to 17 cm. in width and calls for 85 Kv.P.

Let us make a series of four radiographs of the lateral skull with 85 Kv.P. The milliamperage may be any factor we choose. The time factors should be what is thought to be normal, twice normal, one-half normal, and one-fourth normal. Develop the four radiographs and select the one thought to be the most informative. The factors used to produce the desired radiograph will hold true for the skull that is 14, 15, 16, or 17 cm. wide. This procedure is followed for each projection.

Example

Lateral skull   Cone: To area
15 cm.   Kv.P.: 85
Distance: 40 inches   Ma.S.: No. 1–20
Bucky: 8-to-1   No. 2–40
Dev.: automatic   No. 3–10
                                No. 4–5

Suppose radiograph No. 3 is the one selected. Then all lateral skull radiography measuring from 14 to 17 cm. in width will be done at

85 Kv.P.
10 Ma.S.
Below 14 cm. width the Ma.S. value should be reduced by $1/2$
Above 17 cm. width the Ma.S. should be doubled.

The physiologic or disease state of the patient requires some adjustment of the Ma.S. values. When an increase in tissue absorption occurs, a corresponding increase in overall radiographic density is required. Doubling the Ma.S. is often sufficient compensation in the presence of

1. Sclerosis;
2. Fluid or pus;
3. Contrast media.

Conditions which cause a decrease in tissue absorption require a corresponding decrease in radiographic density. Halving the Ma.S. often compensates for

1. Destructive bone disease;
2. Malignant metastases;
3. Malnutrition;

Fixed Kilovoltage System

4. Atrophy;
5. Emphysematous tissue.

EXPOSURE GUIDE: FIXED KILOVOLTAGE TECHNIQUES (Adult)

Projection: Proj.
Centimeters: Cm.
Distance: FFD (Focus-film)
Videx cone: V
Cylinder cone: C
Tube: Rotating anode

Cardboard and regular film: F
Screens: Medium: S
Screens and 8-to-1 grid: SG
Filter: 2 mm. al.
Development: 5 minutes at 68° or automatic
Film: Regular

THE SKULL

Region	Proj.	Cm. Range	FFD	Guide Ma.S.	Ma.	Time	Ma.S.	Kv.P.	Cone and Film
Skull	Lat.	8–12	36"	10 SG				85 SG	V-12 10 x 12
		12–17		15 SG					
		17–22		20 SG					
	P.A.	13–17		15 SG					V-8 8 x 10
		17–21		25 SG					
		21–26		35 SG					
	A.P. 20°	13–17		20 SG					
		17–23		30 SG					
		23–27		40 SG					
	Axial	15–19		40 SG					
		19–25		50 SG					
		25–29		70 SG					
	Towne 35°	13–17		40 SG					C 8 x 10
		17–24		60 SG					
		24–29		75 SG					
	Mastoid Law	9–12		10 SG					
		12–17		15 SG					
		17–20		20 SG					
	Stenvers	14–17	30"	15 SG					
		17–21		25 SG					
		21–25		35 SG					
	Optic P.A.	13–17		15 SG					
		17–21		25 SG					
		21–26		35 SG					

Note: Automatic processing will require some adjustment in exposure factors (Ma.S.).

FORMULATING X-RAY TECHNIQUES

Region	Proj.	Cm. Range	FFD	Guide Ma.S.	Ma.	Time	Ma.S.	Kv.P.	Cone and Film
	Facial Bones P.A.	13–17	36"	15 SG				85 SG	V-8 8 x 10
		17–21		25 SG					
		21–26		35 SG					
Nose	Lat.	1.5–4		70 F 2.5 S				50 F 70 S	C 8 x 10
Mandible	Lat.	6–10		2.5 S				70 S	
		10–14		5 S					
Sinuses	P.A.	10–14	30"	5 SG				85 SG	
		14–17		10 SG					
	Lat.	9–12		2.5 S 2.5 SG				70 S 85 SG	
		12–17		7.5 S 10 SG				70 S 85 SG	
		17–21		10 S 15 SG				70 S 85 SG	
	P.A. Front P.A. Max.	14–17		20 S 15 SG				70 S 85 SG	
		17–21		25 S 25 SG				70 S 85 SG	
		21–25		30 S 30 SG				70 S 85 SG	
	Open Mouth Sphenoid	14–17		20 S 20 SG				70 S 85 SG	
		17–22		30 S 30 SG				70 S 85 SG	
		22–26		40 S 40 SG				70 S 85 SG	

THE CHEST

Region	Proj.	Cm. Range	FFD	Guide Ma.S.	Ma.	Time	Ma.S.	Kv.P.	Cone and Film
Chest	P.A.	14–17	72"	3.33 S				80 S	V-14 14 x 17
		17–20		5 S					
		20–24		6.66 S					
		24–28		10 S					

Fixed Kilovoltage System

Region	Proj.	Cm. Range	FFD	Guide Ma.S.	Ma.	Time	Ma.S.	Kv.P.	Cone and Film
Chest	P.A.	28–31	72″	15 S				80 S	V-14 14 x 17
		31–35		20 S					
	Obl.	15–19		3.33 S				85 S	
		19–23		6.66 S					
		23–29		13.33 S					
		29–34		20 S					
	Lat.	22–26		13.33 S				90 S	
		26–31		15 S					
		31–35		20 S					
	P.A.	19–24		10 SG				100 SG	
		24–28		15 SG					
		28–31		25 SG					
		31–36		40 SG					
	Obl.	19–24		10 SG				100 SG	
		24–29		20 SG					
		29–35		40 SG					
	Lat.	24–27		15 SG				110 SG	
		27–30		20 SG					
		30–35		30 SG					
		35–40		50 SG					

THE SPINE AND PELVIS

Region	Proj.	Cm. Range	FFD	Guide Ma.S.	Ma.	Time	Ma.S.	Kv.P.	Cone and Film
Cervical	Lat. and obl.	6–9	72″	6.5 S				85 S	V-8 8 x 10
		9–13		15 S					
		13–18		20 S					
	Lat. Soft tissue	6–9		3.2 S					
		9–13		5 S					
		13–18		10 S					

FORMULATING X-RAY TECHNIQUES

Region	Proj.	Cm. Range	FFD	Guide Ma.S.	Ma.	Time	Ma.S.	Kv.P.	Cone and Film
Cervical	A.P.	8–11		10 SG				80 SG	V-8 8 x 10
		11–15		15 SG					
		15–20		20 SG					
Thoracic	A.P.	16–19		40 SG				75 SG	V-7 7 x 17 or 11 x 14
		19–24		60 SG					
		24–29		80 SG					
	Lat.**	26–30		50 SG				80 SG	
		30–34		100 SG					
		34–39	36"	150 SG					
Lumbar	A.P.	13–17		60 SG				70 SG	V-11 11 x 14
		17–22		80 SG					
		22–27		100 SG					
	Obl.	15–18		60 SG				75 SG	V-8 8 x 10
		18–22		80 SG					
		22–27		100 SG					
	Lat.	23–26		100 SG				85 SG	V-11 11 x 14
		26–32		200 SG					
		32–37		275 SG					
Pelvis	A.P.	12–15		50 SG				65 SG	V-14 14 x 17
		15–20		80 SG				70 SG	
		20–25		100 SG					
		25–29		125 SG					
Hip	A.P.	14–17		40 SG				80 SG	V-10 8 x 10
		17–21		60 SG					
		21–25	36"	80 SG					
	Lat. (Rotation)	15–19		50 SG					
		19–23		60 SG					
		23–26		80 SG					

**LAT. THORACIC: Patient breathing. Use a low Ma. station and long exposure time. Example: Technique calls for 100 Ma.S. Use 25 Ma. and 4 seconds exposure.

Fixed Kilovoltage System

Region	Proj.	Cm. Range	FFD	Guide Ma.S.	Ma.	Time	Ma.S.	Kv.P.	Cone and Film
Hip	Lat. (True)	17–20	36"	125 SG				80 SG	C 8 x 10
		20–25		150 SG					
		25–30		175 SG					
Abdomen	A.P.	14–19		75 SG				70 SG	V-14 14 x 17
		19–23		100 SG					
		23–26		125 SG					
		26–31		150 SG					
Gallbladder	P.A.	14–17		20 SG				75 SG	V-10 10 x 12
		17–22		30 SG					
		22–25		60 SG					
		25–30		100 SG					

GASTRO-INTESTINAL: COLON AND PELVIMETRY

Region	Proj.	Cm. Range	FFD	Guide Ma.S.	Ma.	Time	Ma.S.	Kv.P.	Cone and Film
Colon	A.P.	15–18	36"	5 SG				100 SG	V-14
		18–21		10 SG					
		21–25		20 SG					
	P.A.	25–29		40 SG					
		29–33		80 SG					
	Chassard Lapine	19–22		50 SG					14 x 17
		22–26		75 SG					
		26–30		100 SG					
G.I.	A.P.	15–20		20 SG				90 SG	V-10
		20–23		40 SG					
	P.A. Oblique	23–26		75 SG					
		26–30		90 SG					10 x 12
		30–34		100 SG					

FORMULATING X-RAY TECHNIQUES

Region	Proj.	Cm. Range	FFD	Guide Ma.S.	Ma.	Time	Ma.S.	Kv.P.	Cone and Film
Esophagus	P.A. Oblique	15–20		10 SG				90 SG	V-11 or V-7 11 x 14 7 x 17
		20–23		20 SG					
		23–26		30 SG					
		26–30		40 SG					
		30–34		50 SG					
Pelvimetry	A.P. Supine	20–23	36"	100 SG				75 SG	V-14 14 x 17
		23–28		150 SG					
		28–33		200 SG					
	Thoms A.P.	24–27		100 SG				100 SG	V-10 10 x 12
		27–32		150 SG					
		32–36		200 SG					
	Lat.	23–26		80 SG					V-14 14 x 17
		26–32		100 SG					
		32–25		150 SG					

THE EXTREMITIES

Region	Proj.	Cm. Range	FFD	Guide Ma.S.	Ma.	Time	Ma.S.	Kv.P.	Cone and Film
Hand Wrist	P.A.	–2		50 F				50 F 60 S	V-8 8 x 10
		3–5		70 F 1.66 S					
		5–8		90 F 2.5 S					
	Lat.	7–10		120 F 5 S					
		10–14		150 F 7.5 S					
Forearm	A.P. P.A. Lat.	3–6	36"	60 F 2.5 S				60 F 60 S	V-11 11 x 14
		6–10		70 F 2.5 S					
		11–14		80 F 4.16 S					

Fixed Kilovoltage System

Region	Proj.	Cm. Range	FFD	Guide Ma.S.	Ma.	Time	Ma.S.	Kv.P.	Cone and Film
Elbow	A.P. Lat.	3–6		60 F 1.66 S				60 F	V-8
		6–10		100 F 2.5 S				60 S	8 x 10
		10–14		120 F .5 S					
Shoulder Upper ⅓ Humerus	A.P. Lat.	8–12		7.5 SG				80 SG	V-8
		12–16		12.5 SG					
		16–20		15 SG					8 x 10
		20–24		20 SG					
Foot	A.P. and Obl.	3–6	36"	60 F 1.66 S				60 F	V-10
		6–10		70 F 2.5 S				60 S	
		10–14		80 F 3.5 S					
	Lat.	3–6		80 F 3.33 S					10 x 12
		6–10		100 F 5 S					
		10–14		120 F 7.5 S					
Os calcis	Axial	5–8		75 F				80 F	C
		8–13		100 F					8 x 10
		13–17		125 F					
Tibia Fibula	A.P.	6–8		5 SG				80 SG	V-7
		8–12		10 SG					
		12–15		15 SG					
	Lat.	5–7		2.5 SG					7 x 17
		7–11		3.2 SG					
		11–15		5 SG					
Knee	A.P.	7–9		5 SG					V-8
		9–14		6.5 SG					8 x 10
		14–17		10 SG					

FORMULATING X-RAY TECHNIQUES

Region	Proj.	Cm. Range	FFD	Guide Ma.S.	Ma.	Time	Ma.S.	Kv.P.	Cone and Film
Knee	Lat.	6–8	36"	5 SG				80 SG	V-8 8 x 10
		8–13		6.5 SG					
		13–15		7.5 SG					

THE EXTREMITIES

Screen exposure only

Region	Proj.	Cm. Range	FFD	Guide Ma.S.	Ma.	Time	Ma.S.	Kv.P.	Cone and Film
Hand	P.A. or Obl.	2–5		1.66 S					
		5–8		2.5 S					
									To part
Wrist	P.A. Lat. Obl.	2–5		1.66 S					
		5–10		2.5 S					
Forearm	A.P. Lat.	3–6		1.66 S				60 S	
		6–10		2.5					
		10–15		4.16					
Elbow	A.P. Lat. Obl.	3–5	36"	1.66 S					
		5–10		2.5 S					
		10–15		5 S					
Ankle	A.P. Lat. Obl.	4–8		3.33 S					
		8–12		6.6 S					
		12–15		10 S					
Leg	A.P. Lat.	4–8		3.33 S					
		8–13		6.66 S					
		13–17		10 S					
Knee	A.P. Lat.	4–8		3.33 S					
		8–13		6.66 S					
		13–17		10 S					

Note: Cast, add 10 Kv.P.

Fixed Kilovoltage System

EXPOSURE GUIDE: FIXED Kv.P. TECHNIQUE (Infants and Children)

S — Screens. average speed
SG — Screens and grid (8-to-1)
F — Regular film and cardboard holder
Filter — 2.5-mm Al.

C — Cylinder cone
V — Videx
Dev. 5 min. at 68 degrees or automatic

Region	Proj.	Cm. Range	FFD	Guide Ma.S.	Ma.	Time	Kv.P.	Cone
Chest (premature)	A.P.	5–9	40″	3.3 S	200	$1/60$	60	C
Chest (table top)	A.P.	10–14	60″	2.5 S	50	$1/20$	75	To part
		15–18		4 S	125	$1/30$	70	
		19–21		6 S	125	$1/20$	70	
	Obl.	12–15		4 S	125	$1/30$	75	
		16–18		6 S	125	$1/20$		
		19–21		8 S	125	$1/15$		
	Lat.	12–15		4 S	125	$1/30$	80	
		16–19		6 S	125	$1/20$		
		20–22		8 S	125	$1/15$		
Chest (upright)	P.A.	14–17	72″	3.33 S	100	$1/30$	80	To part
		18–20		5 S	100	$1/20$		
	Obl.	12–15		6 S	125	$1/20$	75	
		16–18		8 S	125	$1/15$		
		19–21		6.7 S	200	$1/30$	85	
		22–25		8.5 S	125	$1/15$		
	Lat.	12–15		3.3 S	100	$1/30$	90	
		16–19		5 S	100	$1/20$		
		20–23		6.7 S	200	$1/30$		
		24–26		8.5 S	125	$1/15$		

Note: For automatic processing reduce Kv.P. or adjust the Ma.S.

FORMULATING X-RAY TECHNIQUES

Region	Proj.	Cm. Range	FFD	Guide Ma. S.	Ma.	Time	Kv.P.	Cone
Skull	A.P.	9–12	36"	3.3 SG	50	$1/15$	85	V-8
		12–15		6.6 SG	100	$1/15$		
		16–20		13.3 SG	200	$1/15$		
		21–22		20 SG	200	$1/10$		
	Lat.	9–12		2.5 SG	25	$1/10$		
		13–17		7.5 SG	50	$3/20$		
		18–21		10 SG	100	$1/10$		
	Mento-vertex	12–16		15 SG	100	$3/20$		
		17–21		25 SG	100	$1/4$		
		22–25		40 SG	200	$1/5$		
		26–29		60 SG	200	$3/20$		
	Petrous A.P.	9–12		10 SG	100	$1/10$		C
		12–15		20 SG	200	$1/10$		
		16–20		30 SG	200	$3/20$		
		21–25		50 SG	200	$1/4$		
	Stenvers	12–16		15 SG	100	$3/20$		
		17–23		20 SG	200	$1/10$		
	Optic	10–14		5 SG	50	$1/10$		
		15–18		10 SG	100	$1/10$		
		19–22		20 SG	200	$1/10$		
	Mastoid Lat.	6–9	30"	2.5 SG	25	$1/10$	75	
		10–13		5 SG	50	$1/10$		
		14–17		7.5 SG	50	$3/20$		
	Sinuses P.A.	11–16		10 SG	100	$1/10$	85	
		17–23		20 SG	200	$1/10$		
	Sinuses Lat.	4–8		2.5 S	25	$1/10$	80	
		9–12		5 S	50	$1/10$		
		13–16		7.5 S	50	$3/20$		

Fixed Kilovoltage System

Region	Proj.	Cm. Range	FFD	Guide Ma.S.	Ma.	Time	Kv.P.	Cone
Skull	Mandible P.A.	4–8	30"	2.5 SG	50	$1/20$	85	C
		9–13		5 SG	100	$1/20$		
		14–18		10 SG	200	$1/20$		
	Mandible Lat.	4–8		1.2 S	25	$1/20$	70	
		9–11		2.5 S	50	$1/20$		
		12–15		5 S	100	$1/20$		
Cervical Spine	Lat. & Obl.	3–6	72"	5 S	100	$1/20$	85	
		7–11		10 S	200	$1/20$		
		12–15		15 S	300	$1/20$		
	A.P.	3–6		5 SG	50	$1/10$	80	
		7–11		10 SG	100	$1/10$		
		12–15		20 SG	200	$1/10$		
Thoracic	A.P.	10–15		10 SG	100	$1/10$	75	
		16–19		20 SG	200	$1/10$		
		20–23		40 SG	200	$1/5$		
	Lat.	14–19		7.5 SG	50	$3/20$	80	
		20–24		10 SG	25	$4/10$		
		25–28		20 SG	50	$4/10$		
Lumbar & Pelvis, & Abdomen	A.P. & Obl.	7–11	36"	10 SG	100	$1/10$	65	
		12–15		25 SG	100	$1/4$		
		16–19		40 SG	200	$1/5$		
		20–24		60 SG	200	$3/10$		
Extremities (Premature)	All			3.33 S	100	$1/30$	45	To part
Extremities	Wrist, Elbow, Forearm A.P. & Lat.	3–5		1.66 S	50	$1/30$	55	
		6–10		2.5 S	50	$1/20$		
		11–15		3.33 S	100	$1/30$		
	Ankle, Leg, Knee A.P. & Lat.	4–8		3.33 S	100	$1/30$		
		9–13		6.6 S	200	$1/30$		
		14–17		10 S	200	$1/20$		

FORMULATING X-RAY TECHNIQUES

Region	Proj.	Cm. Range	FFD	Guide Ma.S.	Ma.	Time	Kv.P.	Cone
Knee	A.P. Lat. Obl.	4–9		2.5 SG	25	$1/10$		
		10–15		5 SG	50	$1/10$		
		16–18		10 SG	100	$1/10$	80	To part
Shoulder	A.P. Lat.	4–9	36″	2.5 SG	25	$1/10$		
		10–14		5 SG	50	$1/10$		
		15–17		10 SG	100	$1/10$		

Thickness ranges

The thickness ranges of body parts in the adult patient are always measured along the course of the central ray. In most instances, three thickness ranges are specified. The first comprises a thickness range for *thin* parts; the second, the *average* thickness range, which includes the majority of thicknesses for a given projection; and the third, the thickness range for the *heavy* parts.

Some projections, such as those for the chest, require a greater breakdown in thicknesses to attain the desired uniformity in radiographic quality.

Focus-film distance (FFD)

In the guide, the focus-film distances are standardized at 30–36 and 72 inches. If the FFD is to be changed at any time, the inverse square law should be used to effect the required change in Ma.S. (see pages 91–93).

The following techniques are based on the use of 2-mm. aluminum external filtration.

Guide Ma.S. values

As a starting point in adapting the Guide to your requirements, Guide Ma.S. values are listed for the various projections. These are trial values, but they are quite close to a corrected value that should be employed. In the column listing fixed kilovoltages, the kilovoltages listed have been attained by extensive experiment and are premised upon the following criteria:

1. That the wave length generated by the kilovoltage will provide radiation that will penetrate a given part when a practical Ma.S. value is used.
2. That the level of secondary radiation fog is such that it will not interfere with the diagnostic quality of the radiographic image.
3. That the image will exhibit a long scale of contrast to assure the rendition of maximum image detail.
4. That the final Ma.S. value selected for the average thickness will provide sufficient overall image silver to reveal essential details. Since all factors but Ma.S. are constant, it can readily be seen that the level of radiographic density must be regulated by Ma.S. The kilovoltage should not be used for this purpose.
5. That the focus–film distances listed will assure satisfactory image sharpness.

Fixed Kilovoltage System

The last column of the Guide indicates the appropriate size of film required and the size of the cone needed to enclose the anatomic area specifically required.

Use of the Guide

Select the projection that is to be standardized. Choose a patient or phantom whose thickness is a median in the average thickness range. This thickness should be measured along the course of the central ray. Once the thickness category into which the part falls is determined, note the Guide Ma.S. listed for that particular thickness range. Make an exposure of the patient or phantom employing the indicated Ma.S., FFD, Kv.P., size of film, and cone. If the over-all density of the radiograph is greater than desired, repeat the exposure using the Guide Ma.S. value for the next lower thickness category. If the density is less than desired, use the Guide Ma.S. value listed for the next higher thickness. Further small adjustments in Ma.S. can be made to arrive at the exact density level desired. Once the density level for the average thickness is determined, the *percentage* increase or decrease in Ma.S. can be easily determined and the other Ma.S. values corrected accordingly. Simplification of this procedure can be effected by classifying radiography into these three types: (1) direct exposure, (2) screen exposure, and (3) screen-grid exposure. By this means, only three adjustments in the Guide Ma.S. values need be made for each class of radiography.

Example: In radiography at 85 Kv.P. of the lateral skull, measuring between 12 and 17 cm., the *guide Ma.S.* for the average thickness range will be found to be 15, employing screens and grid. Suppose the exposure is made and the resultant density is insufficient. Then another exposure should be made, employing 20 Ma.S., with screens and grid (the Ma.S. value needed for thicker skulls), and if the resultant density is satisfactory, the percentage increase in Ma.S. to be applied to all screen grid exposures in the preceding charts, with the exception of children's and infants' exposures, may be obtained in the following manner.

Lateral skull (see Exposure Guide "The Skull"). The Guide Ma.S. proposed is 15 Ma.S. with screens and grid. The corrected trial Ma.S. is 20 with screens and grid. Now $20/15 = 1.33\frac{1}{3}$; i.e., 133 per cent adjustment for other screen-grid exposures listed in the Guide Ma.S. values.

In the example of the lateral skull we would then multiply the first class, 10 Ma.S. by 1.33, the second class by 1.33 for 20 Ma.S. and the third class (20 Ma.S.) by 1.33. The result is 13.3 Ma.S.— or, rounded off, 15 Ma.S. This would give us the adjusted factors. This procedure would be followed throughout the entire chart on the Ma.S. values listed for screens and grid.

See alternative method, page 225, and Chapter 8, pages 104–5.

Example 2: If we make a radiograph of the P.A. hand and find that the 70 Ma.S. recommended in the Guide under "Extremities" for regular film in the cardboard holder, with 50 Kv.P., produces excessive density, we make another radiograph at 50 Ma.S. If this radiograph is adequate, we then make a percentage correction for all techniques in the guide.

Hand — cardboard holder
Guide Ma.S.: 70
Corrected trial Ma.S.: 50
$50/70 = 5/7 = .715$ = about 70 per cent

We would then multiply all techniques listed for cardboard holder by .715 and this would be the corrected Ma.S. value for every such exposure of a part.

Fixed voltage technique is dependent upon a rigid application of the following factors:

1. Focus-film distance —
    a. Influences the sharpness and magnification of the radiographic image.

FORMULATING X-RAY TECHNIQUES

    b. Influences radiographic density.
2. Kilovoltage (Kv.P.) —
    a. Regulates wave length of radiation.
    b. Determines degree of penetration.
    c. Influences production of secondary radiation fog.
    d. Regulates scale of radiographic contrast.
    e. Determines degree of exposure latitude.
    f. Influences radiographic density.
3. Milliampere seconds (Ma.S.) —
    a. Regulates the quantity of x-radiation emitted by the x-ray tube.
    b. Regulates radiographic density.

The physiological or diseased state of the patient requires some adjustment of the Ma.S. values when an increase in tissue absorption occurs. A corresponding increase in over-all radiographic density is required. Doubling the Ma.S. is often sufficient compensation for

1. Sclerosis
2. Fluid or pus
3. Contrast media

Conditions which cause a decrease in tissue absorption require a corresponding decrease in radiographic density. Halving the Ma.S. often compensates for

1. Destructive bone disease
2. Malignant metastases
3. Malnutrition
4. Atrophy
5. Emphysematous tissue

Example: In the posteroanterior adult chest to visualize the bronchi with opaque media, we find that the 17–20-cm. technique calls for 80 Kv.P. and 5 Ma.S. Since an opaque medium has been added, our initial procedure would be to double the Ma.S. (10 Ma.S.) and leave all other factors constant. If the new Ma.S. produces more density than desired, we go "in between" 5 and 10 Ma.S. and use 7.5 Ma.S. See Figure 12.6, oblique bronchogram exposure.

When a chest (or any other part) measures greater than average, the only change that need be made in the technical factors is in the Ma.S. The increased thickness requires more radiation. The Kv.P. is held constant since it has been established that 80 Kv.P. provides the necessary quality of radiation to penetrate any adult chest of normal size.

If we were to use the basic Ma.S. (6.66) for a 15-cm. chest, the density would be excessive. A satisfactory result can be obtained, however, by using $1/2$ x Ma.S. To balance the densities for the 17- and 20-cm. chest, $3/4$ x Ma.S. may be used. For chests that are 10–14 cm., $1/4$ x Ma.S. may be used.

It is impossible to formulate a technique chart that will produce identical results in Durham, North Carolina, and Detroit, Michigan, and unless all machines in a particular department are calibrated the same and all cones and grids are identical, a separate chart must be worked out for each.

The following techniques are designed for use *only* with full-wave rectified equipment, a cone and/or collimator, 8-to-1 grid, and a rotating-anode tube. The exposure factors are the factors that produce excellent radiographs in

Fixed Kilovoltage System

one department. The factors, however, may be adapted to the equipment in your department by a simple adjustment in exposure.

Adapting exposure charts to your equipment

Choose a patient of average build whose thickness falls into the average or middle class. Let us select the knee for a starting point. Measure the knee and use the *Guide Ma.S.* listed for the knee in the A.P. projection. Be sure to use the *Guide Ma.S., Focus–film distance, Kv.P., size of film*, and *cone* as listed. Repeat the exposure using the *Guide Ma.S.* value listed for the first class. Repeat the exposure using the *Guide Ma.S.* for the third or large class. Develop the three films at 68° for 5 minutes. Observe the three radiographs to find the desired density level for the average thickness. The percentage increase or decrease in Ma.S. can now be determined and the other Ma.S. values corrected accordingly. This correction factor will hold true for all radiography of parts with *similar density* (i.e., knee, leg). This procedure is followed for all groups; skull, sinuses, the lateral cervical spine, the lumbar spine, etc.

Example 1: For an A.P. radiograph of the knee employing an 8-to-1 grid, the Guide Ma.S. for the average thickness range (10–14 cm.) is 6. Make a second exposure employing the Guide Ma.S. for the first class (–9 cm.), 4 Ma.S., and a third exposure employing the Guide Ma.S. for the large class (14-cm.), 8 Ma.S. See Figure 8.1A, B, C. We find upon inspection of the three radiographs that 8 Ma.S. gives us the desired density. We now *divide the listed Guide Ma.S.* into the *corrected Ma.S.* to find the percentage or correction factor.

Thus

$$6 \overline{\smash{\big)}\ 8.0} \quad \begin{array}{r} 1.3 \\ \underline{6} \\ 20 \\ \underline{18} \\ 2 \end{array}$$

Therefore our correction factor is 1.3. We now multiply the Guide Ma.S. of *each class* by 1.3.

We now have 5 Ma.S. for the first class, 8 Ma.S. for the second class, and 10.4 or 10 Ma.S. for our large class. Make *no other changes*.

If by chance radiograph number 2, made with 4 Ma.S., is better, we would divide 6 into 4.

$$6 \overline{\smash{\big)}\ 4.0} \quad \begin{array}{r} .66 \\ \underline{3\ 6} \\ 40 \\ \underline{36} \\ 4 \end{array}$$

We then would use .66 times the listed guide Ma.S. values. Or, we could say, $4/6 = 2/3$; therefore $2/3$ times the guide Ma.S. values.

Example 2: In radiography of the skull in the A.P. projection (16–23 cm.), the guide Ma.S. will be found to be 30. If the resulting density is excessive, another exposure should be made employing 20 Ma.S., the value needed for a smaller skull. If the resulting density is satisfactory, the percentage reduction in Ma.S. needed is obtained in the following manner:

Guide Ma.S.	30
Corrected Trial Ma.S.	20

$20/30 = 2/3$ or $66 2/3$ per cent adjustment for the other Guide Ma.S. values listed for skull radiography. This procedure should be followed for other parts of similar density, with screens and grid (S.G.).

$$30 \overline{\smash{\big)}\ 20.00} \quad \begin{array}{r} .66\, 2/3 \\ \underline{180} \\ 20/30 = 2/3 \end{array}$$

FORMULATING X-RAY TECHNIQUES

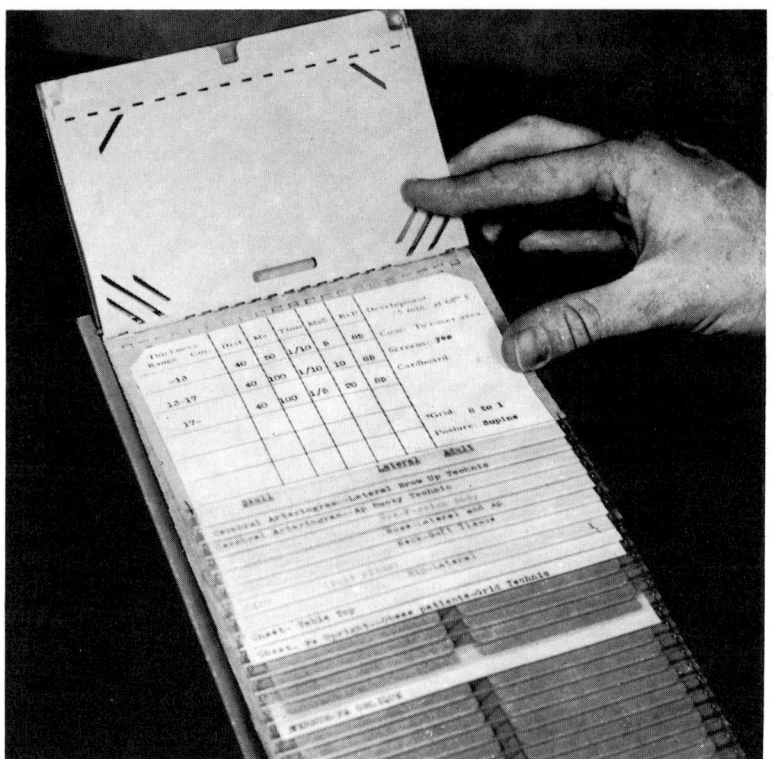

Figure 12.2. A Kardex technique file; below, a specimen card.

Thickness range: Cms.	FFD	Guide Ma.S.	Ma.	Time	Ma.S.	Kv.P.	Legend
Infant —							F — Cardboard
Child —							Ⓢ — Screens, aver. speed
8–12	36	10	100	$1/10$	10	85	Ⓖ — Grid
12–17	36	15	100	$3/20$	15	85	Cone no. V-10 Development: 5 min. 68° F.
17–21	36	20	100	$1/5$	20	85	or automatic
—							
SKULL			Lateral			Film size 10 x 12	Projection no. 15

A Kardex-type technique chart may be set up and each projection recorded; see Figure 12.2. The 4 x 6 cards in the Kardex technique file may be arranged as in Table 12.2.

226

Fixed Kilovoltage System

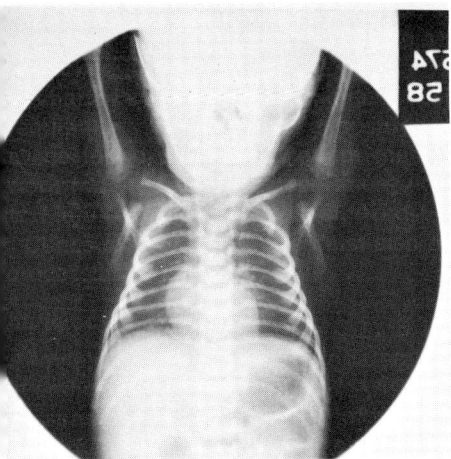

Figure 12.3. Chest of premature infant at 60 Kv.P.

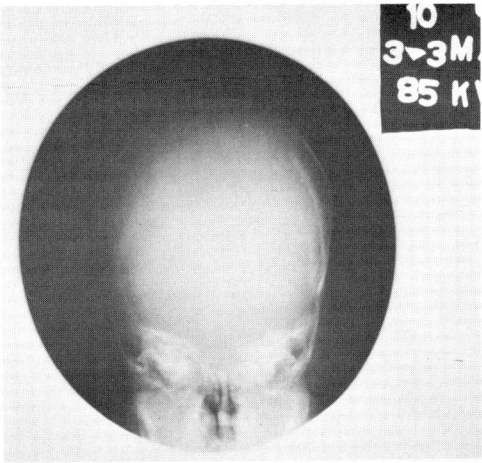

Figure 12.4. Anteroposterior view of skull of premature infant at 85 Kv.P.

Table 12.2 ARRANGEMENT OF KARDEX FILE

Chest	P.A. Oblique Lateral Stretcher Table Bucky P.A.-Grid—Upright Oblique-Grid—Upright Lateral-Grid—Upright	Pelvis	A.P. Lateral
		Hip	A.P. Lateral
		Gallbladder	P.A. Upright Decubitus
Skull	Lateral A.P.-P.A.—Waters Brow Up Petrous Mentovertex Mastoid—Lateral Stenvers—P.A. Optic—P.A. Mandible—P.A. Mandible—Lateral	Colon	Regular Air Contrast Chassard—Lapine
		Pelvimetry	A.P. A.P. Inlet Lateral Placenta
		Extremities	Hand Forearm Elbow Humerus Shoulder Foot Os Calcis Tibia—Fibula Knee
Sinuses	Lateral Frontal Sphenoid—Maxillary		
Spine	Cervical—A.P. Cervical—Lateral Cervical—Oblique Neck—Soft Tissue Dorsal—A.P. Lumbar—A.P. Lumbar—Oblique Lumbar—Lateral Lumbar—Spot, L-5		
		Extremities-screens	Adult Child Infant
		G.I. Series	P.A.—Oblique

FORMULATING X-RAY TECHNIQUES

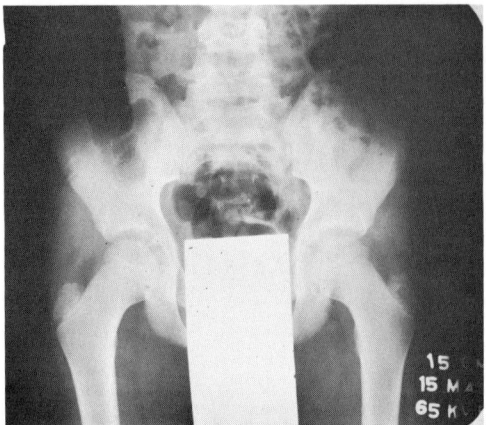

Figure 12.5. Anteroposterior view of pelvis of an 8-year-old child at 65 Kv.P.

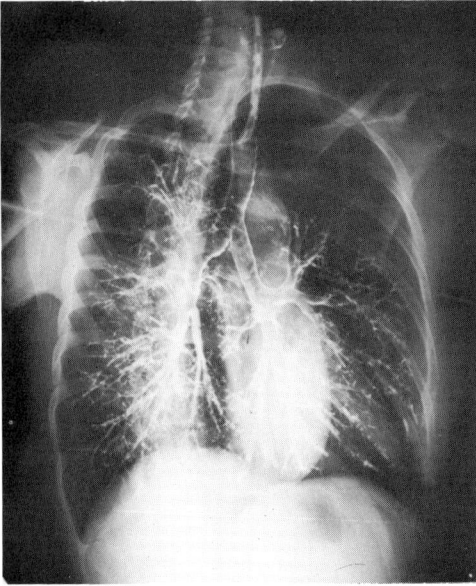

Figure 12.6. Bronchogram at 100 Kv.P.

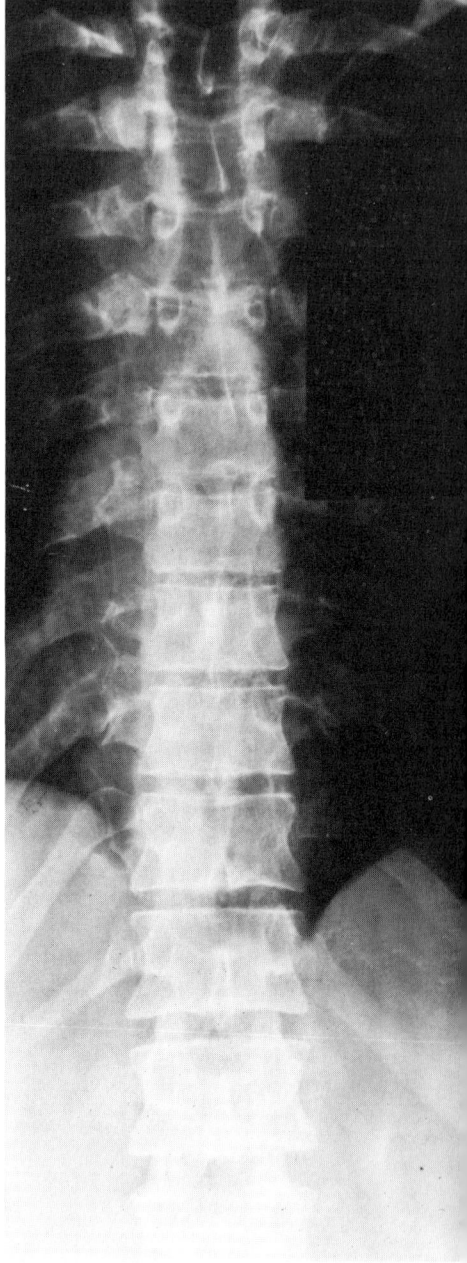

Figure 12.7. Anteroposterior view of dorsal and lumbar spine.

SPECIAL PROCEDURES

Contrary to some opinion, not all chest radiography with fixed kilovoltage is done at 80 Kv.P. Figure 12.3 is a radiograph of a chest of a premature infant at 60 Kv.P. The actual exposure factors were 40-inch focus-film distance,

Fixed Kilovoltage System

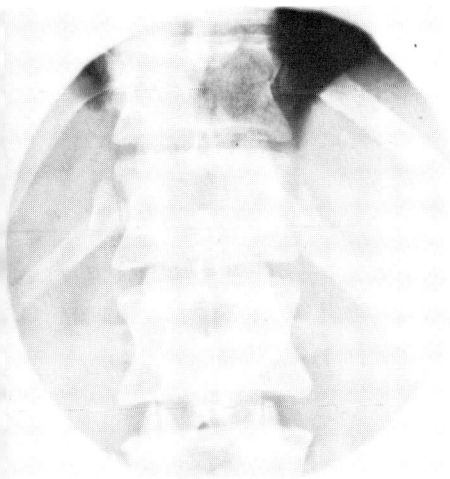

Figure 12.8. Spot film showing pathology in spine of Figure 12.7.

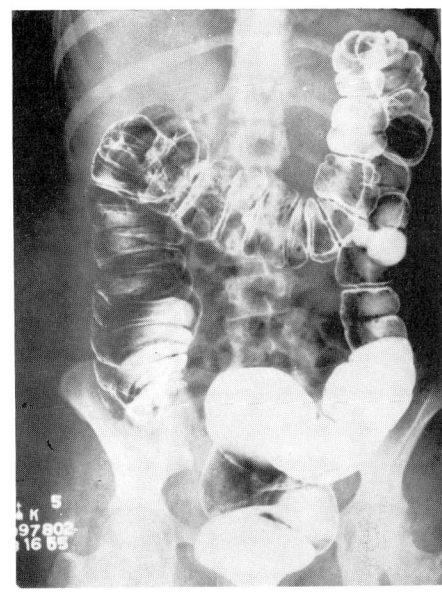

Figure 12.9. Air-contrast colon.

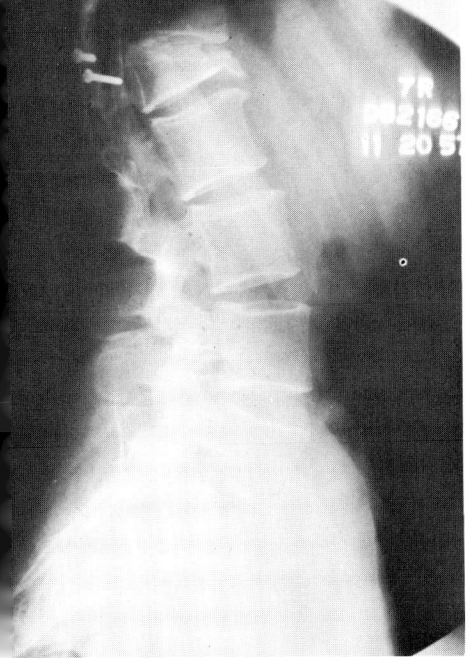

Figure 12.10. Note the pathology at the level of the first lumbar vertebra.

medium screens, cylinder cone, 60 Kv.P., 3.33 Ma.S. (200 Ma for $1/60$ second).

Figure 12.6 illustrates an oblique bronchogram radiograph exposure at 100 Kv.P., 13.33 Ma.S., 72-inch FFD, 8-to-1 grid.

Figure 12.7 is an anteroposterior radiograph of the thoracic-lumbar spine. Since pathology was present, a spot-film for more detail and contrast was

FORMULATING X-RAY TECHNIQUES

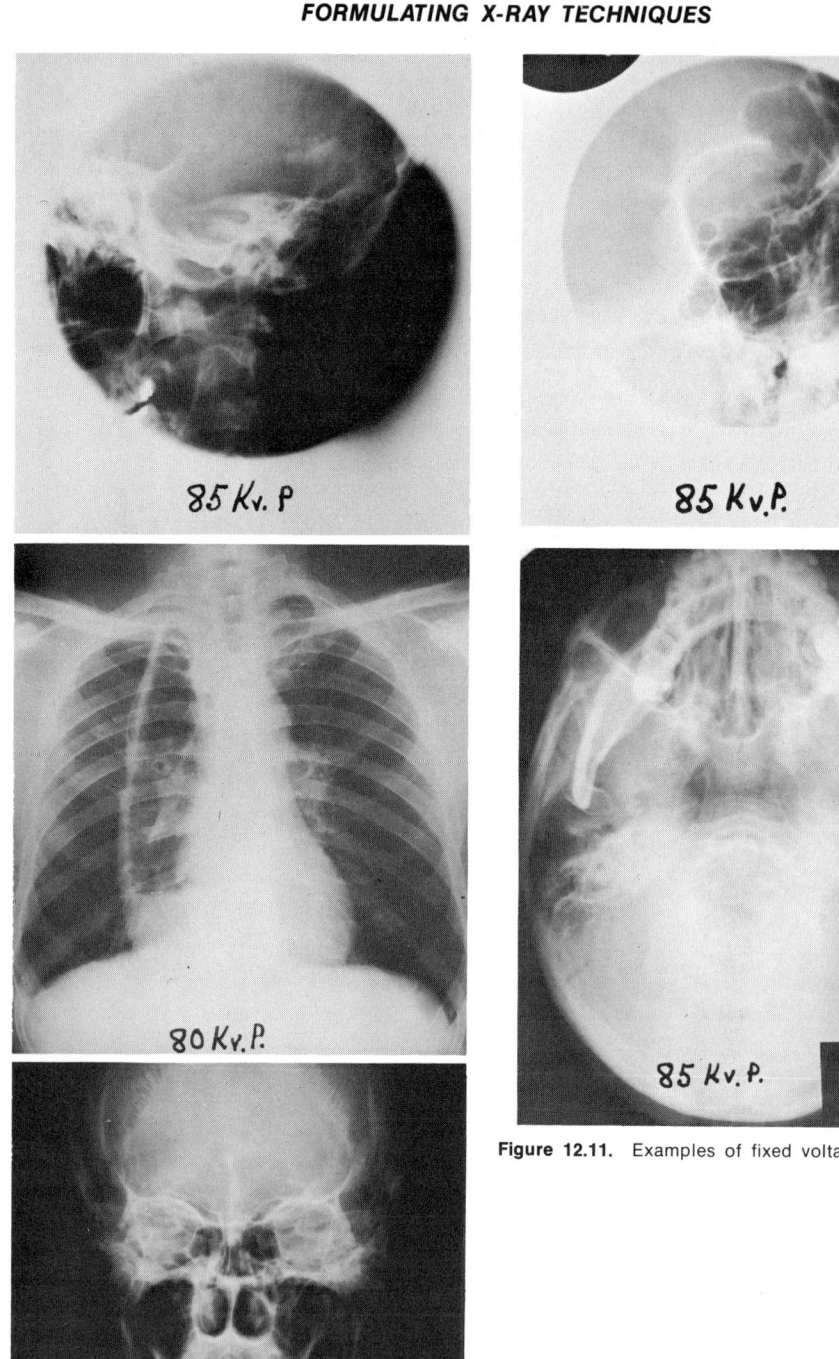

Figure 12.11. Examples of fixed voltage technique.

Fixed Kilovoltage System

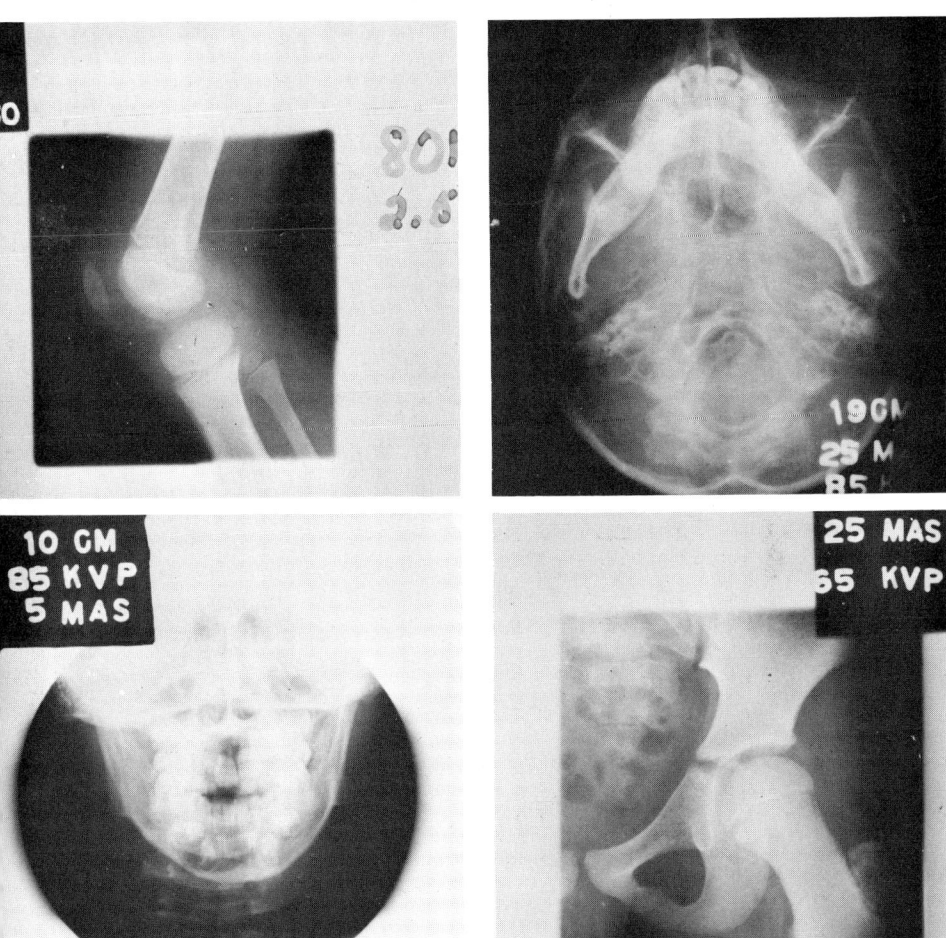

Figure 12.12. Examples of fixed voltage technique with children.

requested. By using the same exposure factors, reducing the distance from 36 to 30 inches and using a cylinder cone, we obtained the radiograph shown in Figure 12.8.

Figure 12.9 is a radiograph of an air-contrast colon employing 100 Kv.P., 15 Ma.S., 36-inch FFD, 8-1 grid.

Figure 12.10 shows pathology at the level of the first lumbar vertebra. Note the detail and contrast shown at the level of L-1 and 2 and L-4 and 5. The exposure factors were 85 Kv.P. and 150 Ma.S.

Other examples of fixed voltage are shown in Figure 12.11, and of fixed voltage technique for children in Figure 12.12.

HIGH-KILOVOLTAGE TECHNIQUE

It is possible to produce films of as good quality with high kilovoltage as

FORMULATING X-RAY TECHNIQUES

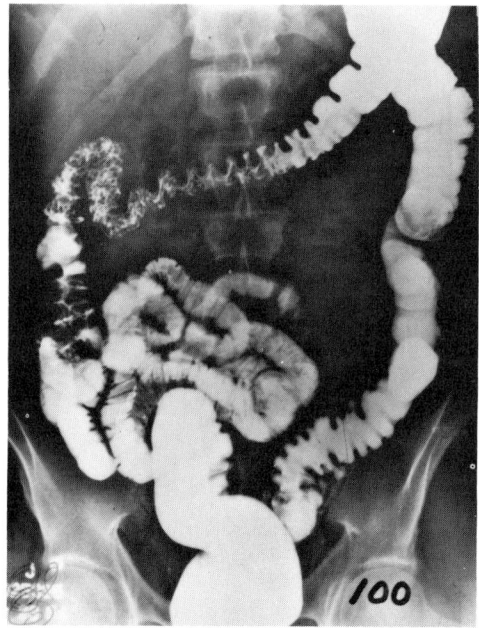

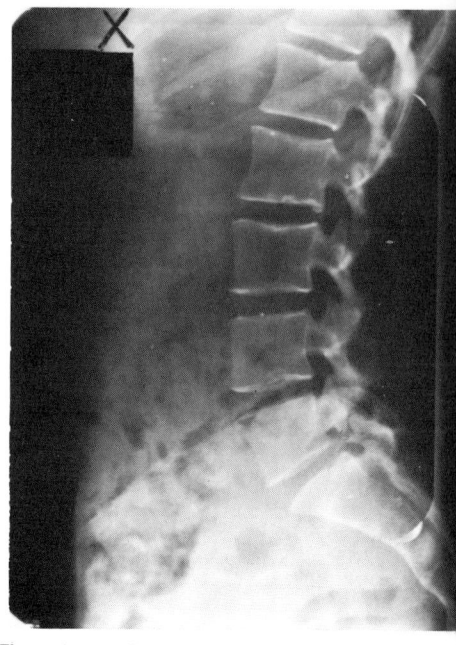

Figure 12.13. Examples of high kilovoltage technique

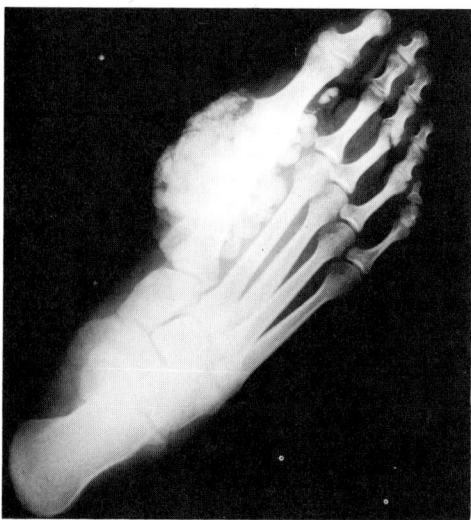

with low or medium kilovoltage. It is not necessarily a fact that radiographs produced by high kilovoltage are gray and flat. Inappropriate selection and control of milliampere seconds have been the most common errors when employing higher kilovoltages. The use of a 12-to-1 or a 16-to-1 grid and limiting the area of exposure are of primary importance.

Actually the only limit imposed on the amount of kilovoltage that might be employed in medical radiography is the limitation of contrast (long-scale). The limit of course is the point at which the contrast scale becomes so long that diagnosis becomes doubtful. To maintain contrast at the higher kilovolt-

Fixed Kilovoltage System

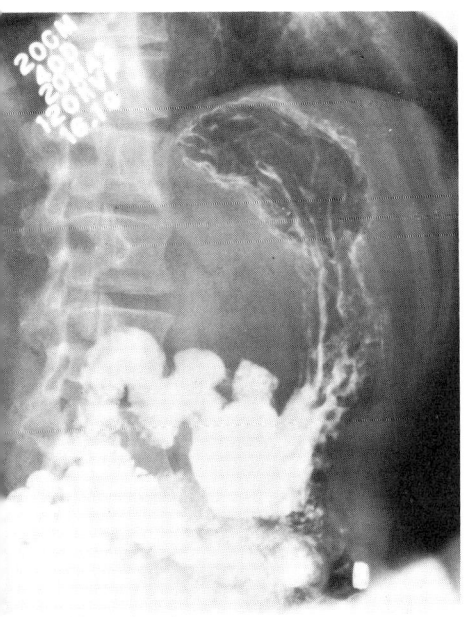
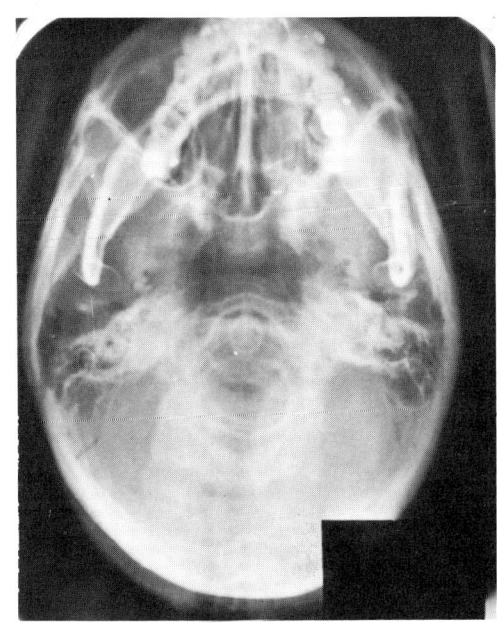

Figure 12.13 continued.

ages the use of a 12-to-1 or a 16-to-1 grid is essential; however, chest radiography may be done up to 150 Kv.P. with a 7-to-1 or 8-to-1 grid.

In the United States many departments use up to 130 Kv.P. There has been a general acceptance of an increase in the average voltage used in routine radiography. Voltage above 100 Kv.P. is being used for various radiographic examinations—notably, radiographic examinations of the gastro-intestinal tract, colon, air-contrast colon, pelvimetry, and lateral lumbar-sacral spine, and also non-screen grid exposures.

Supervoltage technique in chest radiography to visualize lesions overshadowed by bone have been done by Pendergrass, Tuddenham, and others.

See Figures 12.13 and 12.14.

Figure 12.14. Examples of high kilovoltage technique.

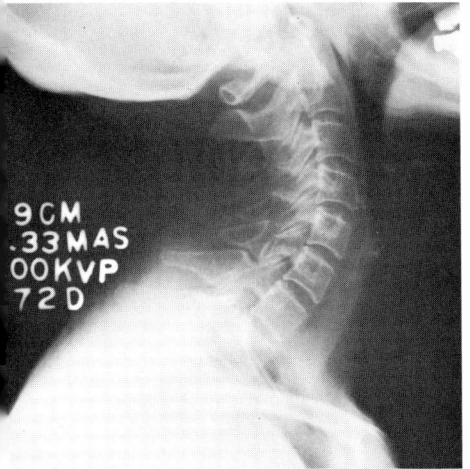
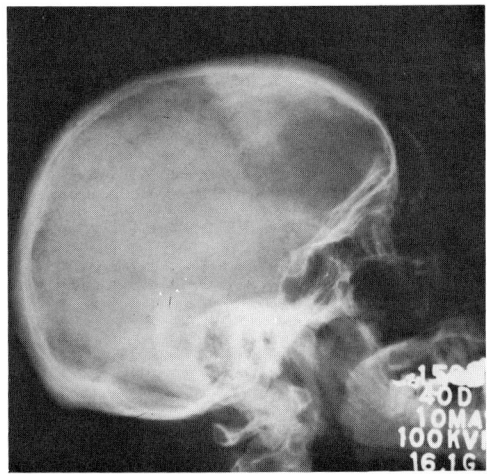

FORMULATING X-RAY TECHNIQUES

EXPOSURE GUIDE FOR FIXED HIGH-KILOVOLTAGE TECHNIQUE AT 100–120 Kv.P.

Tube: Super Dynamax rotating-anode
Grid: 16-to-1 ratio
Cone: Double diaphragm Videx (V) and/or collimator Cylinder cone (C)
Filter: 3 mm. external, ½ mm. internal
Projection: Proj.
Thickness: Cm.
Distance: FFD
Regular film with cardboard holder: F
No-screen film: NS
Screens, medium: S
Screens and grid: SG (16-1)
Development: 5 minutes at 68° or automatic

Region	Proj.	Cm. Range	FFD	Guide Ma.S.	Ma.	Time	Ma.S.	Kv.P.	Cone
Skull	Lat.	12–17	40"	10 SG				100 SG	V-10
		17–20		12.5 SG					
	P.A. A.P.	17–21		17.5 SG					V-8
		21–25		25 SG					
	Towne	17–24		30 SG					C
		24–28		40 SG					
	Vertex	19–25		30 SG					V-8
		25–29		40 SG					
Cervical	A.P.	11–15	72"	10 SG					V-8
		15–18		15 SG					
	Lat.	9–13		8.33 S					
		13–15		12.5 S					
	Lat. Soft tissue	10–15		3.3 S					
		15–18		5 S					
Thoracic	A.P.	19–24	40"	25 SG					V-7
		24–29		30 SG					
	Lat.	30–34		40 SG					7 x 17
		34–38		50 SG					
Lumbar	A.P.	17–22		20 SG					V-11
		22–25		25 SG					11 x 14
	Obl.	17–22		25 SG					V-10
		22–25		30 SG					8 x 10

Note: Automatic processing will require some adjustment in exposure factors.

Fixed Kilovoltage System

Region	Proj.	Cm Range	FFD	Guide Ma.S.	Ma.	Time	Ma.S.	Kv.P.	Cone
Lumbar, cont.	Lat.	26–32		50 SG				120 SG	V-11
		32–38		60 SG					11 x 14
Pelvis	A.P.	19–23		25 SG					V-14
		23–27		30 SG					
Abdomen	A.P.	23–26		25 SG					14 x 17
		26–32		50 SG					
Gallbladder	P.A.	22–25	40"	25 SG				100 SG	V-10
		25–31		30 SG					10 x 12
		31–33		40 SG					
Pregnancy	A.P.	23–28		30 SG				120 SG	V-14
		28–34		50 SG					14 x 17
Pelvimetry	A.P. Thoms	24–27		50 SG					V-10
		27–32		75 SG					10 x 12
		32–36		100 SG					
	Lat.	23–26		40 SG					
		26–32		50 SG					
		32–37		75 SG					
Placenta	Lat.	Small		15 SG					V-14
		Medium		20 SG					14 x 17
		Large		30 SG					

G.I. series and colon

Region	Proj.	Cm. Range	FFD	Guide Ma.S.	Ma.	Time	Ma.S.	Kv.P.	Cone
G.I. and colon	P.A. Obl. Lat.	13–17	40"	6.66 SG				120	To Film
		17–22		10 SG					
		22–27		20 SG					
		27–32		33.3 SG					

FORMULATING X-RAY TECHNIQUES

Bronchogram — with grid cassette

Region	Proj.	Cm. Range	FFD	Guide Ma.S.	Ma.	Time	Ma.S.	Kv.P.	Cone
Lungs	P.A.	20–24	72"	10 SG				100	V-14 14 x 17
		24–27		15 SG					
		27–30		20 SG					
		30–34		30 SG					
	Obl.	19–23		10 SG					
		23–30		20 SG					
		30–35		40 SG					
	Lat.	24–27		15 SG					
		27–29		25 SG					
		29–33		30 SG					
		33–40		60 SG					

P.A. chest six-inch air-gap technique (see p. 229)

Region	Proj.	Cm. Range	FFD	Guide Ma.S.	Ma.	Time	Ma.S.	Kv.P.	Cone
Chest	P.A.	26–30	120"	5 S				125	To part 14 x 17
		30–35		8.3 S					
		35–40		15 S					

Extremities

Part	Position	Avg. Cm. Thickness	Kv.P.	Suggested Ma.S. Cb. H.*	Suggested Ma.S. Screen	Selected Ma.S. Cb. H.	Selected Ma.S. Screen	Dist.	Grid
Hand	P.A.-Obl.	3–5	76	20	.83			40	No
Wrist	P.A.	4–6	76	25	1			40	No
Wrist	Lateral	5–8	76	50	2.08			40	No
Forearm	All	6–9	76	50	2.08			40	No
Elbow	A.P.	6–9	76	50	2.5			40	No
Elbow	Lateral	7–10	76	50	2.5			40	No
Humerus	All	7–10	100		7.5			40	16:1
Shoulder	A.P.	13–16	100		7.5			40	16:1

Fixed Kilovoltage System

Part	Position	Avg. Cm. Thickness	Kv.P.	Suggested Ma.S. Cb. H.*	Suggested Ma.S. Screen	Selected Ma.S. Cb. H.	Selected Ma.S. Screen	Dist.	Grid
Clavicle	A.P.	13–16	100		7.5			40	16:1
Foot	A.P.-Obl.	7–9	76	25	2.08			40	No
Foot	Lateral	7–9	76	50	2.5			40	No
Os calcis	Axial	8–13	76	40	2.08			40	No
Ankle	A.P.	7–10	76	75	3.33			40	No
Ankle	Lateral	6–9	76	50	2.5			40	No
Leg	A.P.	9–12	76		3.33			40	No
Leg	Lateral	8–11	76		2.5			40	No
Knee	A.P.	11–14	100		7.5			40	16:1
Knee	Lateral	10–13	100		6.67			40	16:1
Patella	Axial		100		.83			40	No
Femur	A.P.	14–17	100		7.5			40	16:1
Femur	Lateral	13–16	100		6.67			40	16:1

*Cb. H.: Cardboard holder and regular filter.

EXPOSURE GUIDE FOR FIXED KILOVOLTAGE TECHNIQUE AT 150 Kv.P.

Part	Position	Avg. Cm. Thickness	Kv.P.	Suggested Ma.S.	Selected Ma.S.	Dist.	Screen	Grid
Pelvis	A.P.	17–20	150	5		40	Yes	16:1
Lumbar spine	A.P.	17–21	150	7.5		40	Yes	16:1
Lumbar spine	Oblique	18–22	150	10		40	Yes	16:1
Lumbar spine	Lateral	24–26	150	15		40	Yes	16:1
Lumbar spine	Lateral	27–30	150	20		40	Yes	16:1
Lumbar spine	Lateral	31–34	150	30		40	Yes	16:1
Lumbar spine	Lateral	35–38	150	40		40	Yes	16:1
Dorsal spine	A.P.	21–24	150	4		40	Yes	16:1
Dorsal spine*	Lateral	30–34	150	2		40	Yes	16:1
Cervical spine	A.P.	11–14	150	2.5		40	Yes	16:1
Cervical spine	Oblique	10–13	150	1		72	Yes	No
Cervical spine	Lateral	11–14	150	1		72	Yes	No
Atlas & axis	A.P.	12–16	150	3.33		40	Yes	16:1

FORMULATING X-RAY TECHNIQUES

Part	Position	Avg. Cm. Thickness	Kv.P.	Suggested Ma.S.	Selected Ma.S.	Dist.	Screen	Grid
Lumbo-sacral jt.	Lateral	30–34	150	40		40	Yes	16:1
Lumbo-sacral jt.	Lateral	35–38	150	50		40	Yes	16:1
Lumbo-sacral jt.	Lateral	39–42	150	60		40	Yes	16:1
Hip	A.P.	17–21	150	5		40	Yes	16:1
Hip	Lateral	20–24	150	7.5		40	Yes	16:1

*Slow breathing.

Part	Position	Avg. Cm. Thickness	Kv.P.	Suggested Ma.S.	Selected Ma.S.	Dist.	Screen	Grid
Skull	Lateral	16–18	150	1.5		40	Yes	16:1
Skull	P.A.	18–21	150	3		40	Yes	16:1
Skull	Occiput	18–21	150	3.75		40	Yes	16:1
Skull	Sub-mentovert.	23–26	150	6.25		40	Yes	16:1
Sinuses	Maxillary	18–22	150	5		30	Yes	16:1
Sinuses	Frontal	18–22	150	5		30	Yes	16:1
Sinuses	Open-mouth	21–24	150	5		30	Yes	16:1
Sinuses	Lateral	11–14	150	1		30	Yes	16:1
Mastoid	Lateral	14–17	150	1.5		30	Yes	16:1
Mandible	P.A.	12–15	150	.83		40	Yes	16:1
Mandible	Lateral	10–13	76	2.5		30	Yes	No
Nose	Lateral		76	20		40	No	No

Part	Position	Avg. Cm. Thickness	Kv.P.	Suggested Ma.S.	Selected Ma.S.	Dist.	Screen	Grid
Esophagus	P.A.	20–25	150	2.08		40	Yes	16:1
Esophagus	Lateral	28–32	150	5		40	Yes	16:1
Stomach	P.A.	18–22	150	7.5		40	Yes	16:1
Colon	P.A.	18–22	150	7.5		40	Yes	16:1
Colon post evac.	P.A.	18–22	150	5		40	Yes	16:1
Gallbladder	P.A.	18–22	150	7.5		40	Yes	16:1
Abdomen	A.P.	17–21	150	6.67		40	Yes	16:1

Fixed Kilovoltage System

Chest	P.A.	–14	150	.83		72	Yes	10:1
Chest	P.A.	15–17	150	1.67		72	Yes	10:1
Chest	P.A.	18–22	150	2		72	Yes	10:1
Chest	P.A.	23–25	150	3		72	Yes	10:1
Chest	P.A.	26–29	150	6		72	Yes	10:1
Chest	P.A.	30	150	8.33		72	Yes	10:1
Chest	Lateral	–26	150	4		72	Yes	10:1
Chest	Lateral	27–32	150	6		72	Yes	10:1
Chest	Lateral	33	150	8.33		72	Yes	10:1
Chest	Oblique	19–23	150	3		72	Yes	10:1
Chest	Oblique	24–30	150	5		72	Yes	10:1
Chest	Oblique	31–35	150	6.67		72	Yes	10:1
Ribs**	A.P.-P.A. A.D.	21–24	150	2.08		40	Yes	16:1
Ribs	A.P. B.D.	17–22	150	7.5		40	Yes	16:1

**Suspend respiration.

Pregnancy	A.P.	Average	150	7.5		40	Yes	16:1
Pregnancy	Lateral	34–38	150	12.5		40	Yes	16:1

All technical factors are based on the use of regular film and medium speed intensifying screens.
Radiation should be confined to an area no larger than the size of film.
To radiograph a part smaller than the indicated average centimeters – halve Ma.S.
To radiograph a part larger than the indicated average centimeters – double Ma.S.
Technical factors are based on 5 min. development at 68° in supermix chemicals. If 3 min. development is preferred, increase developer temperature to 75° or use automatic processing.
Caution: Carefully observe tube rating chart when using 150 Kv.P.
Courtesy of X-ray Department, General Electric, Milwaukee 1, Wisconsin.

HIGH-KILOVOLTAGE AIR-GAP TECHNIQUE

It has been well established that the part to be radiographed should be as near to the film as possible in order to obtain sharpness in the radiographic image.

As stated previously, definition or detail is good or bad according to the contrast in the radiographic image. Contrast depends partly on the amount of scattered radiation reaching the film, and a means must be provided for reducing the scatter to the film. Scattered radiation can be reduced by cones, diaphragms, and grids. Scattered radiation can also be reduced by an air gap such as used in fractional-focus radiography. Watson has used an air-gap technique for radiography of the chest in large patients without a grid by increasing the part-film distance by six inches and employing a 10-foot focus-film distance (Figures 12.15 and 12.16).

FORMULATING X-RAY TECHNIQUES

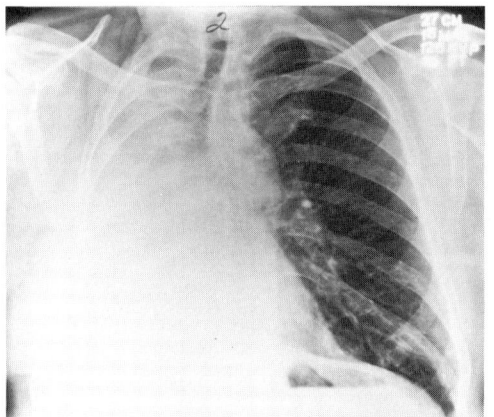

Figure 12.15. High kilovoltage air-gap technique, with pathology: 125 Kv.P.

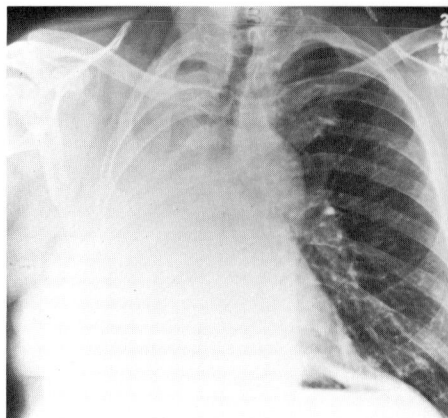

Figure 12.16. High kilovoltage air-gap technique 150 Kv.P.

Table 12.3 AIR GAP CHEST TECHNIQUE

Measuring reference: With the patient in position, measure the thickness through the thorax at the level of the sixth thoracic vertebra.

Intensifying screens, non-grid, 120-inch focus-film distance, 6-inch air gap.

Kv.P. 125

Anterior

Cm. range	Ma.S.
16–17	1.6
18–19	2.5
20–21	3.3
22–23	5
24–25	6.6
26–27	7.5
28–29	8.3

Oblique

Cm. range	Ma.S.
22–23	6.6
24–25	8.3
26–27	10
28–29	13.3
30–31	16.6
32–33	20
34–35	25

Lateral

Cm. range	Ma.S.
22–23	3.3
24–25	5
26–27	6.6
28–29	8.3
30–31	10
32–33	13.3
34–35	16.6
36–37	20
38–39	25
40–41	30

Lordotic

Cm. range	Ma.S.
18–19	6.6
20–21	8.3
22–23	10
24–25	13.3
26–27	16.6

ADDITIONAL EXPOSURE GUIDES

To adapt any technique to another machine, make a radiograph of any one part. Process the film under standard conditions and study the film on a standard illuminator. Make the necessary change in Kv.P. or Ma.S. to produce a film of the quality desired. This change will hold true for all parts of that group.

Fixed Kilovoltage System

BRONCHOGRAM WITH GRID CASSETTE (5-TO-1 RATIO)

Position	Cm. thickness	Ma.	Time	Ma.S.	Kv.P.	Distance	Cone
Lateral	24–27	300	1/20	15	100	72	V-14
	28–29	300	1/12	24–	100	72	V-14
	30–34	300	1/10	30	100	72	V-14
Oblique	19–23	100	1/15	6.5	100	72	V-14
	24–30	300	1/15	20	100	72	V-14
	31–35	300	1/10	30	100	72	V-14
P.A.	20–24	100	1/15	6.5	100	72	V-14
	25–27	300	1/30	10	100	72	V-14
	28–30	300	1/20	15	100	72	V-14
	31–34	300	1/15	20	100	72	V-14

COLON—AIR-CONTRAST TECHNIQUE (8-TO-1 GRID)

Position	Cm. thickness	Ma.	Time	Ma.S.	Kv.P.	Distance	Cone
A.P.-P.A.	16–19	100	1/10	5	100	36	V-14
	20–24	100	3/20	15	100	36	V-14
	25–30	200	1/10	20	100	36	V-14

ANGIOCARDIOGRAPHY

Radiographic technique

Regardless of the apparatus used, angiocardiograms must exhibit maximum detail, contrast, and latitude. The exposure requires an increase in density over that of the average chest radiograph, and it is wise to make a "control radiograph" prior to the actual procedure.

POSITIONS FOR ANGIOCARDIOGRAPHY

Anomalous pulmonary vein	P.A.
Aorta	L.A.O.–P.A.
Pulmonary disease	P.A.
Cor pulmonale	P.A.–Lat.
Eisenmenger's	L.A.O.–Lat.
Interatrial defect Interventricular defect	L.A.O.–P.A.
Left ventricular enlargement	L.A.O.–P.A.
Mediastinal tumors	P.A.–Lat.
Patent ductus	L.A.O.
Effusion	P.A.
Pulmonary artery aneurysm	Lat.–P.A.
Pulmonary stenosis	Lat.–P.A.
Rheumatic heart disease	L.A.O.–R.A.O.
Right aortic arch	P.A.
Right ventricular enlargement	L.A.O.–P.A.–R.A.O.
Superior vena cava	P.A.
Tetralogy	P.A.–Lat.–L.A.O.
Transposition	Lat.–P.A.
Tricuspid atresia	P.A.–Lat.

FORMULATING X-RAY TECHNIQUES

NORMAL TIME OF OPACIFICATION AFTER BEGINNING OF INJECTION

Structure		Structure	
Sup. vena cava	0.5 – 1.5 sec.	Pulmonary veins	5.0 – 7.0 sec.
Right atrium	1.0 – 2.0 sec.	Left atrium	5.0 – 8.0 sec.
Right ventricle	1.5 – 2.5 sec.	Left ventricle	7.0 – 10.0 sec.
Pulmonary artery		Thoracic aorta	7.0 – 10.0 sec.
and branches	2.0 – 3.5 sec.	Abdominal aorta	9.0 – 12.0 sec.

ANGIOCARDIOGRAPHIC EXPOSURE

	Ma.	Ma.S.	Time	Kv.P.	
Adult					
A.P.	300	5	1/60	100	
Obl.	300	10	1/30	100	8-to-1 Grid
Lat.	300	20	1/15	100	
Child					
A.P.	300	5	1/60	75	
Obl.	300	5	1/60	85	
Lat.	300	5	1/60	95	
Premature					
A.P.	300	5	1/60	70	
Obl.	300	5	1/60	80	
Lat.	300	5	1/60	85	

CEREBRAL ARTERIOGRAM

Short-scale contrast technique

Adult – Lateral	Adult – A.P.
Grid cassette	*Grid:* 8-to-1
Ma.S.: 40	*Ma.S:* 40
Kv.P.: 65	*Kv.P.:* 75
Dist.: 36 inches	*Dist.:* 36 inches

CEREBRAL ARTERIOGRAM

Long-scale contrast technique

–12 cm.	7.5 Ma.S.	85 Kv.P.	
13–17	15 Ma.S.	85 Kv.P.	Lateral
17–20	20 Ma.S.	85 Kv.P.	
Grid: 8-to-1	*Cone:* To part		
–15 cm.	15 Ma.S.	85 Kv.P.	
16–21	30 Ma.S.	85 Kv.P.	A.P.
22–26	40 Ma.S.	85 Kv.P.	

VENOGRAM ADULT

Proximal femur and lower leg	Distal femur and lower leg
Dist.: 60 inches	*Dist.:* 60 inches
Film: 36 inches	*Film:* 36 inches
Screens: medium	*Screens:* medium
Grid: 8-to-1	*Grid:* none
Ma.S.: 30	*Ma.S.:* 15
Kv.P.: 75	*Kv.P.:* 75
Barium plastic or aluminum filter	No additional filter

Fixed Kilovoltage System

MAGNIFICATION TECHNIQUE (30-INCH 30-INCH)

No grid	Regular film	Par-speed screens	
		Ma.S.	Kv.P.
Hip		70	85
Mandible lat.		50	55
Mastoid			
Law		50	80
Stenvers		50	75
Nose		20	50
Optic foramen		100	80
Shoulder		25	75
Sinuses			
frontal		50	80
Waters		100	80
lateral		50	70
skull lat.		50	80
Towne		125	85
Cervical, A.P.		50	65
Odontoid		50	72
Lateral		50	65
Thoracic, A.P.		70	85
Lumbar, A.P.		70	85
Extremities		10 $-$ 2 times cm., plus 40 Kv.P.	
no-screen		50 $-$ 3 times cm., plus 45 Kv.P.	

Courtesy — Clark R. Warren, R.T.

Appendix A. THE APPLICATION OF RADIOGRAPHIC FUNDAMENTALS

A general review

A good radiograph is the net result of favorable conditions with respect to two basic physical factors; *contrast* and *definition* (detail). Contrast is determined by the *relative intensities* in the x-ray image pattern which reaches the film. These are determined primarily by subject contrast, the ratio of relative opacity to x-rays between parts of the object under consideration. This in turn, determines how this pattern will be rendered as radiographic densities.

Definition or detail is affected by *screen resolution* (which is determined by the size of the crystals in the intensifying screens), *graininess* in the emulsion on the film, unsharpness due to *motion* of the body part, and *penumbra* due to geometric conditions.

It cannot be said that definition is more important than contrast or vice versa, for in a radiograph with insufficient contrast, brightnesses over the area are too nearly the same for satisfactory discrimination, while with poor definition, areas of different densities merge into one another so gradually that the diffuse image cannot be interpreted.

Experiment

A number of radiographs of the skull in lateral projection were made with various changes in order to study the affects of *detail, density, distortion,* and *contrast*. The same subject was used in all examinations, as well as the same cassette and screens.

Figures A.1 to A.15. Radiographs of the skull. To be correlated with the film numbers in Table A.1.

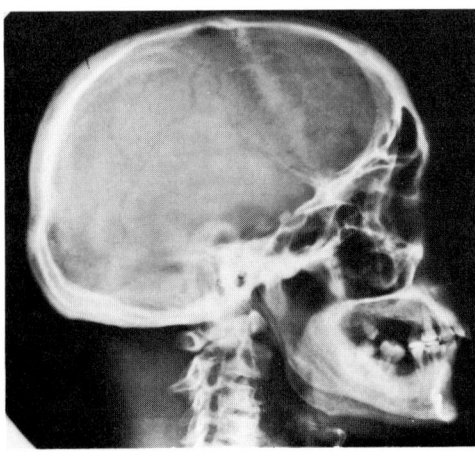

Figure A.1

Appendix A

Densitometer readings were made for all radiographs and as a check, additional radiographs were made to substantiate the original data. It should be noted, the illustrations do not indicate the true contrast and density of the original radiographs.

A satisfactory lateral radiograph of the skull, Figure A.1 was made employing the following factors:

1 mm focal spot	36-inch focus-film distance	Regular film
Medium screens	100 Ma.	Cone: to part
8-to-1 ratio Bucky	$1/_{10}$ second (10 Ma.S.)	2 mm Al filter
	85 Kv.P.	

Development: 5 minutes at 68 degrees F.

A number of changes in the *above factors,* to be made one at a time *without compensation* are suggested below. Opposite each suggested change, indicate the effect you believe it would have on each of the radiographic qualities listed.

Table A.1 CHANGES TO BE MADE

Film no.	Change	Detail	Density	Density reading	Contrast	Magnification or distortion	Measurement of nickel
1.	Normal			.65			2.8 cm
2.	Develop 5 minutes at 75 degrees	−	+	.77	−	0	2.8
3.	Use 48 inch focus-film distance	−	−	.4	−	−	2.7
4.	Increase object-film distance, 4 inches	−		.62	−	+	3.2
5.	Use 2-mm focal spot (at 10 Ma.S.)	−	+	.78	−	0	2.8
6.	Tabletop non-Bucky	−	+	2	−	−	2.75
7.	Use 58 Kv.P.	−	−	.27	−	0	2.8
8.	Use cylinder cone	−	−	.62	−	0	2.8
9.	200 Ma.	−	+	1.1	−	0	2.8
10.	16-to-1 ratio Bucky	−	−	.49	−	0	2.8
11.	100 Kv.P.	−	+	1.32	−	0	2.8
12.	3.33 Ma.S.	−	−	.25	−	0	2.8
13.	4-mm Al filtration	−	−	.55	−	0	2.8
14.	Develop 2 minutes at 68 degrees	−	−	.31	−	0	2.8
15.	Use 30-inch focus-film distance	−	+	.95	−	+	2.9

FORMULATING X-RAY TECHNIQUES

If any quality is *decreased* indicate by marking the appropriate square with a minus mark (−).

If any quality is *increased* indicate by marking the appropriate square with a plus mark (+).

If there is no change in a quality, mark with a zero (0).

Results:

The radiographs, reproduced as Figures A.2 through A.15, show the changes that occur with each suggested change in the chart. The densitometer reading for radiograph A.1 is .65. The density reading for radiographs A.2 through A.15 are shown in the chart.

To check on magnification, either increasing or decreasing, a nickel was measured and found to be 2.6 cm. A radiograph was then made with the nickel placed on a 2-inch square of paraffin. The radiographic image was then measured and found to be 2.8 cm. This was then used as a guide for evaluating the skull radiographs, regarding magnification and distortion.

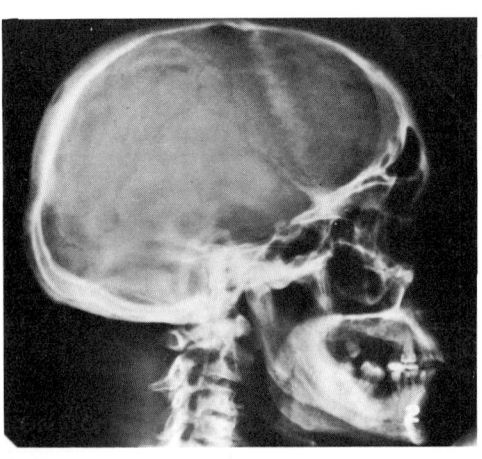

Figure A.2

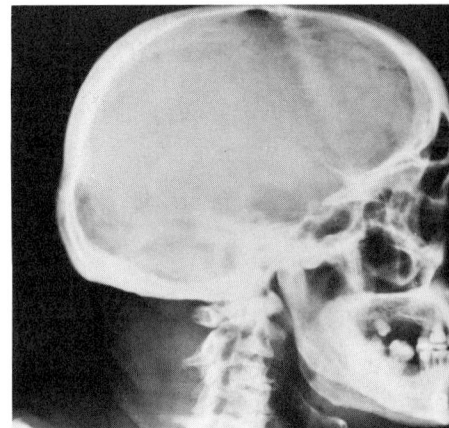

Figure A.3

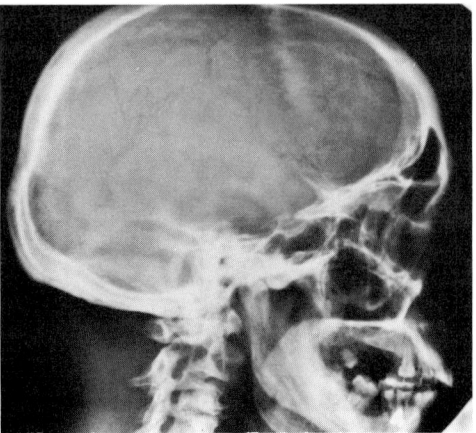

Figure A.4

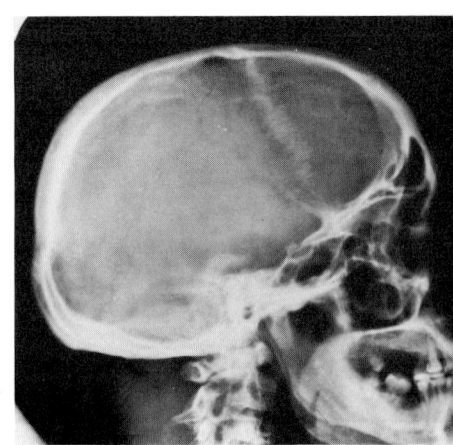

Figure A.5

Appendix A

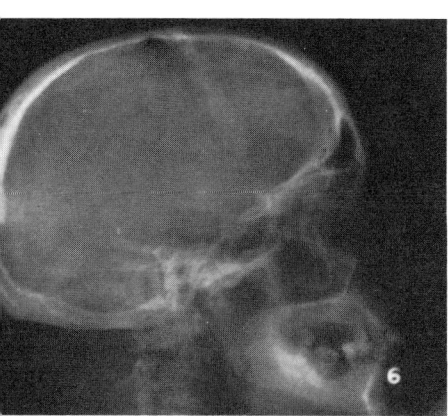

Figure A.6

Figure A.7

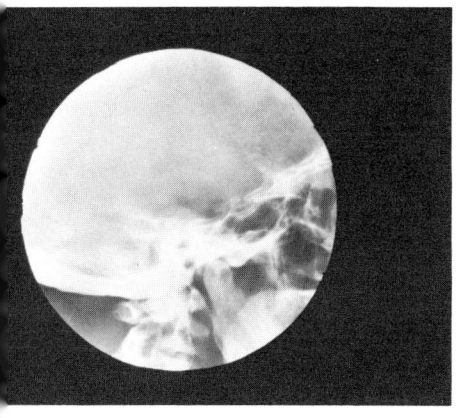

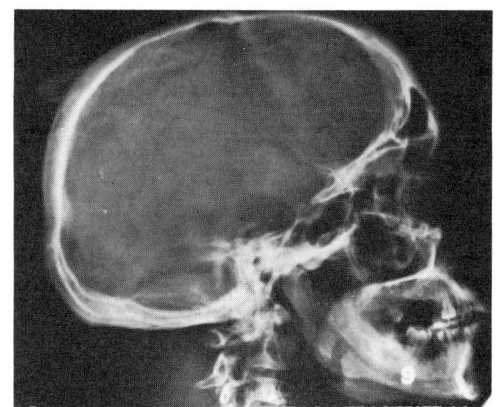

Figure A.8

Figure A.9

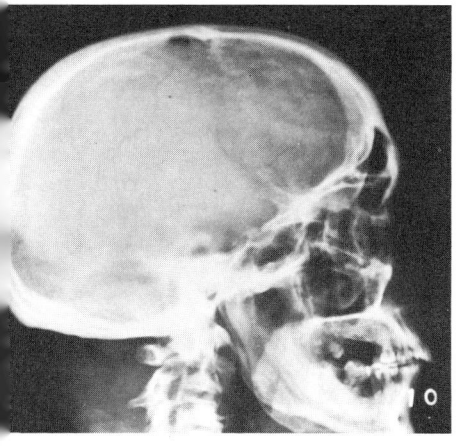

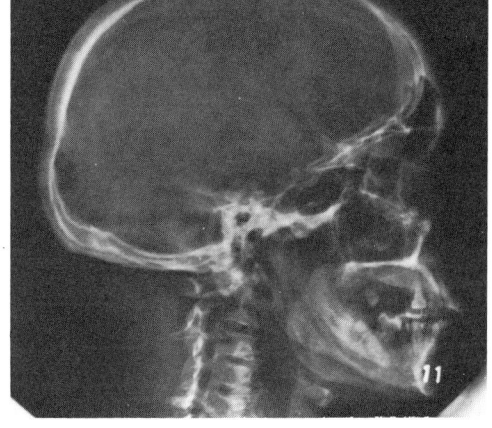

Figure A.10

Figure A.11

247

FORMULATING X-RAY TECHNIQUES

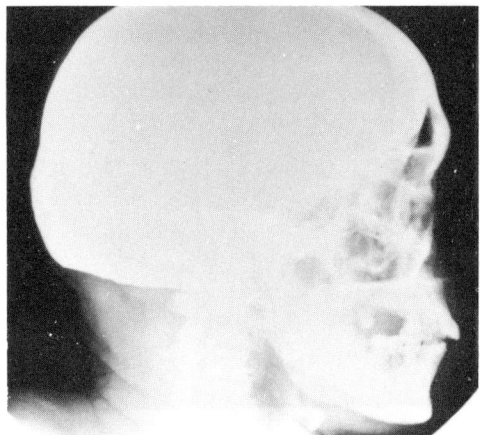

Figure A.12

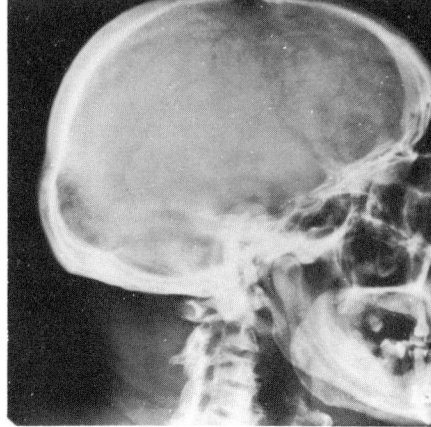

Figure A.13

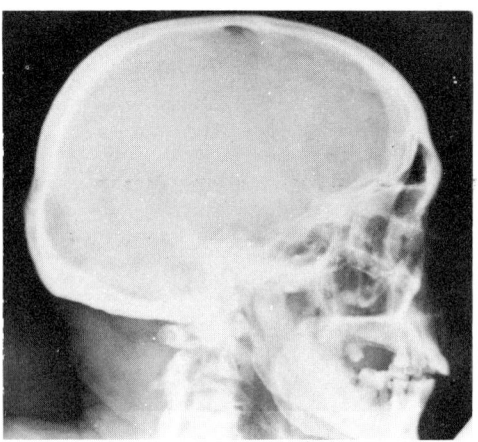

Figure A.14

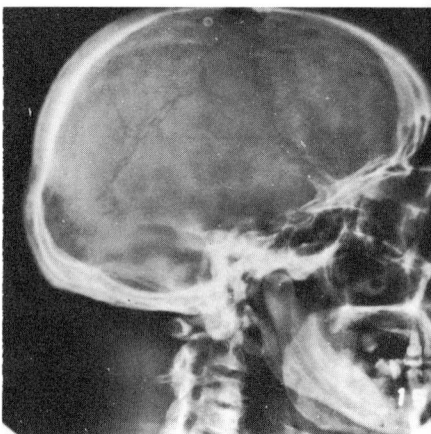

Figure A.15

Appendix B. SENSITOMETRY

Everyone engaged in radiologic technology or radiology wants to know how a particular film in use will react to x-rays, especially its sensitivity, its contrast, and the stability of these properties in practice.

When we are evaluating the quality of an x-ray film we generally test it in comparison with another type of x-ray film whose properties we already know. If we want to make an accurate comparison between two or more films to decide which would be best to use for a particular purpose — that is, we want to assign them quantitative values — we have to use a sensitometric method with bands or steps of density. This procedure consists of exposing successive stepped areas on the film, starting with the fog density, "no exposure," and going up to the maximum density obtainable. These exposures are so produced that the amount of radiation used can be accurately measured and varied as required.

After the film is processed the different degrees of blackening, or photographic densities, are measured, using a densitometer. A graph is drawn from these values, with the incident x-radiation plotted along the abscissa (the division of the horizontal scale). When the points so plotted are joined by a smooth curve, a "characteristic curve" of the film is obtained. This enables one to establish, by simply reading, the blackenings of the film in question and the amounts of radiation necessary to produce them. This curve will not be valid for exposure and development conditions which are markedly different from those used to make it. The shape of the characteristic curve, its slope, its horizontal position relative to the axis, and as a consequence, the values which it gives will vary considerably according to the conditions of development, the duration of exposure (reciprocity failure), and the tube voltage.

A characteristic curve is, in its production and its interpretation, much like a patient's temperature chart, which is also a graph with a horizontal axis (abscissa) and a vertical axis (ordinate). In the temperature chart, the hours of the day are set up along the abscissa and the patient's temperature is set up along the ordinate. When the points that have been plotted on the chart are joined with a line, we have the temperature curve. It is not necessary for the doctor to examine each individual point on the graph; a glance at the complete curve tells him instantly how the patient is progressing. It is much the same with the *characteristic curve*. Along the abscissa are plotted the x-ray dosages, while the densities produced are plotted in the vertical direction. The scale used along the abscissa can be graduated in several different ways: it can be divided into "r" units, in Ma.S. of exposure time for a given tube voltage, or thicknesses of an absorbent material such as aluminum, copper, or paraffin, to obtain an "absorption scale." In all cases successive steps of the film receive increasing amounts of x-radiation according

FORMULATING X-RAY TECHNIQUES

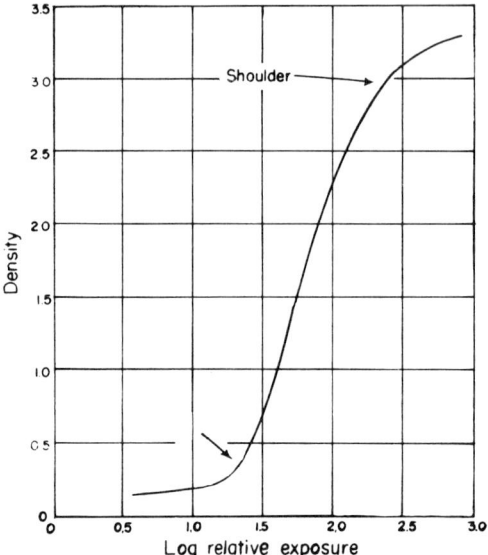

Figure B.1. The characteristic curve of a typical medical x-ray film, exposed with intensifying screens of calcium tungstate.

to a predetermined series. After development the film strip, a "stepped" set of densities is obtained—a sensitometric strip.

The simplest method is based on a time scale, that is, successive areas on the film are exposed for regularly increasing times, while all other factors are kept constant. The blackenings (densities) of the successive steps are measured on a *densitometer*. (Note that "fog" is density without any exposure; speed is expressed by the lateral position of the curve; and film contrast is determined by the slope of the curve.)

Qualitatively, the two basic factors that affect the density of a film are (1) exposure factors and (2) processing conditions. Each specific type of film has various characteristics, only one of which is its sensitivity to light or x-rays. If the film has a high sensitivity, then for a given rate of exposure the exposure time will be small; and the film is referred to as being *fast* or having a high speed. The speed of the film, or the efficiency with which the film responds to exposure, is determined by the amount of exposure that is necessary to produce a certain density after controlled processing. The sensitivity of the film to light or x-rays determines in turn the density of the finished product. Thus, the quantitative relationship between exposure, processing, and the inherent density qualities of film is determined by the measurement of the sensitivity of the film, i.e., the sensitometry. Sensitometry is defined as the "science of controlling exposure and processing and measurement of the resultant density." Those properties which influence the relationship between exposure, processing, and density are known as the sensitometric properties.

Appendix B

While a thorough understanding of sensitometery is not necessary to the radiologic technologist, a working knowledge of the sensitometric properties of all types of films is essential before undertaking any changes in radiographic techniques, making quantitative measurements, or determining which brand of film is best suited for individual departments.

Appendix C. RADIATION DOSE TO THE SKIN: OPTIMUM KILOVOLTAGE TECHNIQUE

Region	Projection	Thickness Range (cm.)	Mas.	Kv. Peak	Film Size	FFD (in.)	Skin Dose in (r) No Filter (corrected)	1 mm. Al	2 mm. Al	
Chest	Posteroanterior	18-20	3.33 S	80	14 × 17	72	.017	.009	.006	.C
		21-24	5 S	80	14 × 17	72	.025	.013	.009	.C
		25-27	6.66 S	80	14 × 17	72	.037	.019	.013	.C
	Oblique	19-23	5 S	80	14 × 17	72	.017	.013	.009	.C
		24-30	10 S	80	14 × 17	72	.056	.028	.019	.C
		31-35	15 S	80	14 × 17	72	.107	.054	.037	.C
	Lateral	-26	10 S	90	14 × 17	72	.064	.031	.021	.C
		27-32	13 S	90	14 × 17	72	.094	.044	.029	.C
		33-	15 S	90	14 × 17	72	.119	.052	.037	.C
Chest bronchi (w/opaque media)	Posteroanterior	20-24	10 SG	100	14 × 17	72	.074	.041	.026	.C
		25-27	15 SG	100	14 × 17	72	.115	.062	.040	.C
		28-30	20 SG	100	14 × 17	72	.159	.080	.055	.C
	Oblique	19-23	6.5 SG	100	14 × 17	72	.047	.025	.016	.
		24-30	20 SG	100	14 × 17	72	.157	.082	.055	.C
		31-35	30 SG	100	14 × 17	72	.292	.130	.092	.
	Lateral	24-27	15 SG	100	14 × 17	72	.115	.062	.041	.C
		28-29	25 SG	100	14 × 17	72	.199	.101	.069	.C
		30-34	30 SG	100	14 × 17	72	.291	.132	.092	.C
Chest bronchi (w/opaque media)	Posteroanterior	Child 2 to 10 yrs.	10 SG	76	11 × 14	60	.0670	.0327	.0222	.
	Oblique		10 SG	82	11 × 14	60	.0697	.0354	.0244	.C
	Lateral		10 SG	90	11 × 14	60	.0830	.0430	.0300	.
Chest bronchi (w/opaque media)	Posteroanterior	Infant	10 SG	70	8 × 10	60	.0562	.0265	.0155	.
	Oblique		10 SG	78	8 × 10	60	.0645	.0320	.0218	.
	Lateral		10 SG	86	8 × 10	60	.0727	.0374	.0259	.
Skull	Lateral	12	10 SG	85	10 × 12	36	.385	.177	.13	.
		13-17	15 SG	85	10 × 12	36	.563	.346	.214	.
		18	20 SG	85	10 × 12	36	.924	.458	.310	.
	Posteroanterior	17	15 SG	85	8 × 10	36	.676	.330	.227	.
		18-21	25 SG	85	8 × 10	36	1.21	.605	.398	.
		22	35 SG	85	8 × 10	36	1.85	.912	.580	.
	Anteroposterior	15	20 SG	85	8 × 10	36	.858	.406	.284	.
		16-23	30 SG	85	8 × 10	36	1.44	.725	.476	.
		24	40 SG	85	8 × 10	36	2.16	1.10	.698	.
	Towne	17	40 SG	85	8 × 10	36	1.80	.885	.605	.
		18-24	50 SG	85	8 × 10	36	2.56	1.26	.812	.
		25 Cylinder cone	60 SG	85	8 × 10	36	3.39	1.40	1.06	.

Appendix C

Region	Projection	Thickness Range (cm.)	Mas.	Kv. Peak	Film Size	FFD (in.)	Skin Dose in (r)			
							No Filter (corrected)	1 mm. Al	2 mm. Al	3 mm. Al
	Mento-Vertex	19	40 SG	85	8 × 10	36	1.90	.951	.634	.456
		20-25	50 SG	85	8 × 10	36	2.66	1.31	.835	.642
		26	60 SG	85	8 × 10	36	3.43	1.76	1.08	.810
oid	Law	12	10 SG	85	8 × 10	30	.539	.240	.148	.115
		13-17	15 SG	85	8 × 10	30	1.02	.593	.285	.203
		18 Cylinder cone	20 SG	85	8 × 10	30	1.58	.665	.440	.320
	Stenvers	17	15 SG	85	8 × 10	30	1.017	.593	.285	.203
		18-21 Cylinder cone	20 SG	85	8 × 10	30	1.58	.665	.440	.320
c	Posteroanterior	17	10 SG	85	8 × 10	30	.676	.395	.190	.135
		18-21	20 SG	85	8 × 10	30	1.58	.665	.440	.320
		22 Cylinder cone	25 SG	85	8 × 10	30	2.27	.925	.600	.432
dible	Posteroanterior	17	10 SG	85	8 × 10	30	.676	.395	.190	.135
		18-21	15 SG	85	8 × 10	30	1.20	.497	.330	.240
		22 Cylinder cone	20 SG	85	8 × 10	30	1.81	.740	.500	.360
	Lateral	9	2.5 S	70	8 × 10	30	.094	.036	.023	.014
		10-14 Cylinder cone	5 S	70	8 × 10	30	.212	.085	.052	.035
es	Lateral	12	2.5 S	70	8 × 10	30	.097	.039	.024	.016
		13-17	5 S	70	8 × 10	30	.242	.092	.059	.039
		18 Cylinder cone	7.5 S	70	8 × 10	30	.451	.170	.105	.075
	Caldwell	17	20 S	70	8 × 10	30	.968	.368	.236	.156
		18-21	25 S	70	8 × 10	30	1.49	.565	.350	.250
		22 Cylinder cone	30 S	70	8 × 10	30	2.14	.780	.498	.360
	Sphenoid	17	20 S	70	8 × 10	30	.968	.368	.236	.156
		18-22	30 S	70	8 × 10	30	1.80	.678	.420	.300
		23 Cylinder cone	40 S	70	8 × 10	30	2.86	1.04	.665	.480
	Maxillary	17	20 S	70	8 × 10	30	.968	.368	.236	.156
		18-22	30 S	70	8 × 10	30	1.80	.678	.420	.300
		23 Cylinder cone	40 S	70	8 × 10	30	2.86	1.04	.665	.480
ical spine	Anteroposterior	11	10 SG	80	8 × 10	36	.325	.148	.102	.077
		12-15	15 SG	80	8 × 10	36	.566	.261	.171	.128
		16	20 SG	80	8 × 10	36	.805	.388	.254	.176
	Lateral	9	6.5 S	85	8 × 10	72	.040	.016	.012	.087
		10-13	15 S	85	8 × 10	72	.084	.038	.027	.019
		14	20 S	85	8 × 10	72	.108	.051	.034	.026
	Oblique	9	7.5 S	85	8 × 10	72	.047	.018	.014	.010
		10-13	15 S	85	8 × 10	72	.084	.038	.027	.019
		14	20 S	85	8 × 10	72	.108	.051	.034	.026

FORMULATING X-RAY TECHNIQUES

Region	Projection	Thickness Range (cm.)	Mas.	Kv. Peak	Film Size	FFD (in.)	Skin Dose in (r)			
							No Filter (corrected)	1 mm. Al	2 mm. Al	3 mm. Al
Dorsal spine	Anteroposterior	19	40 SG	75	7 × 17	36	1.56	.685	.462	.31
		20-24	60 SG	75	7 × 17	36	2.55	1.163	.733	.50
		25	80 SG	75	7 × 17	36	3.78	1.710	1.040	.74
	Lateral	30	50 SG	80	7 × 17	36	3.76	1.55	1.07	.75
		31-34	100 SG	80	7 × 17	36	8.25	3.37	2.32	1.60
		35	150 SG	80	7 × 17	36	14.3	6.0	3.75	2.62
Lumbar spine	Anteroposterior	17	60 SG	65	10 × 12	36	1.74	.625	.456	.29
		18-22	80 SG	70	10 × 12	36	2.90	1.23	.784	.52
		23	100 SG	70	10 × 12	36	4.02	1.74	1.050	.73
	Oblique	17	60 SG	75	8 × 10	36	2.15	.940	.638	.43
		18-22	80 SG	75	8 × 10	36	3.22	1.58	.940	.64
		23	100 SG	75	8 × 10	36	4.51	2.12	1.27	.90
	Lateral	26	100 SG	85	10 × 12	36	6.60	3.12	2.10	1.50
		27-32	200 SG	85	10 × 12	36	17.6	7.00	4.88	3.50
		33	250 SG	85	10 × 12	36	25.19	10.3	6.85	4.80
	Lateral L-5	26	125 SG	85	8 × 10	36	7.15	3.67	2.25	1.75
		27-32	225 SG	85	8 × 10	36	18.59	7.88	5.50	3.94
		33 Cylinder cone	275 SG	85	8 × 10	36	27.72	10.3	7.80	5.28
Pelvis	Anteroposterior	15-19	80 SG	70	14 × 17	36	2.76	1.17	.768	.50
		20-23	100 SG	70	14 × 17	36	3.80	1.66	.99	.69
		24	125 SG	70	14 × 17	36	5.00	2.15	1.32	.91
Hip	Anteroposterior	15-19	80 SG	70	10 × 12	36	2.76	1.17	.768	.50
		20-23	100 SG	70	10 × 12	36	3.80	1.66	.99	.69
		24	125 SG	70	10 × 12	36	5.00	2.15	1.32	.91
	Lateral	19	125 SG	80	8 × 10	36	5.34	2.43	1.68	1.04
		20-24	150 SG	80	8 × 10	36	7.18	3.36	2.31	1.50
		25	175 SG	80	8 × 10	36	9.13	4.28	2.73	2.05
Abdomen	Anteroposterior	15-19	75 SG	70	14 × 17	36	2.58	1.10	.720	.47
		20-23	100 SG	70	14 × 17	36	3.80	1.66	.99	.69
		24-26	125 SG	70	14 × 17	36	5.00	2.15	1.32	.91
	Lateral	26	75 SG	80	14 × 17	36	3.87	1.83	1.17	.88
		27-32	100 SG	80	14 × 17	36	7.53	3.10	2.14	1.50
		33	125 SG	80	14 × 17	36	11.33	4.38	3.05	2.09
Gallbladder	Posteroanterior	14-17	20 SG	75	10 × 12	36	.720	.314	.213	.14
		18-22	30 SG	75	10 × 12	36	1.21	.594	.352	.24
		23-25	60 SG	75	10 × 12	36	2.70	1.27	.765	.54
Colon	Posteroanterior; anteroposterior	15-17	20 SG	85	14 × 17	36	.88	.420	.294	.21
		18-22	40 SG	85	14 × 17	36	1.98	.983	.642	.47
		23-25	80 SG	85	14 × 17	36	4.35	2.21	1.39	1.09
	Air contrast	15-17	5 SG	95	14 × 17	36	.280	.142	.097	.07
		18-21	10 SG	95	14 × 17	36	.620	.334	.212	.17
		22-25	20 SG	100	14 × 17	36	1.45	.860	.520	.41

Appendix C

Region	Projection	Thickness Range (cm.)	Mas.	Kv. Peak	Film Size	FFD (in.)	Skin Dose in (r)			
							No Filter (corrected)	1 mm. Al	2 mm. Al	3 mm. Al
	Chassard Lapine	Small	50 SG	100	14 × 17	36	3.75	2.26	1.28	1.13
		Medium	80 SG	100	14 × 17	36	8.58	4.16	2.80	2.16
		Large	100 SG	100	14 × 17	36	13.75	6.10	4.14	2.95
vis lvimetry)	Anteroposterior; supine	20-23	100 SG	75	14 × 17	36	4.46	1.94	1.22	0.84
		24-28	150 SG	75	14 × 17	36	7.09	3.21	1.95	1.43
		29-33	200 SG	75	14 × 17	36	13.64	5.24	3.68	2.52
vis Thoms	Anteroposterior Thoms	Small	100 SG	100	10 × 12	36	7.21	3.94	2.45	2.05
		Medium	150 SG	100	10 × 12	36	11.28	6.79	3.83	3.39
		Large	200 SG	100	10 × 12	36	21.45	10.40	7.00	5.40
	Lateral	Small	80 SG	100	14 × 17	36	5.80	3.44	2.08	1.64
		Medium	100 SG	100	14 × 17	36	9.62	4.87	3.32	2.47
		Large	150 SG	100	14 × 17	36	18.15	8.26	5.80	4.20
centa	Lateral	Small	12.5 SG	100	14 × 17	36	.907	.538	.325	.256
		Medium	25 SG	100	14 × 17	36	2.41	1.22	.830	.620
		Large	40 SG	100	14 × 17	36	4.84	2.20	1.54	1.12
nd	Posteroanterior	2	40 F	50	8 × 10	36	.588	.168	.092	.074
		3 - 5	50 F	50	8 × 10	36	.761	.225	.125	.100
		6	60 F	50	8 × 10	36	.957	.287	.162	.126
	Lateral	7-10	120 F	50	8 × 10	36	1.958	.61	.36	.264
		11	150 F	50	8 × 10	36	2.68	.88	.51	.36
ulder	Anteroposterior	9-11	7.5 SG	80	8 × 10	36	.249	.108	.075	.053
		12-16	12.5 SG	80	8 × 10	36	.478	.217	.146	.105
		17-18	15 SG	80	8 × 10	36	.640	.291	.201	.132
	Lateral	5	60 F	60	10 × 12	36	1.15	.36	.24	.18
		6 - 9	70 F	60	10 × 12	36	1.46	.455	.336	.228
		10	80 F	60	10 × 12	36	1.64	.687	.384	.256
calcis	Axial	4 - 8	60 F	80	8 × 10	36	1.95	.75	.55	.398
		9-13	100 F	80	8 × 10	36	3.52	1.56	1.13	.75
		14-18	125 F	80	8 × 10	36	5.02	2.30	1.60	1.10
a-fibula	Anteroposterior	8	5 SG	80	7 × 17	36	.170	.065	.05	.034
		9-12	10 SG	80	7 × 17	36	.33	.144	.100	.070
		13	15 SG	80	7 × 17	36	.574	.261	.176	.126
	Lateral	7	2.5 SG	80	7 × 17	36	.077	.031	.022	.017
		8-11	3.2 SG	80	7 × 17	36	.105	.046	.032	.023
		12	5 SG	80	7 × 17	36	.574	.078	.056	.038
e	Anteroposterior	9	5 SG	80	8 × 10	36	.170	.065	.05	.034
		10-14	6.5 SG	80	8 × 10	36	.229	.101	.073	.049
		15	10 SG	80	8 × 10	36	.401	.184	.128	.088
	Lateral	8	5 SG	80	8 × 10	36	.170	.065	.05	.034
		9-13	6.5 SG	80	8 × 10	36	.229	.101	.073	.049
		14	7.5 SG	80	8 × 10	36	.301	.138	.096	.066
nach vith barium)	Right anteroposterior	15-17	20 SG	90	10 × 12	36	1.02	.500	.340	.262
		18-22	40 SG	85	10 × 12	36	2.02	.982	.641	.477
		23-26	80 SG	85	10 × 12	36	4.34	2.21	1.38	1.09

Appendix D. RADIATION DOSE TO THE SKIN: TISSUE MEASUREMENT TECHNIQUE

Region	Projection	Thickness Range (cm.)	Mas.	Kv. Peak	Film Size	FFD (in.)	Skin Dose in (r)			
							No Filter (corrected)	1 mm. Al	2 mm. Al	3 mm. Al
Chest	Posteroanterior	18	10 S	62	14 × 17	72	.037	.017	.011	.00
		21	10 S	68	14 × 17	72	.045	.021	.014	.01
		27	10 S	78	14 × 17	72	.054	.027	.018	.01
	Oblique	19	20 S	64	14 × 17	72	.079	.037	.024	.01
		24	20 S	74	14 × 17	72	.097	.047	.032	.02
		31	20 S	90	14 × 17	72	.137	.071	.050	.03
	Lateral	26	20 S	78	14 × 17	72	.109	.054	.037	.02
		29	20 S	84	14 × 17	72	.122	.062	.043	.03
		32	20 S	90	14 × 17	72	.137	.071	.050	.03
Chest bronchi (w/opaque media)	Posteroanterior	18	10 S	67	14 × 17	72	.043	.020	.013	.01
		21	10 S	73	14 × 17	72	.046	.022	.015	.01
		27	10 S	83	14 × 17	72	.058	.030	.020	.01
	Oblique	19	20 S	70	14 × 17	72	.090	.042	.028	.02
		24	20 S	82	14 × 17	72	.116	.059	.040	.03
		31	20 S	95	14 × 17	72	.144	.076	.052	.0
	Lateral	26	20 S	85	14 × 17	72	.119	.061	.042	.03
		27	20 S	90	14 × 17	72	.130	.068	.048	.0
		32	20 S	98	14 × 17	72	.152	.080	.057	.0
Skull	Lateral	12	60 SG	56	10 × 12	36	1.17	.432	.258	.14
		14	60 SG	60	10 × 12	36	1.36	.540	.318	.2
		18	60 SG	68	10 × 12	36	1.98	.842	.546	.3
	Posteroanterior	17	100 SG	66	8 × 10	36	3.00	1.26	.81	.5
		19	100 SG	70	8 × 10	36	3.53	1.53	.98	.6
		22	100 SG	76	8 × 10	36	4.32	2.02	1.28	.8
	Anteroposterior	15	100 SG	62	8 × 10	36	2.53	1.00	.62	.4
		19	100 SG	70	8 × 10	36	3.53	1.53	.98	.6
		24	100 SG	80	8 × 10	36	4.96	2.32	1.50	1.1
	Towne	17	125 SG	66	8 × 10	36	3.75	1.57	1.01	.6
		19	125 SG	70	8 × 10	36	4.42	1.91	1.10	.8
		25	125 SG	82	8 × 10	36	6.55	3.34	1.74	1.6
	Mento-Vertex	19	125 SG	70	8 × 10	36	4.43	1.91	1.10	.8
		21	125 SG	74	8 × 10	36	5.09	2.30	1.45	.9
		26	125 SG	84	8 × 10	36	8.35	3.49	2.15	1.7
Mastoid	Law	12	60 SG	56	8 × 10	30	1.75	.60	.336	.2
		14	60 SG	60	8 × 10	30	2.18	.770	.462	.2
		17 Cylinder cone	60 SG	66	8 × 10	30	2.88	1.056	.661	.4

Appendix D

Region	Projection	Thickness Range (cm.)	Mas.	Kv. Peak	Film Size	FFD (in.)	Skin Dose in (r)			
							No Filter (corrected)	1 mm. Al	2 mm. Al	3 mm. Al
oid	Stenvers	17	80 SG	66	8 × 10	30	3.85	1.408	.881	.576
		18	80 SG	68	8 × 10	30	4.20	1.58	.994	.680
		21 Cylinder cone	80 SG	74	8 × 10	30	5.49	2.18	1.375	.978
c	Posteroanterior	17	80 SG	66	8 × 10	30	3.85	1.408	.881	.576
		18	80 SG	68	8 × 10	30	4.20	1.58	.994	.680
		21	80 SG	74	8 × 10	30	5.49	2.18	1.375	.978
dible	Posteroanterior	15	100 SG	62	8 × 10	30	3.97	1.40	.86	.53
		18	100 SG	88	8 × 10	30	5.25	1.98	1.24	.85
		21	100 SG	74	8 × 10	30	6.85	2.73	1.72	1.22
	Lateral	9	10 S	50	8 × 10	30	.226	.067	.036	.022
		10	10 S	52	8 × 10	30	.245	.074	.072	.026
		12 Cylinder cone	10 S	56	8 × 10	30	.294	.100	.096	.035
ses	Lateral	9	20 S	36	8 × 10	30	.303	.074	.034	.012
		13	20 S	44	8 × 10	30	.520	.142	.072	.044
		16 Cylinder cone	20 S	50	8 × 10	30	.560	.168	.096	.050
	Caldwell	17	80 S	66	8 × 10	30	3.85	1.408	.881	.576
		18	80 S	68	8 × 10	30	4.20	1.58	.994	.680
		22 Cylinder cone	80 S	76	8 × 10	30	6.02	2.30	1.52	1.04
	Maxillary	17	80 S	66	8 × 10	30	3.85	1.408	.881	.576
		18	80 S	68	8 × 10	30	4.20	1.58	.994	.680
		22	80 S	76	8 × 10	30	6.02	2.30	1.52	1.04
ical spine	Anteroposterior	10	100 SG	52	8 × 10	36	1.83	.59	.32	.23
		13	100 SG	58	8 × 10	36	2.15	.81	.48	.34
		16	100 SG	64	8 × 10	36	2.68	1.12	.70	.48
	Lateral	9	40 S	50	8 × 10	72	.096	.041	.023	.015
		12	40 S	56	8 × 10	72	.121	.053	.032	.022
		14	40 S	60	8 × 10	72	.136	.062	.039	.027
	Oblique	9	40 S	50	8 × 10	72	.096	.041	.023	.015
		12	40 S	56	8 × 10	72	.121	.053	.032	.022
		14	40 S	60	8 × 10	72	.136	.062	.039	.027
al spine	Anteroposterior	19	100 SG	70	7 × 17	36	3.53	1.53	.98	.64
		21	100 SG	74	7 × 17	36	4.07	1.84	1.16	.79
		25	100 SG	82	7 × 17	36	5.23	2.67	1.65	1.29
	Lateral	30	150 SG	66	7 × 17	36	4.50	1.89	1.21	.797
		32	150 SG	70	7 × 17	36	5.30	2.30	1.47	.960
		35	150 SG	76	7 × 17	36	6.48	3.03	1.92	1.32
bar spine	Anteroposterior	17	100 SG	66	10 × 12	36	3.00	1.26	.81	.53
		19	100 SG	70	10 × 12	36	3.53	1.53	.98	.64
		23	100 SG	78	10 × 12	36	4.72	2.17	1.39	.99

FORMULATING X-RAY TECHNIQUES

Region	Projection	Thickness Range (cm.)	Mas.	Kv. Peak	Film Size	FFD (in.)	Skin Dose in (r)			
							No Filter (corrected)	1 mm. Al	2 mm. Al	3 mm Al
Lumbar Spine	Oblique	17	100 SG	66	10 × 12	36	3.00	1.26	.81	.53
		19	100 SG	70	10 × 12	36	3.53	1.53	.98	.64
		23	100 SG	78	10 × 12	36	4.72	2.17	1.39	.99
	Lateral	26	200 SG	84	10 × 12	36	11.12	5.84	3.60	2.96
		28	200 SG	88	10 × 12	36	15.80	7.50	5.10	3.50
		33	200 SG	98	10 × 12	36	25.3	11.50	9.90	5.72
	Spot L-5	26	250 SG	84	8 × 10	33	21.2	9.05	6.20	4.33
		28	250 SG	88	8 × 10	33	26.0	10.4	7.22	5.73
		33	250 SG	98	8 × 10	33	38.7	18.20	12.7	9.85
Pelvis	Anteroposterior	15	100 SG	62	14 × 17	36	2.49	1.0	.62	.43
		20	100 SG	72	14 × 17	36	3.74	1.66	1.05	.70
		24	100 SG	80	14 × 17	36	4.98	2.32	1.50	1.10
Hip	Anteroposterior	15	100 SG	62	14 × 17	36	2.49	1.0	.62	.43
		20	100 SG	72	14 × 17	36	3.74	1.66	1.05	.70
		24	100 SG	80	14 × 17	36	4.98	2.32	1.50	1.10
	Lateral	19	100 SG	70	8 × 10	36	3.53	1.53	.98	.64
		22	100 SG	76	8 × 10	36	4.30	2.02	1.28	.88
		25	100 SG	82	8 × 10	36	5.22	2.67	1.65	1.29
Abdomen	Anteroposterior	15	80 SG	62	14 × 17	36	1.99	.80	.496	.34
		20	80 SG	72	14 × 17	36	3.99	1.33	.842	.56
		25	80 SG	82	14 × 17	36	4.18	2.13	1.32	1.03
	Lateral	26	80 SG	78	14 × 17	36	3.78	1.74	1.10	.79
		28	80 SG	82	14 × 17	36	5.65	2.60	1.68	1.16
		32	80 SG	92	14 × 17	36	8.35	3.70	2.56	1.84
Gall bladder	Posteroanterior	14	80 SG	60	10 × 12	36	1.82	.720	.424	.30
		19	80 SG	70	10 × 12	36	2.83	1.23	.784	.51
		23	80 SG	78	10 × 12	36	3.78	1.74	1.11	.79
Colon (air contrast)	Anteroposterior; posteroanterior	16	20 SG	88	14 × 17	36	.979	.468	.320	.24
		21	40 SG	88	14 × 17	36	2.13	1.08	.70	.53
		27	80 SG	90	14 × 17	36	5.75	2.84	1.92	1.38
Pelvis (Pelvimetry)	Anteroposterior; supine	20	100 SG	72	14 × 17	36	3.74	1.66	1.05	.70
		28	100 SG	88	14 × 17	36	7.76	3.75	2.54	1.75
		33	100 SG	98	14 × 17	36	13.1	5.62	3.90	2.85
Pelvis	Anteroposterior Thoms	24	200 SG	80	10 × 12	36	9.94	4.64	3.00	2.20
		30	200 SG	92	10 × 12	36	18.7	8.60	5.80	4.30
		35	200 SG	100	10 × 12	36	27.5	12.2	8.28	5.80
	Lateral	26	200 SG	84	10 × 12	36	11.1	5.84	3.60	2.96
		30	200 SG	92	10 × 12	36	18.7	8.60	5.80	4.30
		34	200 SG	100	10 × 12	36	27.5	12.2	8.28	5.80
Hand	Posteroanterior	2	50 NS	36	8 × 10	36	.403	.10	.04	.02
		4	50 NS	40	8 × 10	36	.515	.14	.06	.03
		6	50 NS	44	8 × 10	36	.625	.18	.10	.06

Appendix D

Region	Projection	Thickness Range (cm.)	Mas.	Kv. Peak	Film Size	FFD (in.)	Skin Dose in (r)			
							No Filter (corrected)	1 mm. Al	2 mm. Al	.3 mm. Al
...d	Lateral	7	50 NS	46	8 × 10	36	.678	.20	.10	.06
		11	50 NS	52	8 × 10	36	.915	.29	.16	.12
...lder	Anteroposterior	9	50 NS	52	8 × 10	36	.915	.29	.16	.12
		12	50 NS	56	8 × 10	36	.975	.36	.215	.145
		17	50 NS	66	8 × 10	36	1.50	.63	.405	.265
...calcis	Axial	7	50 NS	46	8 × 10	36	.678	.20	.10	.06
		10	50 NS	52	8 × 10	36	.915	.29	.16	.12
		15	50 NS	62	8 × 10	36	1.24	.50	.31	.215
...a-fibula	Anteroposterior	8	10 S	48	7 × 17	36	.150	.045	.024	.016
		11	10 S	52	7 × 17	36	.184	.059	.032	.023
		13	10 S	58	7 × 17	36	.216	.081	.048	.034
	Lateral	7	10 S	46	7 × 17	36	.136	.040	.021	.013
		10	10 S	52	7 × 17	36	.184	.059	.032	.023
		12	10 S	56	7 × 17	36	.196	.072	.043	.029
...e	Anteroposterior	9	10 S	48	8 × 10	36	.150	.045	.024	.016
		11	10 S	56	8 × 10	36	.208	.073	.047	.031
		15	10 S	62	8 × 10	36	.248	.100	.062	.043
	Lateral	8	10 S	48	8 × 10	36	.150	.045	.024	.016
		10	10 S	52	8 × 10	36	.184	.059	.032	.023
		14	10 S	60	8 × 10	36	.228	.090	.053	.038
...ach (w/barium)		18	40 SG	82	10 × 12	36	1.76	.862	.577	.392
		21	80 SG	88	10 × 12	36	4.27	2.16	1.40	1.07
		25	100 SG	86	10 × 12	36	6.75	3.25	2.18	1.55

F = Regular film with cardboard holder.
S = Medium speed screens, regular film.
G = 8:1 Lysholm grid and/or 8:1 Bucky grid.
SG = Medium speed screens and 8:1 Lysholm grid and/or 8:1 Bucky grid.
Technical Factors: Development, 5 min. at 68° F.; 2 mm. Al filtration; 4 valve tube full wave machine; cone to film.
F = Regular film with cardboard holder.
NS = Non-screen film with cardboard holder.
S = Medium speed screens.
SG = Medium speed screens and 8:1 Lysholm and/or 8:1 Bucky grid.
Technical Factors: Development, 5 min. at 68° F.; 2 mm. Al filtration; rotating anode tube; 4 valve tube full wave machine; cone to film.
The kilovoltage variation per centimeter thickness was determined by the formula kv. peak = 2×cm. thickness + 30

Appendix E. X-RAY UNIT TROUBLE SYMPTOMS

Symptoms	Probable causes	What to do
1. No x-ray (lights and meters on control do not indicate)	Line switch open	Check wall switch.
	Main fuse out	Have electrician check and replace fuse.
	Auxiliary fuse out in control	Same as above
2. No x-rays (lights and meters indicate but contactor does not close; no thump or noise in control)	Auxiliary fuse out in control	Same as above
	Timer motor not turned on	Check timer scale switch and setting.
	Timer set above safe exposure time (if equipped with safety limit switches)	Same as above
	Circuit breaker not pushed in	Check.
	Bucky not latched	Check and latch.
	Bucky electrical release defective	Set Bucky for longer time, attach string to manual release on Bucky, and release manually.
	Interlocking safety switches not properly set.	Recheck setting of all switches.
3. No x-ray (contactor closes but MA meter does not indicate)	Defective MA meter	Check for x-rays from tube by placing open cassette on table, darkening room and making exposure with tube directed toward screen. If no fluorescence is seen, follow checks below.
	X-ray tube filament not lighted	1. Check filament meter setting if there is one. 2. Observe tube filament through port with main switch on. 3. Check position of over-under table switch. 4. Check setting of focus selector switch if there is one. 5. Make sure that shockproof cables are properly attached at both x-ray tube and transformer.

Appendix E

Symptoms	Probable causes	What to do
		6. Flex cathode cable and observe tube filament with control turned on to check for broken lead in cable.
	KV selector on dead button or making poor contact	Check KV selectors and line compensation selector switch.
4. MA meter fluctuates	Loose connection of cathode cable either at x-ray tube or transformer	Check for loose connection of cable.
	Manual over-under table high tension switch making poor contact because of improperly meshed switch blades	Check and reset high-tension switch.
	Gassy x-ray tube Note: Slightly gassy x-ray tube can be operated at reduced MA temporarily, if MA meter holds constant at lower MA values.	Put mirror on table and direct x-ray tube toward it. Make exposure and watch for bluish-green fluorescence in x-ray tube.
	Varying power line. Observe KV line comp. and filament meters.	Consult power company and have one of its electricians make test with recording voltmeter.
	Improperly set focus switch if machine is equipped with one.	Check and reset switch.
5. MA meter indicates too low.	Improper filament setting	Check and reset switch.
	Valve filament burned out. Meter approx. $1/2$ value	If machine is equipped with valve tube filament meter, find out what proper indication should be. Low (25%) filament amperes means burned out valve filament. If no valve-filament meter is provided but valve tubes can be observed, check that all are lighted. If one valve is out, consult x-ray tube rating chart. (Caution! Use half-wave or self-rectified ratings and operate at reduced MA until valve tube is replaced.)
	Poor connection of cathode cable at x-ray tube or transformer	Check connections at both ends of cathode cable and make sure that they are tight.

FORMULATING X-RAY TECHNIQUES

Symptoms	Probable causes	What to do
6. MA meter indicates too high.	Defective MA meter or wrong meter scale	Recheck filament setting and scale if provided with manual switch.
	Filament setting too high	Check and reset filament control.
	Wrong meter scale	Check position of MA meter scale, change switch if machine is so equipped.
	Gassy x-ray tube (meter flicks up)	Place mirror on table and direct x-ray tube toward it. it. Make exposure and watch for bluish green fluorescence in x-ray tube.
	Improper filament setting due to aging of x-ray tube	Reduce filament setting until proper MA is obtained.
7. Circuit breaker pops or jumps out and opens up exposure circuit.	Filament setting too high resulting in excessive MA	Recheck filament setting.
	KV set too high	Recheck setting.
	Punctured shockproof cable	Examine both shockproof cables carefully over entire length for any evidence or odor of burning.
	Gassy x-ray tube	Examine x-ray tube with mirror as described previously.
	Gassy valve tube	Call for service.
8. Inconsistent radiographic results	Error in setting of technical factors	Recheck settings for MA.-Kv. Exposure time, distance, use or non-use of cones, grids, filters, angulation of x-ray tube.
	Error in measurement or estimation of size of part to be examined	Remeasure patient, taking into consideration variations in patient types.
	Variations in film speeds	
	Variations in screen speeds (screen contact)	
	Failure to observe time and temperature development	
	Exhausted developing solutions	Change solutions frequently.
	Erratic exposure timer	Check with spin top.

Appendix E

Symptoms	Probable causes	What to do
	Line voltage variation	Observe all meters on control panel during day to check for variations.
	Poor connecting in filament circuit	Check connections at both ends of cathode cable to make sure they are right.
	Partial shockproof cable puncture	Observe MA meter during long exposure (2 to 3 sec.). If it fluctuates rapidly examine both shockproof cables carefully over entire length for any evidence or odor of burning.
9. Synchronous grid lines — handlatch Buckys	Bucky time dial set too long	Adjust Bucky time dial to slightly different setting.
	Bucky time dial set too short	Adjust Bucky time dial to slightly different setting.
	Exposure time too short	
	Air in Bucky timing device	Aim x-ray tube away from table, remove cassette tray, make long (2–3 sec.) Bucky exposure while holding hand on grid to check for smooth operation.
	Identification marker catching on grid	
10. Grid lines — reciprocating Buckys	Selected exposure times too close to initial travel time	
	Identification marker catching on grid	

Present generators and how they relate to radiographic quality

The most widely used type of generator operates on a single-phase power line. When provided with full-wave rectification, its kilovoltage output fluctuates between zero and a peak value in a manner that produces two impulses per cycle.

A second type of generator operates on a three-phase power line. It uses twelve rectifiers and a full-wave circuit, and produces a pattern of six impulses per cycle.

A third type of generator also operates on the three-phase power line, and it uses twelve rectifiers and a full-wave circuit, that produces a power of twelve impulses per cycle. With this type of rectification, the kilovoltage can be considered to be almost constant.

GENERAL QUESTIONS

1. When making films to be viewed in a standard stereoscope, the amount of shift required is determined by the
    a. Focus-skin distance
    b. Focus-film distance
    c. Bucky-film distance
    d. Object-film distance
2. Magnification can be decreased by
    a. Increasing object-film distance
    b. Decreasing object-film distance
    c. Increasing Ma.S.
    d. Decreasing focus-film distance
3. Poor screen contact results in
    a. Half-moon shadows on the film
    b. Black streaks on the film
    c. Blurring of the radiographic image
    d. Decreased time in the developer
4. The greatest density would be obtained by using
    a. 25 Ma. and $1/15$ second
    b. 50 Ma. and $1/30$ second
    c. 100 Ma. and $1/60$ second
    d. 10 Ma. and $1/5$ second
5. The quantity of x-rays is dependent upon
    a. Kv.P.
    b. Ma.S.
    c. Ma.
    d. Time
6. When going from an 8-to-1 grid to a 16-to-1 grid, you should increase the Kv.P. by
    a. 4 Kv.P.
    b. 6 Kv.P.
    c. 12 Kv.P.
    d. 16 Kv.P.
7. When a 16-to-1 grid is employed, the distance that should be used is
    a. 36 inches
    b. 48 inches

General Questions

   c. 40 inches
   d. 72 inches

8. Artifacts on a finished radiograph result from
   a. Poor screen contact
   b. Rough handling of the film
   c. Insufficient Ma.S.
   d. Exhausted hypo

9. Which of the following directly influences the radiographic contrast?
   a. Ma.
   b. Ma.S.
   c. Kv.P.
   d. Time

10. Which of the following directly influences the radiographic density?
    a. Kv.P.
    b. Ma.
    c. Ma.S.
    d. Time

11. Which item below will increase the exposure to the patient's skin?
    a. Using the collimator
    b. 3 mm. of aluminum
    c. Low Kv.P. and High Ma.S.
    d. High Kv.P. and Low Ma.S.

12. Gamma radiation is measured by
    a. Voltmeter
    b. Ammeter
    c. Geiger counter
    d. Galvanometer

13. Which of the following would not require a sterile technique?
    a. Myelogram
    b. Urography
    c. Planogram
    d. Arteriogram

14. The quality of the x-ray beam is determined by
    a. The kilovoltage
    b. The Ma.S.
    c. The size of the focal spot
    d. The size of the target

15. A patient comes into your department with a foreign body of the abdomen. It would be better to
    a. Fluoroscope first
    b. Take a flat film of the abdomen first
    c. Operate first
    d. Put the patient to sleep first

265

FORMULATING X-RAY TECHNIQUES

16. Like poles of a magnet
    a. Repel each other
    b. Attract each other
    c. Do not affect each other
    d. Heat each other

17. When heat is applied to the filament of an x-ray tube
    a. Electrons are emitted
    b. X-rays are emitted
    c. Protons are emitted
    d. Neutrons are emitted

18. The time required to develop a film (manual processing) is dependent upon
    a. The amount of developer in the tank
    b. The size of the developing tank
    c. Temperature of the developer
    d. Temperature of the hypo

19. When doing a barium enema, the barium fluid should always be
    a. At least 6 feet above the table
    b. At least 3 feet above the table
    c. At least 9 feet above the table
    d. At least 12 feet above the table

20. The Ma. for a routine fluoroscopy should be
    a. 0.2 to 0.4 Ma.
    b. 3 to 5 Ma.
    c. 10 to 20 Ma.
    d. 5 to 8 Ma.

21. An arthrogram is a study of the
    a. Skull
    b. Kidneys
    c. Knee
    d. Eye

22. The primary purpose of a filter used in the diagnostic x-ray machine is
    a. To reduce contrast in the radiograph
    b. To reduce scattered radiation
    c. To reduce the skin dosage
    d. To increase the x-ray beam wave length

23. What is a *rad*?
    a. A unit of electrical pressure
    b. The basic measurement of radiation absorbed by living tissue
    c. A measurement of a designated portion of the primary x-ray beam
    d. A unit of electrical resistance

24. The chief advantage of high Kv.P. (over 100) in radiographs of heavy people is
    a. To reduce the exposure time
    b. To decrease latitude

General Questions

    c. To increase penetration
    d. To improve contrast

25. Density in a radiograph is
    a. Differences between the black and whites
    b. Over-all blackness of the radiograph
    c. The amount of distortion of the object
    d. Clearness and sharpness of the image

26. What is a teleoroentgenogram?
    a. A.P. view of the right hip
    b. P.A. chest film taken at 72" distance
    c. Lateral view of the odontoid
    d. Lateral view of the chest at 36" distance

27. Which of the following is not a portion of the colon?
    a. Cecum
    b. Transverse colon
    c. Sigmoid
    d. Ilium

28. Which of the following terms is not used to measure radiation?
    a. Rads
    b. Milliroentgen
    c. Milliamperes
    d. Roentgen

29. Name the tissue that is more sensitive to radiation
    a. Brain
    b. Skin
    c. Muscle
    d. Gonads

30. The primary function of Ma.S. is to
    a. Increase detail
    b. Increase penetration
    c. Improve contrast
    d. Regulate density

31. Long exposures are used to the best advantage during an examination of the
    a. Chest and heart
    b. A.P. abdomen
    c. Lateral cervical spine
    d. Lateral dorsal spine

32. In the A.P. projection of the lumbar-sacral articulation, the central ray is projected
    a. Caudad 10°
    b. Caudad 15° to 35°
    c. Cephalad 15° to 35°
    d. Cephalad 5°

FORMULATING X-RAY TECHNIQUES

33. In the P.A. Caldwell projection of the frontal sinuses, the central ray is angled caudad
    a. 10°
    b. 15°
    c. 23°
    d. 30°

34. In order to flatten and straighten the spine, an A.P. projection of the lumbar-sacral spine is taken with
    a. The knees and feet together
    b. The knees flexed and feet flat on the table
    c. The knees extended and toes internally rotated
    d. The patient sitting up

35. Elon has what function in the developer (manual)?
    a. As preserver
    b. As restrainer
    c. As alkali or activator
    d. As developing or reducing agent

36. Potassium bromide has what function in the developer (manual)?
    a. Fixing
    b. Washing
    c. Restraining
    d. Activating

37. What is the optimum time-temperature for the development of maximum contrast in the radiograph in manual processing?
    a. 3 minutes at 68°
    b. 4 minutes at 63°
    c. 5 minutes at 68°
    d. 6 minutes at 69°

38. What type of filter is used over the safelights in the darkroom?
    a. Wratten 5-B
    b. Wratten 10-B
    c. Wratten 6-B
    d. Bratten 6-B

39. What is the purpose of potassium alum in the fixer solution (manual)?
    a. To acidify the solution
    b. To preserve the film
    c. To fix the film
    d. To harden the film

40. How often should you change the developer (manual)?
    a. When you are told to do so
    b. When you run out of replenisher
    c. When fixation occurs
    d. When oxidation occurs

General Questions

41. Chemical fog is caused by
    a. Overexposure to x-rays
    b. Light leaks
    c. Aged developer
    d. Improper coning

42. Stains on intensifying screens caused by darkroom chemicals (manual)
    a. Will have no effect on the finished radiograph
    b. Will cause light spots on the finished radiograph
    c. Will cause black spots on the finished radiograph
    d. Will not affect the quality of the intensifying screens

43. What is the purpose of the stop bath (manual)?
    a. To activate the developer
    b. To stop the developing process
    c. To add acetic acid to the fixer
    d. To preserve the film

44. A grayish yellowish strip at one end of the film is caused by
    a. High developing level
    b. High hypo level
    c. Low developing level
    d. Low hypo level

45. Small white marks on the finished radiograph may be caused by
    a. Static because of impact
    b. Dirty cassettes
    c. Inadequate washing after hypo
    d. Hot solutions

46. A strip of transparent film at one end of the film (manual) is caused by
    a. Low hypo
    b. Low hypo and high developer
    c. High hypo and low developer
    d. Low hypo and low developer

47. Transfer of image from one film to another is caused by
    a. Old developer
    b. Excessive heating of wet emulsion during processed drying
    c. Slight contact of emulsion surfaces of two films in the developer
    d. Slight contact of emulsion surfaces of two films in the hypo

48. Excessive density throughout the finished radiograph is caused by
    a. Underexposure
    b. Overexposure
    c. Cold solution
    d. Defective screens

49. The current flowing between the transformer and the rectifier is
    a. Direct current
    b. Alternating current

FORMULATING X-RAY TECHNIQUES

    c. Pulsating current
    d. High-frequency current

50. Electrical pressure, or potential difference, is measured in
    a. Amperes
    b. Volts
    c. Watts
    d. Ohms

51. X-rays travel at a speed of
    a. 189,000 miles per hour
    b. 186,000 miles per second
    c. 198,000 miles per second
    d. 186,000 miles per hour

52. If one is checking the timer of a full-wave rectified x-ray machine, the number of dots recorded on the film should be as follows:

    a. At $1/10$ of a second: d. At $1/20$ of a second:
       6   2
       12   3
       3   6
       16   4
    b. At $1/60$ of a second: e. At $1/120$ of a second:
       2   2
       4   1
       6   3
       8   4
    c. At $1/30$ of a second:
       2
       4
       5
       6

53. The safe tolerance amount of whole-body radiation per week is about
    a. 0.6 r
    b. 3.0 r
    c. .001 r
    d. 0.3 r

54. The acetabulum is
    a. The socket for the malleolus
    b. The groove for the optic nerve
    c. Housing for the pituitary gland
    d. The socket for the hip

55. What is the atlas?
    a. 5th L.S. spine
    b. 1st dorsal spine

General Questions

    c. 1st cervical spine
    d. 5th dorsal spine

56. The semicircular canal is located
    a. In the external auditory meatus
    b. In the internal auditory meatus
    c. In the frontal portion of the skull
    d. In the maxillary sinuses

57. The lordotic view of the chest is used to demonstrate the
    a. Heart
    b. Apex of the lungs
    c. Ribs
    d. Diaphragm

58. To judge if your position is correct in the mentovertex view of the skull, on the radiograph you should visualize the
    a. Foramen magnum
    b. Optic foramen
    c. Foramen ovale
    d. Sphenoid sinuses

59. Under 100 Kv.P., the percentage of energy in the cathode stream which is converted into x-rays is
    a. 60 to 100 per cent
    b. Less than 1 per cent
    c. 10 per cent
    d. 3 to 5 per cent

60. A good insulator is
    a. Aluminum
    b. Tin
    c. Water
    d. Oil

61. Following manual development, the film should be placed in a stop bath for at least
    a. 2 minutes
    b. 3 minutes
    c. 1 minute
    d. $1/2$ minute

62. The emulsion on an x-ray film consists of
    a. Silver nitrate and cellulose
    b. Silver bromide and gelatin
    c. Silver nitrate and gelatin
    d. Cellulose and acetate

63. The fixed-voltage technique uses
    a. Fixed Kv.P. and varied Ma.S.

FORMULATING X-RAY TECHNIQUES

    b. Fixed Ma.S. and varied Kv.P.
    c. Fixed Kv.P. and fixed Ma.S.
    d. Varied Ma.S. and varied Kv.P.

64. Which of the following materials is not generally used in x-ray-therapy filters
    a. Aluminum
    b. Tin
    c. Copper
    d. Brass

65. The purpose of the filter used in x-ray therapy is to
    a. Change the quality of radiation
    b. Limit the area of exposure
    c. Increase the average wave length
    d. Increase the amount of radiation

66. The total amount of filtration (including inherent filtration) for the average diagnostic machine is
    a. 1.5 mm. of Al.
    b. 4.2 mm. of Al.
    c. 3.5 mm. of Al.
    d. 2.5 mm. of Al.

67. High speed screens are made with
    a. Small crystals
    b. No crystals
    c. Large crystals
    d. Silver bromide

68. In making a P.A. radiograph of the wrist, the hand should be placed in
    a. Supination
    b. Flexion
    c. Pronation
    d. Extension

69. Rotation of the body in positioning for a radiograph is primarily to overcome
    a. Superimposition
    b. Magnification
    c. Motion
    d. Discomfort

70. The primary purpose of a KUB is to show
    a. The urogenital diaphragms, kidneys, and ureters
    b. Bladder, ureters, and kidneys
    c. Pelvis, femur, and bladder
    d. Chest, diaphragm, and kidneys

71. Match the prefix with the meaning
    Retro-   a. Above
    Dys-   b. After

General Questions

Hyper-   c. Through
Peri-   d. Under
Hypo-   e. Large
Macro- f. Behind
Semi-   g. Across
Trans- h. One
Uni-   i. Half
         j. Around
         k. Difficult

72. Match the landmark to the part

    Glenoid cavity   a. Shoulder
    Radius   b. Scapula
    Styloid process c. Elbow
    Navicular   d. Forearm
    Innominate bone e. Ulna
    Patella   f. Mandible
    Medial malleolus g. Ankle
    Cuboid   h. Skull
    Foramen magnum i. Pelvis
    Lamina   j. Foot
                      k. Knee
                      l. Wrist
                      m. Lumbar spine

73. Match the meanings:

    Arthritis   a. Inflammation of the mastoid
    Carcinoma b. Inflammation of the skin
    Bursitis   c. Cancer
    Dermatitis d. Tumor of bone
    Sinusitis   e. Inflammation of bone
    Mastoiditis f. A piece of dead bone
    Osteoma   g. A tear
    -oma   h. Inflammation of a joint
    -osis   i. Condition or state
    Ostitis   j. Tumor
                 k. Inflammation of a bursa
                 l. Inflammation of the paranasal sinuses

74. The left side of the brain controls the
    a. Left side of the body
    b. Neither side of the body
    c. Right side of the body
    d. Both sides of the body

75. The cystic duct is associated with the
    a. Kidney
    b. Colon
    c. Heart
    d. Gallbladder

FORMULATING X-RAY TECHNIQUES

76. Match the name of the study with the part:
    I.V. cholangiogram   a. Heart
    Bronchogram   b. Cystic duct
    Salpingogram   c. Bronchial tree
    Ventriculogram   d. Gallbladder
    Venogram   e. Parotid glands
    Angiocardiogram   f. Veins of legs
    Cerebral arteriogram   g. Abdominal aorta
    Sialogram   h. Urinary tract
                            i. Colon
                            j. Uterus and tubes
                            k. P.A. chest film
                            l. Fluid-containing space of brain
                            m. Arteries of the brain

77. When necessary, you can decrease your time by one-half if you increase your Kv.P. by
    a. 20 per cent
    b. 15 per cent
    c. 10 per cent
    d. 5 per cent

78. You cannot use planography to its best advantage for
    a. The skull
    b. The L.S. spine
    c. The finger
    d. The chest

79. Magnification distortion is used to advantage in making good radiographs of the
    a. Femoral neck
    b. Gallbladder
    c. Heart
    d. T.M. joints

80. In the examination of the gallbladder, a lateral decubitus view is usually taken to show
    a. Mobility of gallbladder
    b. Layering of gallstones
    c. Dye content of the stones
    d. Increased density of the gallbladder

81. In the P.A. projection of the chest, the shoulders are rolled forward to
    a. Raise the diaphragm
    b. Decrease part-film distance
    c. Give true heart size
    d. Remove the scapulae from the lung field

82. X-rays were discovered in
    a. 1795

General Questions

    b. 1895
    c. 1869
    d. 1902

83. The father of x-rays was
    a. Coolidge
    b. Fuchs
    c. Whithead
    d. Roentgen

84. The first vacuum tube was made by
    a. Coolidge
    b. Crooks
    c. Roentgen
    d. Hudson

85. In order to make any visible change in a radiograph using the fixed-voltage technique you have to increase
    a. 20 Kv.P.
    b. 5 Kv.P.
    c. 10 Kv.P.
    d. 15 Kv.P.

86. High Kv.P. results in
    a. Long wave lengths
    b. Short wave lengths
    c. No wave lengths
    d. Short and long wave lengths

87. Long wave lengths result in
    a. Short scale contrast
    b. Ma.S.
    c. Long scale contrast
    d. No contrast

88. Dental films are available in several sizes, including
    a. Proximal
    b. Periapical
    c. Komberg
    d. Bite-wing

89. The compound most commonly employed in intensifying screens is
    a. Calcium carbonate
    b. Silver bromide
    c. Sodium carbonate
    d. Calcium tungstate

90. Continued fluorescence of a screen after exposure is called
    a. Bucking
    b. Warping
    c. Lag
    d. Large crystals

FORMULATING X-RAY TECHNIQUES

91. The exposure timer cord on a bedside unit should be at least
    a. 2 feet long
    b. 4 feet long
    c. 6 feet long
    d. 8 feet long

92. The amount of radiation received by the patient and the technologist is greatest in
    a. A radiograph of the wrist
    b. A barium enema using 2 minutes fluoro
    c. A P.A. chest taken at 72 inches
    d. A radiograph of the L.S. spine

93. The sharpness of detail of a thin part is increased by the use of
    a. No screens
    b. High-speed screens
    c. High-speed film
    d. A collimator

94. The sharpness of detail in a radiograph is decreased by the use of
    a. A grid
    b. A decrease of 10 Kv.P.
    c. A large focal spot
    d. Increased Ma.S.

95. The following disease is always hard to penetrate:
    a. Carcinoma
    b. Hyperparathyroidism
    c. Paget's disease
    d. Emphysema

96. The structures not shown in a P.A. of the wrist are the
    a. Radial and ulnar styloid process
    b. Metatarsal bones
    c. Metacarpal bones
    d. Navicular

97. In the following, check the items which you believe demonstrate a fracture of the external malleolus:

    A. Part to be radiographed:
    1. Foot
    2. Knee
    3. Hip
    4. Ankle

    B. Central ray directed to the:
    1. Foot
    2. Knee
    3. Ankle
    4. Hip

    C. Position of the part:
    1. Standing
    2. Prone
    3. Supine
    4. Lateral

    D. Accessories to be used:
    1. Screens
    2. Screens and grid
    3. Potter Bucky
    4. Cone

General Questions

98. The ideal views to demonstrate a fracture of the metatarsal bones are
    a. Lateral and P.A.
    b. Standing A.P.
    c. A.P., lateral and oblique
    d. Lateral and oblique

99. The radiographs which may be taken to demonstrate free air in the peritoneal cavity are the:
    a. A.P. upright
    b. Lateral decubitus
    c. A.P. supine
    d. Transabdominal

100. In the lateral projection of the wrist, it is important to
    a. Pronate the wrist 15°
    b. Flex the fingers
    c. Extend the hand
    d. Superimpose the radius and ulna

101. Indicate which of the following is located in the right upper quadrant of the abdomen:
    a. Spleen
    b. Appendix
    c. Hepatic flexure
    d. Descending colon

102. Indicate which of the following is not located in the pelvic area:
    a. Ovaries
    b. Sigmoid
    c. Kidneys
    d. Rectum

103. Which of the following is not used for an anatomical reference point?
    a. Iliac crest
    b. Symphysis pubis
    c. Umbilicus
    d. Suprasternal notch

104. Beta rays consist of high-speed
    a. Neutrons
    b. Electrons
    c. Protons
    d. Atoms

105. In order to show the nasopharynx to its best advantage, we would take a lateral radiograph of the
    a. Chest
    b. Cervical spine
    c. Lateral skull, slow inspiration
    d. Soft tissue of cervical spine

FORMULATING X-RAY TECHNIQUES

106. Medical x-ray film should be kept in a
    a. Wet, cool place
    b. Dry, cool place
    c. Hot, wet place
    d. Hot, dry place

107. In an illuminator the following type of bulb should be used:
    a. 15-watt, daylight-type bulb
    b. 20-watt, incandescent
    c. 100-watt, daylight-type bulb
    d. Any type you have

108. When a cylinder cone is employed, all other factors the same, Kv.P. should be increased
    a. 10 Kv.P.
    b. 15 Kv.P.
    c. 25 Kv.P.
    d. 5 Kv.P.

109. A grid ratio is determined by the relationship of the
    a. Length to the width of the strips
    b. The width to the space
    c. The height to the width of the strip
    d. None of the above

110. The cushion between vertebrae is called the
    a. Intervertebral disc
    b. Spinous process
    c. Transverse process
    d. Intervertebral foramina

111. The coccyx is composed of
    a. 12 vertebrae
    b. 4 fused vertebrae
    c. 8 well-developed vertebrae
    d. None of the above

112. The xiphoid process is located in the
    a. Pelvis
    b. Abdomen
    c. Sternum
    d. Shoulder

113. Loss of the ability to smell most commonly occurs when there is an abnormality of the
    a. Nose
    b. Frontal bone
    c. Cribriform plate
    d. Zygomatic process

General Questions

114. The alveolar border is located in the:
    a. Foot
    b. Temporal bone
    c. Parietal bone
    d. Mandible

115. The crista galli is found in the
    a. Sphenoid bone
    b. Ethmoid bone
    c. Hard palate
    d. None of the above

116. The following is not found in the structure of a healthy tooth:
    a. Crown
    b. Root
    c. Neck
    d. Cavity

117. If you took a film of the bicipital groove, you would have a radiograph of the
    a. Skull
    b. Elbow
    c. Humerus
    d. Foot

118. The two large soft spots at the top of a child's skull at birth are called
    a. Parietals
    b. Lambdoidals
    c. Coronal sutures
    d. Fontanelles

119. In viewing a flat film of the abdomen, the muscle usually visualized is the
    a. Psoas muscle
    b. Deltoid muscle
    c. Triceps muscle
    d. None of the above

120. In the lateral projection of the skull, the interpupillary line is
    a. Angled 5° to the film
    b. Perpendicular to the film
    c. Parallel to the film
    d. None of the above

121. The flow of electricity is
    a. From negative to positive
    b. From positive to negative
    c. 151,000 miles per hour
    d. None of the above

FORMULATING X-RAY TECHNIQUES

122. Match the following:

    Stat.   a. Cardboard
    NPO   b. Focal film distance
    CR   c. Kilovoltage
    FFD   d. Grid
    SWG   e. Central ray
    Kv.P   f. Screens with grid
    16-to-1   g. Nothing by mouth
                h. Rush

123. The orbital-meatal line for the Waters view is at
    a. 20°
    b. 37°
    c. 23°
    d. 30°

124. The epidermis is the name of
    a. The inner layer of skin
    b. The outer layer of skin
    c. Sweat glands
    d. None of the above

125. Match the following:

    Anterior   a. Upper
    Superior   b. Lower
    Internal   c. Front
    External   d. Back
    Posterior   e. Close to
    Proximal   f. Away from
                g. Inside
                h. Outside

126. The type of glass used on an illuminator is
    a. Clear glass
    b. Tinted glass
    c. White opal glass
    d. None of the above

127. In radiography of the L.S. spine for a disc, prior to the myelogram, the views normally taken are
    a. A.P.
    b. Obliques
    c. Lateral
    d. All of the above

128. Complete the following sentences:
    a. The front of a cassette is made of _____.
    b. The light from intensifying screens is _____ in color.
    c. The light from a fluoroscopic screen is _____ in color.

General Questions

d. The type of film that cannot be used with automatic processing is _____.
e. The optimum developing time for hand processing is _____° for _____ minutes.
f. Intensifying screens are made of _____.
g. Fluoroscopic screens are made of _____.
h. Non-screen film is used for _____ parts.
i. Screen "afterglow" is called _____.
j. Poor screen contact results in _____ of the radiographic image.

129. Define:
   a. Medial
   b. Lateral
   c. Anterior
   d. Posterior
   e. Superior
   f. Inferior
   g. Proximal
   h. Distal
   i. Cephalic
   j. Caudad
   k. Plantar
   l. Supine
   m. Prone
   n. Flex
   o. Extend

130. Name the bones comprised in the knee joint.
131. Name the bones of the cranium.
132. How many pairs of ribs are there?
133. What is the acetabulum?
134. What is a sesamoid bone?
135. Name the sections of the spine and the number of vertebra in each.
136. Draw and label the colon.
137. Name the main divisions of the urinary tract.
138. What are the fingers and toes called?
139. Where is the gallbladder located?
140. What joint do the carpals form?
141. What joint do the tarsals form?
142. In what bone are the mastoid cells found?
143. Where is the occipital protuberance?
144. Name the nasal accessory sinuses.

145. Match the following:

   Manubrium   a. Ankle
   Atlas   b. Hand
   Malleolus   c. Pelvis
   Glenoid fossa   d. Shoulder
   Metacarpals   e. Sternum
   Ileum   f. Cervical
   Os calcis   g. Knee
   Patella   h. Hip
   Symphysis pubis   i. Foot
   Olecranon process   j. Small bowel
                        k. Sphenoid
                        l. Elbow

FORMULATING X-RAY TECHNIQUES

146. Draw and label the parts of the stomach.
147. Define the following:
     a. Median plane
     b. Saggital plane
     c. Canthomeatal line
     d. Acanthiomeatal line
     e. Interpupillary line
148. The clavicle articulates with the _____ and _____.
149. The bones of the forearm are _____ and _____.
150. The bones of the lower leg are the _____ and the _____.
151. The styloid process is part of the _____ bone (skull).
152. The term vertex refers to the _____ portion of the skull.
153. The appendix is connected to the _____.
154. Where is the glabella?
155. Where is the xiphoid process?
156. To what joints is the navicular related?
157. Name the four quadrants of the abdomen.
158. Where are the kidneys located?
159. The olecranon is related to what joint?
160. Match:

    Acromion   a. Liver
    Coronoid process   b. Temporal
    Petrous   c. Facial bone
    Gallbladder   d. Spleen
    Lacrimal   e. Scapula
    Sphenoid   f. Mandible
                          g. Ischium
                          h. Sella turcica

161. To what do the following terms refer:
     a. Cephalic   c. Adduction
     b. Extrinsic   d. Abduction
162. Define the following prefixes:
     a. anti-   d. sub-   g. lateral
     b. hypo-   e. supra-   h. antero-
     c. intra-   f. median-   i. postero-
163. Name nine systems of the human body.
164. Define *articulation, lumen, shaft, sinus,* and *symphysis.*
165. What system is the periosteum in?
166. In what extremity is the metacarpal?
167. Where is the talus? The calcaneus? Tibia? Navicular? Scapula? Patella?
168. Where is a disc found?
169. Where is the suprasternal notch?
170. Where is the zygomatic bone?
171. Where is the mastoid process?
172. Where is the mediastinum?
173. What does auditory refer to?

General Questions

174. How many chambers does the normal heart have? Name them.
175. What is the function of a vein?
176. What does the biliary system carry?
177. Name two ways in which the biliary tract can be visualized.
178. What passes through the foramen magnum?
179. In order to show the forearm in the lateral projection, the elbow is flexed at _____° and the thumb must be in the _____ position.
180. In order to show the coronoid process of the elbow, free of superimposition, we must have the elbow in the _____ position.
181. With the elbow in acute flexion, we normally would be showing a clear view of the _____ process.
182. In the medial oblique position of the foot, we rotate the leg medially until the sole of the foot forms an angle of approximately _____° to the plane of the film.
183. In the plantardorsal projection of the os calcis, the patient is in which of the following positions: supine, prone, lateral, or standing?
184. If we were to take a radiograph of the bicipital groove, we would be making a radiograph of the _____.
185. In order to show the lateral thoracic spine to its best advantage, we would use a _____, _____ technique.
186. In the A.P. radiograph of the lumbar spine, the knees and feet are in what position? _____
187. For scoliosis we normally would take an A.P. projection in the _____ position and include from the _____ to the third or fourth thoracic vertebra.
188. In the A.P. projection of the sacrum the central ray is directed approximately _____° towards the _____.
189. In the anteroposterior projection of the coccyx we would normally direct the central ray _____° towards the _____.
190. If you were asked to show the anterior and posterior clinoid processes, you would normally take a radiograph in the lateral projection of the _____.
191. In radiography of the lumbar spine for a possible disc prior to a myelogram study, what three views would we normally take?
192. In the case of spondylolisthesis, we would normally take a spot film of _____.
193. In order to show the nasopharynx to its best advantage we would normally take a lateral radiograph of the _____ on _____.
194. In order to show the abdominal aorta we would normally take a _____ position of the _____.
195. Indicate in the right-hand column whether presence of the pathological state listed on the left makes the part being radiographed easy to penetrate or hard to penetrate.

Pathology	Easy to penetrate	Hard to penetrate
Emphysema		
Arthritis		
Hydrocephalus		
Osteoporosis		
Atrophy		

FORMULATING X-RAY TECHNIQUES

196. An x-ray technique from Hospital A for the A.P. skull calls for 85 Kv.P., 20 Ma.S., 36-inch focus-film distance, medium screens, 8-to-1 grid. It is desired to adapt this technique to your hospital. What procedure would you follow in making this technique work in your department?

197. When secondary radiation and Ma.S. are controlled, kilovoltage becomes a factor of radiographic _____.

198. Exposure latitude is the range between _____ exposure and _____ exposure that can be used to produce a diagnostically acceptable radiograph.

199. Great exposure latitude can be secured by using higher kilovoltage. It also can be secured by the use of _____ and _____ film.

200. The only limit to the kilovoltage that can be used in radiography is the limitation imposed by _____.

201. If you are using a technique at 60 Kv.P. and wish to cut the time in half, how much kilovoltage do you add?

202. The principal factor in controlling the penetration of x-rays is _____.

203. The principal factor in controlling density is _____.

204. The wave length of an x-ray beam is determined by _____.

205. The quantity of x-rays received at a given point is primarily dependent on _____.

206. What factors in an x-ray exposure must be changed to produce increased density?

207. Magnification in a radiograph can be lessened by the use of _____.

208. Cones, stationary grids, and Bucky diaphragms are similar in that their primary function is to _____.

209. The grid ratio of the Potter Bucky diaphragm is the ratio of the _____ of the lead strips to the _____ between the strips.

210. The two types of stationary grids used today are referred to as a _____ grid and a _____ grid.

Fill in the following:

211. Kilovoltage
    a. regulates _____.
    b. determines the degree of _____.
    c. influences the production of _____.
    d. regulates the scale of radiographic _____.
    e. determines the degree of exposure _____.
    f. influences radiographic _____.

212. Focus-film distance
    a. influences the _____ and _____ of the radiographic image.
    b. influences radiographic _____.

213. Milliampere seconds
    a. regulate the _____ of x-radiation admitted by the x-ray tube.
    b. regulate radiographic _____.

214. Formulate a typical technique for radiography of the skull with

General Questions

   a. Variable kilovoltage technique, centimeter part thickness
   b. Fixed kilovoltage technique
   c. High-kilovoltage technique

215. Define:

EMF	HVL	Ohm	Volt
Potential	FFD	Ampere	Kilovolt

216. Intensity of electricity is measured in (circle one):

   Kv.P.   Watts   Amperage   Volts   Ohms

217. The flow of electricity is from _____ to _____.
218. Atoms are composed of _____, _____, and _____.
219. The three basic requirements for the production of x-rays are _____.
220. The current flowing between the transformer and the rectifier is _____.
221. The quantity of electrons in the cathode stream is dependent directly on _____.
222. What is the real advantage of a rotating-anode tube?
223. What portion of the total energy delivered to an x-ray tube at the target is given off as x-rays?
224. What is meant by hard rays? Soft rays?

ANSWERS FOR GENERAL QUESTIONS

1. b 2. b 3. c 4. d 5. b 6. b 7. c 8. b 9. c 10. c 11. c 12. c
13. c 14. a 15. b 16. a 17. a 18. c 19. b 20. b 21. c 22. c 23. b
24. a 25. b 26. b 27. d 28. c 29. d 30. d 31. d 32. c 33. c 34. b
35. d 36. c 37. c 38. c 39. d 40. d 41. c 42. b 43. b 44. d 45. b
46. c 47. c 48. b 49. b 50. b

51. b 52. a. 12, b. 2, c. 4, d. 6, e. 1 53. d 54. d 55. c 56. b 57. b
58. c 59. b 60. d 61. d 62. b 63. a 64. d 65. a 66. d 67. c 68. c
69. a 70. b 71. f, k, a, j, d, e, i, g, h 72. a, d, e or h, l, i, k, g, j, h, m 73. h, c, k, b, l, a, d, j, i, e 74. c 75. d 76. b, c, j, l, f, a, m, e 77. b 78. c 79. d
80. b 81. d 82. b 83. d 84. b 85. b 86. b 87. a 88. b 89. d 90. c
91. c 92. b 93. a 94. c 95. c 96. b 97. A4; B3; C4; D1 and D4 98. c
99. a, b, and d 100. d

101. c 102. c 103. c 104. b 105. c 106. b 107. b 108. d 109. d
110. a 111. b 112. c 113. c 114. d 115. b 116. d 117. c 118. d
119. a 120. b 121. a 122. h, g, e, b, f, c, d 123. b 124. b 125. c, a, g, h, d, e 126. c 127. d

128. a. Radiolucent material, such as Bakelite or Magnelite; b. Blue; c. Greenish-yellow; d. Non-screen film; e. 68° for 5 minutes; f. Calcium tungstate; g. Zinc cadmium sulfide; h. Small (less than 12 cm); i. Lag; j. Blurring.

129. a. Close to the median line or center; b. Away from the median line of the body; c. Towards the front; d. Towards the back; e. The upper part or nearer the head; f. The lower part or away from the head; g. Closest to the point of origin; h. Farthest from the point of origin; i. Of the head; j. Towards the tail end; k. Of the sole of the foot; l. Lying on the back; m. Lying face down; n. To bend; o. To straighten 130. The distal femur and the proximal tibia 131. *Cerebral cranium:* frontal (1), parietal (2), occipital (1), temporal (2), sphenoid (1), ethmoid (1); *Visceral cranium:* maxilla (2), zygomatic (2), nasal (2), lacrimal (2), palatine (2), turbinate (2), vomer (1), mandible (1) 132. 12 pairs 133. The socket at the junction of the three parts of the innominate bone which accommodates the head of the femur to form the hip joint 134. One of the small accessory bones located in the tendons, usually at joints and bony prominences 135. Cervical spine (7), thoracic spine (12), lumbar spine (5), sacrum (5 fused), and coccyx (4 fused) 136. Cecum, ascending colon, hepatic flexure, transverse colon, splenic flexure, descending colon, sigmoid, rectum, anus.

137. Kidneys, ureters, bladder, urethra 138. Phalanges 139. In the upper right quadrant of the abdomen, usually opposite the ninth costal cartilage

Answers for General Questions

140. The intercarpal joint of the wrist   **141.** The intertarsal joint of the foot   **142.** The temporal bone   **143.** On the squamous part of the occipital bone, in the midline, where it helps to form the base of the skull   **144.** Frontal, sphenoid, ethmoid, and maxillary   **145.** e, f, a, d, b, j, i, g, c, l   **146.** Fundus, body, pylorus, duodenum, greater and lesser curvatures.

147. a. A plane through the median line of the body as if a cut were made from front to back through the sagittal suture of the skull and continued down through the body, dividing it into equal parts. The view is of one cut surface.   b. Any plane parallel to or in the same direction as the median plane.   c. An imaginary line connecting the outer canthus of the eye and the external auditory meatus; used as a base line in positioning the skull. It is also called the Radiographic Base Line.   d. An imaginary line running from the acanthion to the external auditory meatus and used as a base line in skull radiography.   e. An imaginary line that traverses the skull from side to side passing through the pupils of the eyes; it is used as a base line for skull radiography.

148. Sternum and the acromion of the scapula   **149.** The ulna and the radius   **150.** The tibia and the fibula   **151.** Temporal   **152.** Superior   **153.** Cecum   **154.** Above the root of the nose and between the supraorbital borders, on the frontal bone   **155.** The lower pointed segment of the sternum   **156.** The joints of the wrist and the foot   **157.** Right upper quadrant, left upper quadrant, right lower quadrant, left lower quadrant   **158.** Inside the posterior abdominal wall, in the upper abdomen, behind the peritoneum, between the twelfth dorsal and third lumbar vertebrae   **159.** The elbow   **160.** e, f, b, a, c, h   **161.** a. Of the head;   b. Having origin outside the structure or organ involved;   c. Motion towards or across the midline;   d. Motion away from the midline   **162.** Against; under; inside; under; above; middle or midline; away from the midline; to the front; to the back

163. Circulatory, digestive, endocrine, muscular, nervous, reproductive, respiratory, skeletal, urinary   **164.** Articulation—the joint surface of a bone. Lumen—the channel of a tubular structure. Shaft—the body or major portion. Sinus—a natural cavity in the bone. Symphysis—the union of two paired bones.   **165.** Skeletal   **166.** The upper extremity—the hand   **167.** Talus—one of the bones of the foot; it helps to form the ankle joint. Calcaneus—the heel bone of the foot. Tibia—one of the bones of the lower leg, lying medially to the fibula. Navicular—can be one of the bones of the wrist or one of the bones comprised in the foot. Scapula—the shoulder blade. Patella—the large sesamoid bone lying in front of the knee joint.

168. Between the bodies of adjacent vertebrae   **169.** In the upper border of the sternum between the two depressions where the clavicles articulate   **170.** Immediately below the orbit; it forms the prominent part of the upper cheek on each side   **171.** The part of the temporal bone which extends down behind the ear and contains air cells   **172.** The partition which divides the two halves of the chest cavity   **173.** The ear or hearing   **174.** Four: left atrium, left ventricle, right atrium, and right ventricle   **175.** It is part of the collecting system that carries blood back to the heart   **176.** Bile   **177.** Operative cholangiography and I.V. cholangiography   **178.** The medulla (hind-

FORMULATING X-RAY TECHNIQUES

brain), which is the beginning of the spinal cord   **179.** 90 degrees; upward   **180.** Oblique   **181.** Olecranon   **182.** 30°   **183.** Supine   **184.** Shoulder   **185.** Shallow-breathing

186. For the best result, the knees should be flexed and the feet should be flat on the table. This straightens the spine and brings it in closer contact with the film   **187.** Sitting or standing; fifth lumbar vertebra   **188.** 15°; head   **189.** 10°; feet   **190.** Sella turcica of the sphenoid bone   **191.** A.P. lumbar, lateral lumbar, and oblique lumbar views   **192.** The affected vertebra, usually the fifth lumbar   **193.** Skull; slow inspiration   **194.** Lateral; abdomen   **195.** Emphysema—easy; arthritis—easy; hydrocephalus—easy; osteoporosis—easy; atrophy—easy

196. Make an exposure at your hospital using the same factors as are listed for Hospital A, and also make an exposure using twice the Ma.S. and half the Ma.S., all other factors remaining the same. From these resulting films, choose the best; if none of these are adequate, make the proper adjustment by halving or doubling again, until the desired exposure is obtained. This will be your adapted technique   **197.** Contrast   **198.** Minimum; maximum   **199.** A cardboard holder; regular   **200.** Radiographic contrast

201. Using the 15 per cent rule, you add 9 Kv.P.   **202.** Kilovoltage   **203.** Milliampere-seconds   **204.** Kilovoltage   **205.** Milliampere-seconds   **206.** Milliampere-seconds or kilovoltage   **207.** A small focal spot, close object-film distance, and increased focus-film distance   **208.** Reduce secondary radiation   **209.** Height; space   **210.** Parallel; focused   **211.** a. contrast; b. penetration; c. radiation fog; d. contrast; e. latitude; f. density   **212.** a. magnification; definition; b. density   **213.** a. quantity; b. density   **214.**—

215. EMF—electromotive force; the electrical pressure of a charge. Potential—in physics, the available pressure of electricity. HVL—half-value layer: the thickness of a given substance which will reduce the intensity of the x-ray beam to one-half its original value.   FFD—focus-film distance: the distance from the target of the x-ray tube to the film.   Ohm—the unit of electrical resistance.   Ampere—the unit of measurement of quantity of an electric current.   Volt—the unit of electrical pressure or electrical potential.   Kilovolt—1000 volts

216. Watts   **217.** Negative; positive   **218.** Protons, neutrons, and electrons   **219.** A source of electrons, target for the electrons to strike, and an electrical force to drive the electrons to the target   **220.** Alternating current   **221.** The amperage applied   **222.** It preserves the life of the anode and allows greater heat capacity   **223.** Less than 1 per cent   **224.** Hard rays are the shorter, more penetrating rays attained at higher Kv.P.; soft rays are the longer, less penetrating rays attained at lower Kv.P.

STUDY QUESTIONS

RADIOGRAPHIC FILM, SCREENS, CASSETTES

Check the statement below which is CORRECT:

Poor screen contact results in:
- ☒ Blurring of the radiographic image
- ☐ Increased object-film distance
- ☐ Black streaks at the edge of the film
- ☐ Magnification of the image

Check the statement below which is CORRECT:

The term "screen lag" refers to:
- ☒ The phosphorescence of the screen after the x-ray exposure stops
- ☐ The distance of the tube from the screens
- ☐ A damaged intensifying screen
- ☐ An intensifying screen in which the fluorescent crystals no longer fluoresce
- ☐ Poor contact between screens

Check the statement below which is CORRECT:

The speed of intensifying screens depends primarily on:
- ☒ The size of the fluorescent crystals
- ☐ The size of the focal spot used
- ☐ The type of film used
- ☐ Good screen contact
- ☐ Materials used in constructing the cassette

Check the statement below which is CORRECT:

Poor screen contact will result in:
- ☐ Increased sharpness of detail in the radiograph
- ☐ Increased contrast in the radiograph
- ☒ Decreased sharpness of detail in the radiograph
- ☐ Increased density in the radiograph
- ☐ Screen lag

Check the statement below which is CORRECT:

The back of a cassette is made of material opaque to x-rays because:
- ☐ It tends to protect the technologist from scattered radiation
- ☐ It tends to reduce distortion in the radiograph
- ☒ It tends to prevent fogging of the film by scattered radiation from behind the cassette

FORMULATING X-RAY TECHNIQUES

☐ It further intensifies the image
☐ It tends to reduce the amount of exposure necessary

Check the statement below which is CORRECT:

The essential chemical in an intensifying screen is:
☐ Silver iodide
☐ Silver bromide
☐ Calcium carbonate
☒ Calcium tungstate

Check the statements below which are CORRECT:

Intensifying screens:
☐ Have less speed when the tungstate crystals are large
☒ Permit a shorter exposure time than without screens
☒ Have less speed when the tungstate crystals are small
☐ Give more detail than without screens

Q. What is an intensifying screen?

A. An intensifying screen is a cardboard backing coated with a layer of chemical material which will fluoresce when penetrated by x-radiation. The chemical, a white crystalline salt called calcium tungstate, has the ability to emit a blue-violet light instantaneously upon the absorption of x-rays. The light emitted exposes the x-ray film, which is sandwiched between two intensifying screens.

Q. What is meant by lag in an intensifying screen?

A. Lag is a condition of the screen when it continues to emit light after the x-ray source has ceased.

Q. How many intensifying screens are usually used in each cassette?

A. Each cassette employs a front and a rear intensifying screen.

Q. Will dirt on the surface of the intensifying screen affect the radiograph?

A. Dust, dirt particles, and stains must not be allowed to collect on the surfaces of the screens because such foreign matter will cause extraneous shadows in the radiographic image.

Q. How would you determine if a spotted radiograph is due to a defect in an intensifying screen, to a defect in the cassette, or to the film itself?

A. A defect in an intensifying screen would produce a light spot. A defect in a cassette is apt to produce a defined shadow. The absence of the spot in a duplicate exposure on a second film would point to the film.

Q. What is meant by good screen contact? How do you test for it? What is its importance? What causes poor screen contact?

A. Screens should be in contact with the film over its entire surface to maintain detail sharpness. Contact is tested by making a radiograph of $1/4$-inch wire mesh. If there are any areas in which contact is not maintained, an obvious loss of image sharpness is apparent in those areas.

Q. Describe a cardboard film holder. Explain its construction. What is the importance of keeping the proper side up?

A. A cardboard film holder is a lightproof container used to envelop the

Study Questions

x-ray film during the exposure. It is composed of two pieces of x-ray transparent paperboard hinged together with binding cloth. One of the cardboard covers contains a thin layer of lead foil which serves to absorb secondary radiation arising from the table top. Hence, this cover should be positioned away from the x-ray tube. The proper side of the cardboard holder which should face the tube is usually identified.

Q. Approximately how long will a pair of intensifying screens last?

A. Indefinitely. It is directly proportional to the amount of care they receive in handling and cleaning.

Q. What causes intensifying screens to deteriorate?

A. Improper handling and inadequate cleaning will reduce the life of the screen.

Check all CORRECT statements below:

Intensifying screen speed increases as:
- ☒ Temperature decreases
- ☒ Crystal size increases
- ☒ Crystal layer thickness increases
- ☒ KVP increases

Check the statement below which is CORRECT:

The phosphor which emits the yellow-green luminescence of the fluoroscopic screen is:
- ☐ Barium lead sulfate
- ☒ Zinc cadmium sulfide
- ☐ Zinc sulfide
- ☐ Calcium tungstate

Q. How does the speed of regular film compare to the speed of non-screen film?

A. Regular film is from 4 to 8 times faster.

Q. How do the speeds of fast screens and medium screens compare according to the adjustment that must be made in exposure.

A. Fast screens require a 50% reduction in Ma.S. over medium-speed screens.

Check the CORRECT statement below:

To reduce exposure of x-ray to the patient, the best screen to use is:
- ☐ Non-screen film
- ☐ Par-speed screen with regular film
- ☒ High-speed screen with high-speed film
- ☐ Slow-speed screen with high-speed film

Check the CORRECT statement below:

A property of gelatin in cool solutions is:
- ☐ It dissolves readily
- ☐ It precipitates
- ☐ It liquefies
- ☒ It swells

FORMULATING X-RAY TECHNIQUES

Check the statement below which is CORRECT:

Gelatin is chemically considered to be:
- ☐ A compound
- ☐ A mixture
- ☒ A colloid
- ☐ An element

PROCESSING AND DARKROOM TECHNIQUE

Q. What is a safelight and why is it used? How would you test a safelight for safety?

A. A "safelight" is a source of illumination, of a color and intensity that will not fog an x-ray film exposed to it for a reasonable time.

The "safelight" can be tested by placing an exposed but not developed film in a position similar to that in which films would be under ordinary working conditions. Then, using strips of cardboard, or other opaque material, about one inch wide, beginning at one end of the film place a strip of cardboard on the film at the end of each one-half minute of exposure. After a test of several minutes has been completed, develop the film. The elapsed time up to any fogged area may be measured by measuring the distance from this clear end of the film.

Q. What is meant by developer (manual processing)? What is it composed of?

A. Developer is the agent that reduces the exposed silver salts of the film emulsion to metallic silver so that when properly fixed it is visible to the human eye. Developer is generally composed of the developing agents hydroquinone and metol, the preservative sodium sulfite and the chemical sodium carbonate, which swells the gelatin in which the silver salts are suspended, so that the reducing agents may reach and act on the exposed silver salts in a minimum time.

Q. What is meant by the term "oxidized developer"? How can oxidation be prevented? What is the effect of oxidized developer?

A. Oxidized developer is developer that has become exhausted due to exposure to light and air. Oxidation can be reduced by placing a cover over the developer when it is not in use. Oxidized developer will generally stain films due to its discoloration (manual processing).

Q. What is chemical fog?

A. Chemical fog is a gray, dull appearance of the films, generally caused by the use of too strong a chemical solution or aged developer.

Q. Can an underpenetrated film be corrected by prolonging the development (manual processing) and vice versa?

A. Only within relatively narrow limits, since overdeveloping cannot bring out anything which underexposure failed to put on the film.

Q. What is the proper height of solution level in tanks? How should it be maintained?

A. The proper level of solutions is such that the film, regardless of size, is fully immersed. Level should be maintained by adding either fresh solution or one of the special replenishing solutions.

Study Questions

Q. What determines the length of time for developing x-ray films and under what conditions should it be varied?

A. The time of development is determined by the temperature and age of the developer. As the solution ages or wears, developing time must be increased.

Q. How long and in what manner should a film be rinsed before putting it into the fixer solution (manual processing)?

A. A film should be rinsed for about 30 seconds in water or a "stop bath" before it is placed in the fixer solution. "Stop baths" are intended to stop the developing process and to remove excess developer so that it will not be carried to the fixer.

Q. How often should the developer and fixer be changed?

A. The developer should be changed when it shows signs of oxidation (brownish color) or when it will no longer bring up the blacks on the film. The fixer should be changed when it no longer hardens the emulsion or when the solution requires more than four times as long to fix a film as when the fixer was new, temperatures being the same.

Q. What is x-ray fog and how can it be prevented?

A. X-ray fog is a hazy or cloudy appearance on the radiograph due to the inadvertent exposure of the x-ray film to primary or secondary x-radiation. It can be prevented by storing films in lead-lined containers.

Q. How can the film be tested for x-ray fog?

A. By developing a film without exposing it first.

Q. How can light fog be prevented?

A. Light fog can be prevented by sealing all cracks in darkroom openings and using tested safelights.

Q. What are the usual causes, mode of differentiation, and means of prevention for fogging of films? staining of films?

A. Films are usually fogged by improper safelights, non-lightproof darkrooms, and x-rays. Safelight and light fogs manifest themselves as sharp, dark shadows, while x-ray fog can be recognized as a general all-over graying of the film. Fogging can be prevented by the use of proper safelights, elimination of all white light in the darkroom, and storage of the film in suitable containers.

Staining of films is caused by old developing or fixing solutions. It can be prevented by establishing routines calling for the changing of the solutions before they have deteriorated to the point where they will stain films.

Q. What sometimes causes streakiness in the light areas of a developed film and how may this be avoided (manual processing)?

A. Streaks on films are generally caused by one of two things. Dirty hangers will cause streaks below the clips, or light areas on the film may have streaks under them if the film was not agitated.

Q. If the following marks are found on an x-ray film, what are they due to and how would you prevent them: crinkle mark? friction mark? pinhole mark? water spot? static mark?

FORMULATING X-RAY TECHNIQUES

A. A crinkle mark is caused by kinking the film. It should be kept flat. Friction marks are a series of static discharges on the film caused by sliding the film across the wrapping paper or other surface. A pinhole mark is a single static discharge point—generally caused by uneven drying, usually in a dryer that is too hot.

Water spots may be due to improper film drying or to water wetting the film in one area and then drying before film development.

A static mark is any indication on the film of static discharge, generally caused by friction.

Q. What precautions must be taken with respect to developing, washing, and fixing "non-screen" films?

A. Non-screen film because of the heavier emulsion should be developed, rinsed, fixed, and washed about 30 per cent longer than the regular film (manual processing only).

Q. What is a penetrometer? How is it used?

A. A penetrometer is a radiographic test device usually made of aluminum and built up in steps of varying thickness. It is used in testing the radiographic efficiency of x-ray equipment and for radiographic calibrations, since minor changes in radiographic density can readily be detected and the proper compensation or adjustment can be made.

Q. If a given exposure causes a certain density when processed 5 minutes at 68 degrees, what developing time must be used to produce the same density when developer temperature (manual processing only) is:
1. 64 degrees?
2. 74 degrees?
3. 80 degrees?
4. 70 degrees?

A. A good rule to follow: If the temperature of the developer is higher than the recommended 68 degrees, subtract approximately $1/4$ minute per degree of the increase in temperature; if the temperature of the developer is lower than the recommended 68 degrees, add approximately $1/4$ minute per degree of decrease in temperature. Therefore the answers to the above variations in temperature would be:
1. $6-6\frac{1}{4}$ min.
2. $3\frac{1}{2}-3\frac{3}{4}$ min.
3. $2-2\frac{1}{4}$ min.
4. $4\frac{1}{2}$ min.

Check the statement below which is CORRECT:

The darkroom safelight should have a 10-watt white light bulb behind a:
- ☐ 2 mm. aluminum filter at 4 feet.
- ☒ Wratten 6-B filter at 3 feet.
- ☐ Red acetate filter at 3 feet.
- ☐ Wratten 10-A filter at 3 feet.

Check the statement below which is CORRECT:

Chemical fog is produced by:
- ☐ Cold developer

Study Questions

- ☐ Incomplete development
- ☐ Hot hypo
- ☒ Prolonged development

Check the statement below which is CORRECT:

If the air in the darkroom is too dry, film is susceptible to:
- ☐ Crescent-shaped markings
- ☐ Fingerprints
- ☐ Chemical fog
- ☒ Static accumulation

Check the statement below which is CORRECT:

The emulsion used in making x-ray film contains:
- ☐ Silver nitrate
- ☐ Sodium sulfite
- ☒ Silver bromide
- ☐ Calcium tungstate

Check the statement below which is CORRECT:

Reticulation on the surface of an x-ray film is the result of:
- ☐ Developer carried into the hypo
- ☒ Sudden changes in the temperatures of the solutions
- ☐ Incorrect mixing of the developer
- ☐ Drying in too warm air

Check the statement below which is CORRECT:

The chemical in the developer which reduces oxidation is:
- ☒ Sodium sulfite
- ☐ Sodium carbonate
- ☐ Potassium bromide
- ☐ Sodium sulfate

Check the statement below which is CORRECT:

The color of chemical fog on an x-ray appears to be:
- ☒ Gray
- ☐ Black
- ☐ Brown
- ☐ Yellow

Check the statement below which is CORRECT:

The latent image is the result of:
- ☐ Action of hydroquinone
- ☐ Films stored in too great heat
- ☒ Exposure to x-ray and processing of film
- ☐ Fixing and washing the film

Check the statement below which is CORRECT:

The compound that is used in intensifying screens as a fluorescent agent is:
- ☐ Silver bromide
- ☒ Calcium tungstate
- ☐ Calcium carbonate
- ☐ Potassium bromide

FORMULATING X-RAY TECHNIQUES

Check the statement below which is CORRECT:
    "Christmas tree-like" density defects on an x-ray film are caused by:
- ☐ Movement of patient
- ☐ Dust
- ☒ Static
- ☐ Overexposure

Check the statement below which is CORRECT:
    Moon-shaped areas of decreased density on x-ray film are caused by:
- ☐ Static
- ☐ Excessive heat
- ☒ Bending of film
- ☐ X-radiation leaking in storage room

In reference to manual processing, match:

_6_	Potassium bromide	1. Preservative
_7_	Sodium thiosulfate	2. Hardening agent
_1_	Sodium sulfite	3. Activator
_5_	Acetic acid	4. Developing agent
_4_	Hydroquinone	5. Acidifier
_3_	Sodium carbonate	6. Restrainer
_2_	Potassium alum	7. Fixing agent
_4_	Elon	

EQUIPMENT AND ACCESSORIES

Check the statement below which is CORRECT:
    Magnification distortion can be lessened by the use of:
- ☐ Cones
- ☐ A Bucky diaphragm
- ☒ A longer focus-film distance
- ☐ The use of filters
- ☐ A shorter target-film distance

Check the statement below which is CORRECT:
    If an ordinary 8-to-1 Potter-Bucky diaphragm is used, how much greater is the exposure than if the Bucky is not used?
- ☐ It is the same
- ☒ 3 times greater
- ☐ 8 times greater
- ☐ 10 times greater
- ☐ 12 times greater

Check the statement below which is CORRECT:
    The grid-ratio of a Potter-Bucky diaphragm is:
- ☒ The ratio of the height of the lead strips to space between strips
- ☐ The ratio between the total thickness of the grid and the space between lead strips
- ☐ The ratio between the speed of travel of the grid and the speed of the timer

Study Questions

☐ The ratio of exposure time without the Bucky to exposure time with the Bucky
☐ The ratio of the width of the lead strip to the depth of the strip

Check the statement below which is CORRECT:
The Potter-Bucky diaphragm and the stationary grid are used to:
☐ Localize foreign bodies in the eye
☒ Eliminate a large portion of secondary radiation
☐ Limit the diameter of the primary beam
☐ Produce radiographs free from distortion
☐ Record movements of various organs of the body

Check the statement below which is CORRECT:
The apparatus used for laminagraphy, planigraphy, or tomography is used for:
☐ Developing films rapidly
☐ Producing bedside radiographs
☐ Examining the bladder with light and lens
☒ Producing body-section radiographs
☐ Recording movements of the heart

Check the statement below which is CORRECT:
Cones and cylinders are used in radiography to:
☐ Permit the use of less kilovoltage
☒ Limit the field of radiation and reduce secondary radiation
☐ Reduce wear and tear on the x-ray tube
☐ Focus the x-ray beam
☐ Shorten the exposure

Check the statement below which is CORRECT:
A Bucky diaphragm should not be used in making radiographs of:
☐ The lateral lumbar spine
☒ The lateral cervical spine
☐ The lateral sacral spine
☐ The anteroposterior dorsal spine
☐ The anteroposterior lumbar spine

Check the statement below which is CORRECT:
Cones, stationary grids, and Bucky diaphragms are similar in that their primary function is to:
☐ Protect the technologist from scattered radiation
☐ Reduce distortion in the radiograph
☒ Reduce secondary radiation
☐ Reduce exposure time
☐ Permit using a longer target-film distance

Check the statement below which is CORRECT:
All other factors being the same, which of the following exposure would produce the greatest radiographic density?
☐ $1/10$ second and 100 Ma.
☐ 1 second and 10 Ma.
☐ $1/20$ second and 200 Ma.
☒ $1/40$ second and 500 Ma.
☐ $1/15$ second and 150 Ma.

FORMULATING X-RAY TECHNIQUES

Check the statement below which is CORRECT:

Contrast in a radiograph is increased by:
- ☐ Greater film distance
- ☐ Increased kilovoltage
- ☒ Decreased kilovoltage
- ☐ Use of non-screen film
- ☐ Full-wave rectification

Check the statement below which is CORRECT:

Detail in a radiograph is not improved by:
- ☐ The use of cones and cylinders
- ☒ Increased object-film distance
- ☐ Increased focus-film distance
- ☐ Immobilization
- ☐ The use of non-screen film

Q. What causes grid lines on a radiograph and how may they be corrected?

A. Lines may be caused by improper centering of the tube, by increasing or decreasing the distance from the proper distance at which the grid is focused, by an improper relationship between the exposure time and the grid travel time, or by beginning the exposure before the grid starts in motion or continuing the exposure after it stops.

Q. Of what use is a cone in radiography and where is it used?

A. A cone restricts the x-ray beam to the immediate area under examination and thus minimizes secondary radiation by limiting the volume of tissue exposed. The result is greatly increased contrast, which makes radiographic detail more plainly visible. For regions such as sinuses, gallbladder, with or without Potter-Bucky diaphragm, a cone should be used to cover the desired area—particularly for heavy parts.

Q. Must the shift of the tube in stereoradiography be accompanied by a tube tilt? Explain your answer.

A. In stereoradiography the shift of the tube must be accompanied by a tube tilt if a small cone is used. Unless this is done, the shifting of the cone circle may result in cut-off of the portion of the part being radiographed. If no cone is used, or if a very long focal-film distance, such as is used in chest work, is employed, the tilt is not necessary. In stereoradiography work on the head, however, where a four-inch cone or one even smaller may be used at 30- or 36-inch focus-film distance, it is necessary to tilt the tube and direct it to the same centering point for both views.

TECHNIQUE

Check the statement below which is CORRECT:

In making radiographs of the gastrointestinal tract it is of utmost importance to use:
- ☐ A long distance
- ☒ A short exposure time
- ☐ A short distance

Study Questions

☐ A high voltage
☐ A low voltage

Check the statement below which is CORRECT:

Generally speaking an increase of 10 Kv.P. may be compensated for by the following change in exposure time:

☐ The time would be cut $1/4$
☒ The time would be cut $1/2$
☐ The time would be doubled
☐ The time would be tripled
☐ The time would be increased 5 times

Q. When and why should compression be used in radiography, and what is the effect, if any, on technical procedure?

A. Compression is used in radiography for two reasons: first, to help eliminate motion, and secondly, in the case of obese patients, to compress the fatty tissue or remove it from the field of radiography as much as possible. By the use of compression, the part is reduced in density, and we may use a somewhat lower amount of the penetrating factor or Ma.S.

Q. What is magnification and what are the factors affecting it?

A. Magnification is that form of distortion which causes an enlargement of the image. Magnification is caused by a short focus-film distance or by a great object-film distance.

Q. What is distortion and what are the factors affecting it?

A. Distortion refers to the change in the shape of an object, either by elongation or foreshortening. Distortion is caused by misalignment of the tube, object, and film.

Check the statement below which is CORRECT:

Under 100 Kv.P. the percentage of energy in the cathode stream which is converted into x-rays is:

☐ 80% to 90%
☐ 10% to 20%
☐ 97% to 99%
☒ Less than 1%
☐ 50%

Check the statement below which is CORRECT:

The intensity of x-radiation at any given distance from the source of radiation varies:

☐ Directly with the distance
☒ Inversely with the square of the distance
☐ Inversely with the distance
☐ Directly with the square of the distance
☐ Distance does not change it

Check the statement below which is CORRECT:

The wave length of an x-ray beam is determined by:

☐ The quantity of electrons in the cathode stream
☐ The milliamperage
☐ The voltage in the filament circuit

FORMULATING X-RAY TECHNIQUES

☒ The kilovoltage
☐ The size of the focal spot

Check the statement below which is CORRECT:
The quantity of x-rays received at a given point is primarily dependent on:
☐ The size of the focal spot
☐ The kilovoltage
☐ The type and size of the target
☐ The use of intensifying screens
☒ The milliampere seconds

Check the statement below which is CORRECT:
An increase in kilovoltage across the tube results in:
☒ Radiation of a shorter wave length
☐ Radiation of a longer wave length
☐ No alteration in wave length
☐ Twice as many impulses per second
☐ Higher milliamperage

Q. State the inverse square law.
A. Intensity of x-radiation varies inversely with the square of the distance.

Q. Define primary and remnant radiation.
A. Primary radiation is the radiation emitted from the tube. Remnant radiation is the radiation that emerges to expose the film.

Match:

2	c	High Kv.P.	1. 10 Ma.S.	a.	high contrast
4	b	High density	2. short wave length	b.	more black metallic silver
3	a	Low Kv.P.	3. long wave length	c.	low contrast
1	d	Low density	4. 200 Ma.S.	d.	little black metallic silver

Check the statement below which is CORRECT:
The principal factor controlling the penetration of x-rays is:
☐ Milliamperage
☐ Time
☐ Distance
☒ Kilovoltage
☐ Wattage

Give the Ma.S. for the following Ma. and time combinations:
1. 100 Ma. for $1/2$ sec.   50
2. 200 Ma. for $3/10$ sec.   60
3. 300 Ma. for $2/5$ sec.   120
4. 50 Ma. for $1/20$ sec.   2.5
5. 100 Ma. for $1/15$ sec.   6.66

Of the ten possible answers below, check the *five* completions which you believe to be correct. As it influences the image in a radiograph, the kilovoltage:

Study Questions

- ✓ Affects radiographic density.
-   Affects distortion.
-   Affects detail.
- ✓ Affects exposure latitude.
-   Increases detail.
- ✓ Affects radiographic contrast.
-   Eliminates the use of cones.
-   Decreases distortion.
- ✓ Affects the degree of penetration of the object.
- ✓ Affects the production of fog from secondary radiation.

Check the statement below which is CORRECT:

The term density' when applied to a radiograph refers to:
- ☐ The sharpness and clearness of the shadow
- ☐ The distortion of the true shape of the object
- ☒ The over-all blackness of the radiograph
- ☐ The degree of difference between the light and dark portions of the film
- ☐ The thickness of the emulsion on the film

Q. What factors in an x-ray exposure must be changed to produce increased density?

A. Increased radiographic density may be produced by increasing milliampere seconds or Kv.P.

Q. When good radiographic detail cannot be secured because of inability to approximate the part close to the film, what change in technique may be employed to obtain better detail?

A. When close approximation of the part to the film cannot be secured, the focus-film distance can be increased in order to obtain better detail.

Q. What is the importance of focus-film distance in radiographic technique?

A. The importance of focus-film distance is the fact that it is the controllable factor of detail. Too close a focus-film distance would produce magnification of a part; too great a focus-film distance would cause undue strain on the equipment. Hence, a proper focus-film distance (30 to 40 inches) for most radiographic work is important. The usual focus-film distance in chest radiography is 72 inches.

Q. What is the reason for using very rapid exposures in the examination of the chest?

A. The reason for using very rapid exposures in examination of the chest is to eliminate motion both from respiration and as much as possible from heart action.

Q. What is the reason for using very rapid exposures in the examination of the stomach?

A. The reason for using very rapid exposures in examination of the stomach is to eliminate or minimize motion caused by the peristaltic action of the stomach.

FORMULATING X-RAY TECHNIQUES

Q. What is the purpose of using a six- or seven-foot focus-film distance in the examination of the heart?

A. The purpose for using a six- or seven-foot focus-film distance in examination of the heart is to minimize magnification which is caused by the increased part-film distance.

Q. What is meant by the following terms and how would you correct the same? Overpenetration? Underpenetration?

A. Overpenetration is the result of using a kilovoltage in excess of the value necessary to produce the desired density in the radiograph. It is corrected by reducing the Kv.P. the necessary amount.

Underpenetration is the result of using a Kv.P. less than the value necessary to produce a satisfactory density. It is corrected by increasing the Kv.P. the necessary amount.

Check the statements below which are CORRECT:

The sharpness of detail in a radiograph is dependent on:
- ☐ The milliampere seconds
- ☒ The size of the focal spot
- ☒ The focus-film distance
- ☒ Immobilization
- ☒ The object-film distance

Check the statement below which is CORRECT:

Magnification distortion is used to advantage in making good radiographs of:
- ☐ The heart
- ☐ The femoral neck in lateral projection
- ☐ The gallbladder
- ☒ The temporomandibular joint
- ☐ The shoulder

Q. What formula might be used to find the size of field to be covered by a cone?

A.

$$\text{Size of field} = \frac{\text{target film distance} \times \text{lower diameter of cone}}{\text{distance from target to lower edge of cone}}$$

Check the statement below which is CORRECT:

When using a technique below 85 Kv.P., if an 8-to-1 grid is replaced by a 16-to-1 grid, the Kv.P. should be increased approximately:
- ☐ 2 Kv.P.
- ☒ 6 Kv.P.
- ☐ 12 Kv.P
- ☐ 16 Kv.P.

Check the statement below which is CORRECT:

High Kv.P. is required when radiographing structures of greater density in the body chiefly because of the:
- ☒ Absorption of radiation that results
- ☐ Electrons absorbed by inherent filtration

Study Questions

☐ Electrons absorbed by the part
☐ Penetrating effect of the longer wave lengths

Check the statement below which is CORRECT:

If I were a patient, I would rather a technologist used the following exposure to radiograph my lumbar spine:

☐ 70 Kv.P., 200 Ma.S.
☐ 84 Kv.P., 100 Ma.S.
☐ 100 Kv.P., 50 Ma.S.
☒ 120 Kv.P., 25 Ma.S.

Check the statement below which is CORRECT:

Useful radiographic densities lie within a range of:

☐ 1 to 3
☐ .1 to .5
☒ .25 to 2.5
☐ 4 and above

Check every statement below which is CORRECT:

True distortion on the radiograph is produced by:

☐ Focal spot size
☐ Focus-film distance
☒ Film, part, tube alignment
☐ Part-tube distance

Q. Will the sharpness of detail *increase, decrease,* or *remain the same* if (a) par speed screens are used instead of high? (b) the part-film distance is 6 inches instead of 3? (c) the Kv.P. is increased by 10? (d) the focal spot is 1 mm instead of 2 mm? (e) focus-film distance is increased from 40 to 72 inches?

A. (a) Increase, (b) decrease, (c) same, (d) increase, (e) increase.

Check every statement below which is CORRECT:

Absorption of x-rays is influenced by:

☒ Atomic weight
☒ Ma. used
☐ Temperature of the screen
☒ Thickness of the part
☐ Speed of the ray employed
☒ Wave length of the radiation produced
☒ Kv.P. used

Check any statement below which is CORRECT:

Radiographic fog increases as:

☒ Tissue volume increases
☐ Part moves closer to film
☐ Total quality of primary radiation is reduced
☒ Body part is predominantly soft tissue

Check every statement below which is CORRECT:

Radiographic contrast is the result of:

☐ Focal spot used
☒ Kv.P. used

FORMULATING X-RAY TECHNIQUES

- ☒ Volume of tissue
- ☒ Condition of tissue

Check the statement below which is CORRECT:

The factor which produces the greatest unsharpness is:
- ☐ Focal spot size
- ☐ Large focus-film distance
- ☒ Motion
- ☐ High-speed screens

CHECKLIST FOR RADIOGRAPHIC QUALITY

Detail

1. *Sharpness* of Detail (Definition)
    A. Motion
        i. voluntary
            a. immobilization
        ii. involuntary
            a. exposure time
    B. Projection
        i. size of focal-spot
        ii. object-film distance
        iii. focus-film distance
    C. Physical Factors
        i. film holder
            a. cardboard holder—direct exposure
            b. cassette and intensifying screens—indirect exposure
                (1) type and speed of screens
                (2) film-screen contact
        ii. film resolution

2. *Visibility* of Detail (Photographic)
    A. Density
    B. Contrast
    C. Processing

Density	Contrast
Ma.S.	Kv.P.
(quantitative)	(qualitative)
Thickness of part	Fog
Tissue opacity	Cone–grid
Pathology	Intensifying screens
Respiration	Filtration
Distance	Film characteristics
	Processing
	Efficiency of equipment

Study Questions

Magnification
      1. Object-film distance
      2. Focus-film distance

Distortion
      1. Alignment of tube-object-film

Superimposition
      1. Opacities of surrounding structures
      2. Alignment of tube-object-film

SPECIAL PROCEDURES

Opposite each procedure in Column A place the number of the region where it is used as listed in Column B:

Column A		Column B
11	Venogram (phlebogram)	1. Fallopian tubes
8	Myelogram	2. Lungs
12	Pneumo-encephalogram	3. Heart chambers
4	Sialogram	4. Salivary ducts
6	Cholangiogram	5. Renal calyces and pelves
10	Cholecystogram	6. Bile ducts
13	Carotid angiogram	7. Aorta
2	Bronchogram	8. Spinal canal
1	Salpingogram	9. Knee joint
5	Excretory urogram	10. Gallbladder
		11. Veins of the extremities
		12. Ventricular system
		13. Arteries of the brain

Opposite each procedure in Column A place the number of the region or purpose for which it is used in radiographic visualization as listed in Column B:

Column A		Column B
12	Cholangiography	1. Fluoroscopic images
4	Bronchography	2. Veins
3	Myelography	3. Spinal canal
5	Uterosalpingography	4. The bronchial tree
13	Ventriculography	5. The uterus and fallopian tubes
1	Photofluorography	6. The gallbladder
2	Venography	7. The birth canal
6	Cholecystography	8. The chambers of the heart
14	Body-section radiography	9. The arteries of the brain
7	Pelvimetry	10. The urinary tract
		11. The abdominal aorta
		12. The biliary ducts
		13. The fluid-containing spaces of the brain
		14. Regions at a predetermined depth

FORMULATING X-RAY TECHNIQUES

Opposite each procedure listed in Column A place the number of the region where it is used as listed in Column B:

Column A		Column B
_13_	Uterosalpingogram	1. Skull
_6_	Angiocardiogram	2. G. I. tract
_11_	Aortogram	3. Chest for heart size
_3_	Teleoroentgenogram	4. Arteries of the brain
_4_	Cerebral angiogram	5. Spinal canal
_7_	Ventriculogram	6. Chambers of the heart
_9_	Bronchogram	7. Ventricles of the brain
_1_	Towne's view or position	8. Veins of the extremities
_10_	Intravenous urogram	9. Bronchial tree
		10. Urinary tract
		11. Aorta
		12. Hip
		13. Female genital tract

Check the statement below which is CORRECT:

Rapid filming methods are advantageous in the following study:
- ☒ Aortography
- ☐ Ventriculography
- ☐ Pneumoarthrography
- ☐ Retro-peritoneal air studies

APPLICATION OF RADIOGRAPHIC FUNDAMENTALS

A satisfactory lateral radiograph of the skull has been taken using the following factors.

1.0-mm focal spot
Par-speed screens
8-to-1 ratio Bucky diaphragm
Developed 5 minutes at 68°
40" distance
100 Ma

Screen-type film
Cone to cover 10" x 12" film
2 mm. aluminum filter
$\frac{1}{2}$ second
65 Kv.P.

A number of changes in these factors, to be made one at a time, are suggested in the chart on the next page. Opposite each suggested change, indicate the effect you believe it would have on each of the radiographic qualities listed.

If any quality is DECREASED indicate by marking the appropriate square with a minus mark (−).

If any quality is INCREASED indicate by marking with a plus mark (+).

If there is no change in a quality, mark with a zero (0).

Study Questions

Change to be made	Detail (sharpness)	Density	Contrast	Magnification or distortion
Developed 5 minutes at 75°				
48" distance				
Increased object-film distance				
2.0-mm. focal spot				
Table-top, non-Bucky				
58 Kv.P.				
Use 3" mastoid cone				
200 Ma				
16:1 ratio Bucky				
25 Ma.S.				
0.75 second				
4-mm. aluminum filtration				
Develop 2 minutes at 68°				
30" focus-film distance				

ANATOMY

Q. To what joints are the following related: malleolus, glenoid fossa, condyles, acetabulum, tuberosities?

A. The malleolus is related to the ankle: the glenoid fossa, to the shoulder; the condyles, to the knee, elbow, and occipital; the acetabulum, to the hip; the tuberosities, to the shoulder and hip.

Q. Where is the atlas? malar bone? mandible? maxillae? manubrium?

A. The atlas is the first vertebra or segment of the vertebral column; the malar bone is located on the left and right side of the face or cheek; the mandible is the body of the lower jaw; the maxillae form the upper jaw; and the manubrium is the upper portion of the sternum.

Q. Where is the axis? petrous portion of the temporal bone? acromion process? ilium? zygoma?

A. The axis is the second cervical vertebra; the petrous portion of the temporal bone is the pyramidal portion of the temporal bone extending inward toward the median plane; the acromion process is the distal portion of the spine of the scapula; the ilium is the larger portion of the innominate or hip bone; and the zygoma is the arch of bone extending from the malar or cheek bone to the temporal bone on either side of the skull.

FORMULATING X-RAY TECHNIQUES

Q. Where is the sacroiliac articulation? brim of the acetabulum? first metacarpal? greater trochanter of the femur? patella?

A. The sacroiliac articulation is located at the junction of the sacrum and the ilium; the superior brim of the acetabulum is located at the edge or border of the cavity that receives the head of the femur; the first metacarpal is between the carpus and the phalanges; the greater trochanter of the femur is located at the upper end of the lateral surface of the femur; the patella is located anteriorly to the knee joint.

Q. Where is the outer canthus of the eye? internal auditory canal? foramen magnum? gallbladder? calcaneus?

A. The outer canthus of the eye is the outer junction of the upper and lower lid of the eye; the internal auditory canal is at the apex of the petrous bone; the foramen magnum is located in the floor of the skull between the occipital bone and the basilar portion; the gallbladder is usually on the right side of the abdomen on the under surface of the liver; and the calcaneus is the heel (also called os calcis).

Q. Where are the kidneys? liver? duodenum? urinary bladder? hepatic flexure?

A. The kidneys are located on the right and left side of the vertebral column, between the eleventh thoracic vertebra and the third lumbar vertebra; the liver is in the upper part of the abdomen, the main portion being on the right side; the duodenum lies between the pylorus and the jejunum; the urinary bladder is in the anterior part of the pelvic cavity; the hepatic flexure is located at the bend of the colon at the junction of its ascending and transverse parts.

Q. Where is the appendix? cecum? spleen? sigmoid flexure? tibia?

A. The appendix is an extension of the cecum; the cecum is the dilated intestinal pouch forming the first part of the large intestine; the spleen is in the upper part of the abdominal cavity and lateral to the cardiac end of the stomach; the sigmoid flexure is the part of the colon between the descending colon and the rectum; and the tibia is the inner and larger bone of the leg below the knee.

Q. Name the bones of the face.

A. The bones of the face are two nasals, two superior maxillae, one mandible, two zygomata, one vomer, two lacrimals, two turbinates, and two palatines.

Q. What are the mastoid cells and in what portion of what bone do they lie? What relation do they bear to a major anatomic landmark?

A. The mastoid cells are the cellular portion of the temporal bone lying at the mid-posterior portion of it. They are usually found posterior to the auditory canal.

Q. How many teeth are in the adult mouth and what are they?

A. There are 32 teeth in the adult mouth. They are eight incisors (four centrals, four laterals), four cuspids, eight bicuspids, and twelve molars.

Q. What is the location of the esophagus? Where does it begin and where does it end?

Study Questions

A. The esophagus is the muscular canal extending from the pharynx to the stomach in the mid-sagittal plane.

Q. Name the three major divisions of the small intestines.

A. The three major divisions of the small intestines are the duodenum, the jejunum, the ileum.

Q. What is meant by the hypochondrium? epigastrium? iliac region? hypogastrium? lumbar area?

A. The hypochondrium is the upper lateral region of the abdomen below the lowest rib; the epigastrium is the upper middle portion of the abdomen over or in front of the stomach; the iliac region is the lower lateral region of the abdomen; the hypogastrium is the lower median anterior portion of the abdomen; the lumbar area is the mid-lateral anterior portion of the abdomen.

Q. Name the main divisions of the urinary tract.

A. The main divisions of the urinary tract are the kidneys, ureters, urinary bladder, and urethra.

Q. Where is the symphysis pubis? xyphoid process? external occipital protuberance? iliac crest? parietal bones?

A. The symphysis pubis is the junction of the pubic bones; the xyphoid process is the extension downward of the sternum; the external occipital protuberance is found on the occipital bone at the junction of the median and nuchal lines; the iliac crest is the lateral, superior portion of the innominate bone; and the parietal bones are the bones which form the posterior and lateral portion of the walls of the neural cranium.

Q. What main anatomical structures lie in the lower right quadrant? upper right quadrant? lower left quadrant? upper left quadrant? pelvis?

A. Lower right quadrant—terminal ileum, cecum, part of ascending colon, appendix. Upper right quadrant—hepatic flexure, liver, right kidney, gallbladder, cystic or common duct, portion of pancreas, occasionally the duodenal cap, second portion of duodenum, some loops of the small bowel, right half of transverse colon. Lower left quadrant—sigmoid colon, portion of descending colon, some loops of small bowel. Upper left quadrant—spleen, left half of transverse colon, greater part of pancreas, stomach, splenic flexure, portion of descending colon, third portion of duodenum, left kidney, portion of jejunum. Pelvis (female)—uterus, ovaries, rectum, and bladder; (male)—rectum and bladder.

Q. Define the following terms: supine, saggital plane, distal, occlusal, thorax.

A. Supine—lying on the back; sagittal plane—a plane running in an antero-posterior direction; distal—farthest from the center, origin, or head; occlusal—the masticating surfaces of molar and bicuspid teeth; thorax—the part of the body between the neck and the abdomen.

Check the statement below which is CORRECT:

The following organ is in the left upper quadrant:
- ☐ Gallbladder
- ☒ Spleen
- ☐ Appendix
- ☐ Hepatic flexure

FORMULATING X-RAY TECHNIQUES

Indicate any of the following terms used to describe anatomical landmarks of the lower extremities:
- ☒ Lesser trochanter
- ☐ Greater tuberosity
- ☒ Medial malleolus
- ☒ Lateral condyle

Indicate any of the following located in the skull:
- ☒ Pineal gland
- ☐ Obturator foramen
- ☒ Lacrimal bone
- ☐ Olecranon process

Check the statement below which is CORRECT:

The xiphoid tip is usually located at the level of the:
- ☐ Third lumbar vertebra
- ☐ Fourth thoracic vertebra
- ☒ Tenth thoracic vertebra
- ☐ Ramus of the mandible

Check the statement below which is CORRECT:

The sella turcica serves as a bed for:
- ☐ The pineal gland
- ☐ The suprarenal gland
- ☒ The pituitary gland
- ☐ The sphenoid sinuses

Indicate any of the following diseases that will cause an increase in the density of the bone tissue:
- ☒ Chronic osteomyelitis
- ☒ Paget's disease
- ☒ Metastatic prostate
- ☐ Senility

Fill in the blank:

In the so-called blue baby—a cyanotic child with a congenital heart deformity—the blood is being shunted from the _____ side to the _____ side of the heart.

    A. Right to left.

Check the statement below which is CORRECT:

When the anterior pituitary gland produces too much growth hormone after puberty, we have a disease called:
- ☐ Hyperthyroidism
- ☐ Turner's disease
- ☒ Acromegaly
- ☐ Cushings disease

Check the statement below which is CORRECT:

With the patient in the anatomical position, the hip joint would be located:
- ☐ 5 cm. medial to greater trochanter
- ☐ 5 cm. lateral to the symphysis

Study Questions

☒ 2 in. below the point midway between the symphysis and the anterior superior spine
☐ 2 in. medial to anterior superior spine

Q. Name the three main anatomical portions of a long bone.
A. Diaphysis, metaphysis, and epiphysis.

Q. Name three main functions of the liver.
A. The liver manufactures bile, secretes heparin, and converts glucose to glycogen.

Q. Distinguish between bronchitis, bronchiectasis, and atelectasis.
A. Bronchitis is inflammation of the bronchus; bronchiectasis is dilatation of the bronchus; and atelectasis is collapse of all or part of a lung.

Q. What is meant by the cranium? Name the principal bones concerned in its formation.
A. The cranium means the brain case or pan. The principal bones concerned in the formation of the cranium are the frontal, parietals, occipital, temporals, sphenoid, and ethmoid.

Q. What is meant by medial, lateral, superior, and inferior?
A. Medial refers to the middle of the body, lateral refers to the side, superior refers to the upper, and inferior refers to the lowermost.

Q. What is meant by nasal accessory sinuses?
A. The nasal accessory sinuses are the associated bony cavities found within the bones of the face and cranium. They consist of the frontal, maxillary, sphenoid, and ethmoid sinuses.

Q. How many ribs are there? To what portion of the spine are they attached?
A. There are twenty-four ribs and they are attached to the thoracic portion of the spine.

Q. Name the divisions of the spine and state how many vertebrae compose each division.
A. The following are the divisions of the spine and the number of vertebrae which compose each division: cervical—seven, thoracic—twelve, lumbar—five, sacral—five, and coccygeal—four.

Check the statements below which are CORRECT:

In an examination of the petrous apices the following projections are commonly used:
☐ Lordotic view
☒ Towne view
☒ Stenvers projection
☒ Law projection

Place the number preceding each part of the body listed in Column A in the space following the region in Column B in which it can be found:

Column A	Column B
1. Foramen magnum	9 Foot
2. Anterior nasal spine	___ Ulna
3. Lunate or semilunar	1 Occipital bone

311

FORMULATING X-RAY TECHNIQUES

4. Ischial spine
5. Atlas
6. Ileum
7. Coracoid process
8. Lesser tubercle
9. Cuboid
10. Internal acoustic meatus

__8__ Humerus
__10__ Petrous process
____ Femur
__7__ Scapula
____ Tibia
__6__ Small bowel
__4__ Pelvis
__3__ Wrist
__2__ Maxilla
__5__ Cervical spine

Match:
__3__ Scapula
__6__ Axis
__5__ Frontal bone
__7__ Wrist
__1__ Maxilla
____ Temporal bone
__2__ Foot
__4__ Pelvis
__8__ Sternum

1. Alveolar ridge
2. Os calcis
3. Coracoid
4. Acetabulum
5. Glabella
6. Odontoid
7. Carpal
8. Xiphoid

Match:
__3__ Temporal bone
__4__ Knee joint
____ Sacrum
__5__ Scapula
__6__ Pelvis
__1__ Occipital bone
__7__ Ankle joint
____ Hand

1. Foramen magnum
2. Manubrium
3. Mastoid cells
4. Patella
5. Glenoid cavity
6. Pubis
7. Malleolus

Match:
__3__ Frontal
__1__ Temporal
__4__ Occipital
__2__ Sphenoid
__8__ Ethmoid
__7__ Maxillae
__6__ Mandible
__5__ Fontanelles
____

1. Petrous
2. Sella turcica
3. Glabella
4. Foramen magnum
5. Lambda
6. Coronoid
7. Antra of Highmore
8. Cribriform plate
9. Coracoid

Study Questions

Match:

_4_	Sternum	1.	Talus
_2_	Atlas	2.	First cervical vertebra
_1_	Ankle	3.	Acromion
_5_	Lumbar	4.	Manubrium
_6_	Axis	5.	Five
_9_	Dorsal	6.	Second cervical vertebra
_8_	Coccyx	7.	Seven
_3_	Scapula	8.	Four fused bones
___		9.	Twelve
___		10.	Ten

Match:

_b_	1. Cuboid	a.	Cervical spine
_f_	2. Internal acoustic meatus	b.	Foot
_d_	3. Foramen magnum	c.	Ulna
_m_	4. Anterior nasal spine	d.	Occipital bone
_l_	5. Lunate or semilunar	e.	Humerus
_k_	6. Ischial spine	f.	Petrous process
_a_	7. Atlas	g.	Femur
_j_	8. Ileum	h.	Scapula
_h_	9. Coracoid process	i.	Tibia
_e_	10. Lesser tuberosity	j.	Small bowel
		k.	Pelvis
		l.	Wrist
		m.	Maxilla

Match:

_j_	11	3rd molar (sample)	a. temporal	1.	Waters
_c_	5	Frontal sinuses	b. occipital	2.	lateral skull
_a_	12	Mastoids	c. frontal	3.	Towne
_d_	6	Optic foramen	d. sphenoid	4.	Fletcher's
_a_	8	Int. aud. meatus	e. maxillae	5.	Caldwell
_b_	3	Foramen magnum	f. mandible	6.	Rhese
_e_	1	Antra of Highmore	g. ethmoid	7.	mento-vertex
_d_	2	Sella turcica	h. palatine bones	8.	Stenvers
_f_	9	Ramus	i. fontanelles	9.	lat. mandible
_g_	6	Cribriform plate	j. teeth	10.	A.P. skull 2
_g_	7	Crista galli	k. zygomatic bones	11.	Dental
				12.	Law

Match:

_4_	Odontoid process	1.	Sacrum
_5_	Glenoid fossa	2.	Colon

FORMULATING X-RAY TECHNIQUES

_7_	Greater trochanter	3.	Pelvis
_3_	Anterior superior iliac spine	4.	Cervical spine
_12_	Alveolar process	5.	Scapula
_14_	Phalanx	6.	Small bowel
_9_	Carpal navicular bone	7.	Femur
_2_	Sigmoid	8.	Sternum
_6_	Jejunum	9.	Wrist
		10.	Elbow
		11.	Tarsus
		12.	Mandible
		13.	Patella
		14.	Finger

Match:

_2_	Beside	1.	Pseudo
_3_	Against	2.	Para
_1_	False	3.	Anti
___	Upon	4.	Pan
_5_	Around	5.	Peri
_4_	All		

Match:

_4_	Towards front	1.	Cephalic
_3_	After	2.	Dorsal
_2_	Towards back	3.	Post
___	Before	4.	Ventral
_1_	Towards head	5.	Caudad
_5_	Towards feet		

Match:

_5_	Head	1.	Caudad
_4_	Lying face up	2.	Prone
___	Turn out	3.	Flex
_1_	Tail	4.	Supine
_3_	Bend	5.	Cephalad
_2_	Lying face down		

Opposite each term in Column A place the number of the correct definition as listed in Column B:

_2_	Anterior	1.	Towards the head
_8_	Medial (mesial)	2.	Front
_11_	Lateral	3.	Lying on the side
_12_	Proximal	4.	With the part bent up
_1_	Cephalad	5.	With the part moved away from the body
_4_	Flexed		

Study Questions

_5_	Abducted	6.	Below
_10_	Prone	7.	Above
_6_	Inferior	8.	Towards the midline
_13_	Sagittal	9.	Towards the tail
_15_	Oblique	10.	Lying on the abdomen
_3_	Lateral decubitus	11.	Away from the midline
_7_	Superior	12.	Near the central point of reference

13. Refers to plane which divides the body into right and left parts
14. Refers to plane which divides the body into anterior and posterior parts
15. View of part rotated from true A.P. or P.A. position

POSITIONING

Check the statement below which is CORRECT:

In the lateral projection of the scapula:
- ☐ The coracoid process is centered to the film
- ☒ The central ray is aligned at 90 degrees to the vertebral border of the scapula
- ☐ The patient is placed in a lateral decubitus position
- ☐ The glenoid cavity is best demonstrated

Check the statement below which is CORRECT:

The best position to show the articular facets of the lumbar spine is the:
- ☒ Oblique
- ☐ A.P.
- ☐ Lateral
- ☐ P.A.

Check the statement below which is CORRECT:

The external auditory meatus is used as a landmark to locate the:
- ☒ Sella turcica
- ☐ Maxilla
- ☐ Frontal sinus
- ☐ Nasion

Check the statement below which is CORRECT:

The best position to demonstrate the clavicle in an adult is the:
- ☐ A.P. position with caudal angulation
- ☐ A.P. position with a perpendicular ray
- ☒ P.A. position
- ☐ Lateral position

Check the statement below which is CORRECT:

The A.P. projection of the skull with a 30–35 degree caudal angulation demonstrates primarily the:
- ☐ Sphenoid bone
- ☐ Frontal bone

FORMULATING X-RAY TECHNIQUES

☒ Petrous ridge
☐ Parietal bone

Check the statement below which is CORRECT:

The anterior superior iliac spine is used as a landmark in locating the point of entry of the central ray when making a radiograph of the:

☒ Sacrum
☐ Shoulder
☐ Sternum
☐ Gallbladder

Check the statement below which is CORRECT:

An occlusal film is placed in the mouth with a portion extending from the mouth. The central ray is projected downward perpendicular to the film. This view best demonstrates:

☒ The nasal bone
☐ The palatines
☐ The mandibular symphysis
☐ Wharton's duct

Check the statement below which is CORRECT:

When the patient is in the frog-leg position, the thighs are placed in:

☐ Full adduction
☒ Full abduction
☐ Full extension with the feet together
☐ Full flexion over the abdomen

Check the statement below which is CORRECT:

In mitral stenosis the position that best demonstrates the left atrium of the heart is the

☐ Right lateral
☐ Left anterior oblique
☐ A.P. position
☒ Right anterior oblique

Check the statement below which is CORRECT:

When radiographing the ankle in the antero-posterior projection on a single film, the

☐ Heel is placed in the center of the film
☒ Inter-malleolar plane is parallel to the film
☐ Ankle is rotated laterally 5 degrees
☐ Central ray is angled 10 degrees cephalad

Six bony prominences are listed below. Opposite each one listed place a YES if it can be felt through the skin and a NO if it cannot.

YES Greater trochanter
NO Body of the ninth thoracic vertebra
NO Lesser trochanter
YES Symphysis pubis
YES Acromion process
YES Manubrium

Study Questions

Check the statement below which is CORRECT:

When radiographing the coccyx in the antero-posterior position, the central ray is directed:
- ☐ Perpendicular to the film
- ☐ Cephalad
- ☒ Caudad
- ☐ To a point 2 inches below the pubis

Check the statement below which is CORRECT:

In the Chamberlain-Towne position, the central ray is directed so that the orbito-meatal line forms an angle with the central ray of:
- ☐ 60°
- ☒ 30°
- ☐ 20°
- ☐ 45°

Check the statement below which is CORRECT:

A long exposure time can be used to advantage in a technique intended to show:
- ☐ The stereoscopic lung field
- ☐ Kidney, pelvis, and ureters in an IVP
- ☐ A stomach with barium
- ☐ The gallbladder
- ☒ The lateral thoracic spine

Check the statement below which is CORRECT:

A routine P.A. chest radiograph is taken at a six-foot target-film distance in order to:
- ☐ Increase contrast
- ☐ Increase magnification
- ☐ Decrease detail
- ☒ Decrease magnification
- ☐ Stop motion

Q. In radiography of the lower dorsal spine in the anteroposterior position, why is it desirable to center to the sixth dorsal vertebra?

A. In order to take advantage of the divergent rays for separating the joint spaces and also to equalize density over the entire section of the spine being examined.

Q. In radiography of certain areas of the body, very close focus-film distance may sometimes be desirable. Name one such area and give the reason.

A. An area of the body where very close focus-film distance might be desirable, at times, is the atlas and axis. Such a procedure may be followed in order to obtain magnification of the part and blur out the superimposed parts.

Q. What is the Waters-Waldron position and where is it used?

A. The Waters-Waldron position is used in examination of the maxillary sinuses. The patient is prone, head resting on the chin, cantho-meatal line forming an angle of 37° to the perpendicular, central ray perpendicular to the film and entering the head at the vertex, passing just in front of the ear and making its exit at a point in line with the junction of the nose and upper lip. The median plane of the head is perpendicular to the table top.

Q. What is the modified Law position and where is it used?

A. The modified Law position is used in examination of the mastoid. The patient is prone, head rotated 15° to either side, central ray is angled 15° toward the face and enters the head about two inches above and behind the unaffected ear to exit through the mastoid closest to the film.

Q. What is the Stenvers position and where is it used?

A. The Stenvers position is used in the examination of the petrous portion of the temporal bone. The patient is in the prone position, median line of the body over the center line of the table. The head is turned at an angle of 45° from the posteroanterior position with the forehead and malar bone touching the cassette. The tube is tilted 12° toward the head, the central ray being directed through the external auditory meatus closest to the film.

Q. What is the Towne position and where is it used?

A. The Towne position is used in the examination of the occipital and petrous bones in an anteroposterior projection. The patient is supine, median line of the head is over center line of the table, the chin is depressed as far as comfortably possible. From the side of the table the film is centered to the occipital protuberance. The tube is angled approximately 30° towards the feet, and the central ray is directed to the center of the film.

Q. What methods are used to secure immobilization of the parts radiographed? Why is immobilization so essential to the successful radiograph?

A. Cloth immobilizing bands, sandbags, padded bricks, or head clamp. Such devices are essential to successful radiography for the elimination or control of motion in order to secure good detail.

Q. What views are ordinarily taken of any part and why?

A. Ordinarily two views at right angles to each other are taken of a part in order to secure proper perspective and relation of the parts to the surrounding tissue or parts. When two views at right angles cannot be secured, we can make stereoscopic views in order to secure depth of vision.

Q. What are spot exposures in gastrointestinal work?

A. Spot exposures are usually from one to four exposures made on a film at intervals of a few seconds for the purpose of obtaining progressive views of stomach or colon peristalsis in gastrointestinal radiography. A special spot-taking device is usually a part of the fluoroscopy unit.

Q. Why is it necessary to have close approximation of the part to the film?

A. It is necessary to have close approximation of the part to the film in order to eliminate an objectionable amount of magnification.

Q. Given a set of exposure factors for an x-ray examination of a co-operative patient, what changes would you make for an unco-operative or irrational patient?

Study Questions

A. Decrease the exposure time to a value sufficiently small to obviate possibility of motion; at the same time increasing the Ma. value by the amount needed to produce the original Ma. value. Alternately, decrease the exposure time to obviate motion and increase the Kv.P. so as to maintain film density.

Q. Describe the effects of inspiration and expiration in radiography of the chest, sternum, dorsal spine, ribs.

A. In radiography of the chest, sternum, ribs, and dorsal spine, films made on inspiration will be more dense than those made on expiration, all other factors being the same. In radiography of the chest, the diaphragm will be lower on inspiration than on expiration.

Check every statement below which is CORRECT:

The positions which may be used most successfully in demonstrating the odontoid process are
- ☒ Conventional lateral view of the cervical spine
- ☒ Exaggerated Waters view ordinarily used for facial bones
- ☒ Open-mouth view
- ☐ Conventional A.P. view of the cervical spine
- ☒ A.P. exposure while moving lower jaw

Check the statement below which is CORRECT:

For a radiograph of the gallbladder of an obese person the central ray is usually directed to enter the body:
- ☐ At a point lower and nearer the spine than for a person of normal weight
- ☐ At a point higher and nearer the mid-line than for a person of normal weight
- ☐ At a point lower and more to the right than for a person of normal weight
- ☒ At a point higher and more to the right than for a person of normal weight
- ☐ At a point behind the spine

Check the statement below which is CORRECT:

The odontoid process is well visualized in the following view:
- ☐ Lateral view of the tarsus
- ☐ Oblique view of the mandible
- ☒ Open-mouth view of the cervical spine
- ☐ Oblique view of the lumbosacral joint
- ☐ Lateral view of the sternum

Check the statement below which is CORRECT:

In an examination of the petrous apices the following projection is not commonly used:
- ☒ Lordotic view
- ☐ Towne position
- ☐ Law projection
- ☐ Arcelin projection
- ☐ Stenvers projection

FORMULATING X-RAY TECHNIQUES

Check the statement below which is CORRECT:

In making a radiograph of the sinuses using the Waters position, the purpose of the position is to:
- ☐ Project the sphenoid sinus away from the maxillary sinuses
- ☒ Project the petrous portions of the temporal bones below the maxillary sinuses
- ☐ Project the petrous portions of the temporal bones above the maxillary sinuses
- ☐ Superimpose the petrous portions of the temporal bones on the maxillary sinuses

Check the statement below which is CORRECT:

In making a P.A. radiograph of the abdomen the patient is in:
- ☒ The prone position
- ☐ The abducted position
- ☐ The supine position
- ☐ The lateral recumbent position
- ☐ The dorsal decubitus position

Check the statement below which is CORRECT:

In taking a P.A. radiograph of the chest the shoulders are rolled forward to:
- ☐ Elevate the clavicles
- ☐ Enlarge the chest
- ☐ Lower the diaphragm
- ☒ Remove the scapulae from the region of the lung field
- ☐ Bring the heart closer to the film

Check the statement below which is CORRECT:

In making a P.A. radiograph of the distal radius and ulna the hand should be placed in:
- ☐ The lordotic position
- ☐ Flexion
- ☐ Supination
- ☐ The 'anatomical' position
- ☒ Pronation

Check the statement below which is CORRECT:

In the Waters sinus position the central ray enters the skull in the midsagittal plane emerging at:
- ☐ The external occipital protuberance
- ☒ The junction of the upper lip and nose
- ☐ The external auditory meatus
- ☐ The base of the nose (glabella)
- ☐ The mastoid tip

Check the statement below which is CORRECT:

The foramen magnum is best demonstrated by the use of:
- ☐ Waters position
- ☐ Stenvers position

Study Questions

    ☐ Granger position
    ☐ Law position
    ☒ Towne position

Check the statement below which is CORRECT:

When one is making a P.A. radiograph of the gallbladder of an average adult patient, the central ray is usually directed so as to enter the body:
    ☐ At the level of the 12th thoracic vertebra
    ☒ Three inches to the right of the 2nd lumbar vertebra
    ☐ Two inches to the left of the 2nd lumbar vertebra
    ☐ Two inches above the crest of the left ilium

Check the statement below which is CORRECT:

The Stenvers position is used in making a radiograph of:
    ☐ The sphenoid sinus
    ☐ The sella turcica
    ☐ The maxillary sinus
    ☐ The symphysis menti
    ☒ The petrous process

Check the statement below which is CORRECT:

When one is making a verticosubmental sphenoid sinus radiograph, the central ray enters at:
    ☒ The top of the skull
    ☐ The outer canthus of the eye
    ☐ The root of the nose
    ☐ The external auditory meatus
    ☐ The center of Reid's base line

Check the statement below which is CORRECT:

When one is making a P.A. radiograph of the duodenal bulb of an average adult patient, the central ray is usually directed so as to enter the body:
    ☐ Two inches to the right of the 12th thoracic vertebra
    ☐ One inch to the right of the 5th lumbar vertebra
    ☐ One inch to the right of the 2nd lumbar vertebra
    ☒ Two inches to the left of the 2nd lumbar vertebra
    ☐ In the midline at the level of the 9th thoracic vertebra

Check the statement below which is CORRECT:

When one is making an x-ray of the hip in the anterior-posterior projection, the following bony landmarks must be noted:
    ☒ The anterosuperior spine
    ☒ The symphysis
    ☒ The greater trochanter
    ☐ The patella
    ☐ The 1st lumbar vertebra

Check the statement below which is CORRECT:

The crest of the ilium is used as a landmark in making:
    ☐ A radiograph of the A.P. thoracic spine
    ☐ An A.P. shoulder radiograph

FORMULATING X-RAY TECHNIQUES

☒ A KUB
☐ A lateral radiograph of the sternum
☐ An A.P. of the os calcis

Check the statement below which is CORRECT:

When making an A.P. radiograph of the wrist the hand should be placed in:
☐ Pronation
☒ The anatomical position
☐ Flexion
☐ Adduction
☐ Eversion

Check the statement below which is CORRECT:

The malleoli are used as landmarks when making a radiograph of:
☒ An A.P. ankle
☐ A P.A. knee
☐ An A.P. shoulder
☐ An A.P. elbow

Check the statement below which is CORRECT:

A long exposure time can be used to advantage in techniques intended to show:
☐ The stereoscopic lung field
☐ Kidney, pelves, and ureters in an IVP
☐ A stomach with barium
☐ The gallbladder
☒ The sternum

Check the statement below which is CORRECT:

In making a radiograph of the gastrointestinal tract it is important to use:
☐ A long target-film distance
☒ A short exposure time
☐ Self-rectified equipment
☐ As low kilovoltage as possible
☐ A thoraesus filter

Check the statement below which is CORRECT:

The amount of tube shift required in making stereoscopic radiographs to be viewed in a standard stereoscope is determined by:
☐ The object-film distance
☐ The milliampere seconds used
☐ The kilovoltage employed
☒ The focus-film distance
☐ The type of x-ray tube used

Check the statement below which is CORRECT:

In a pelvimetry the following is not important in obtaining an accurate measurement:
☐ The part-table distance
☐ The tube-table distance

Study Questions

- ☐ The distance between table top and film
- ☒ The kilovoltage used
- ☐ The centering of the tube

Indicate by number the relative position of the wave lengths of the forms of radiation listed starting with No. 1 for that having the shortest wave length:

- __3__ Ultraviolet
- __5__ Infrared
- __1__ Gamma rays
- __4__ Visible light
- __2__ X-rays

PHYSICS, ELECTRICITY

Q. What is matter?

A. Anything which occupies space. Examples: steam, ice, water.

Q. What is an atom?

A. The smallest part of a molecule. It is made up of electrons, protons, and neutrons.

Q. Define *electron.*

A. The electron is the smallest measurable quantity of negative electricity.

Q. Define *proton.*

A. The proton is the smallest measurable quantity of positive electricity.

Q. Define *neutron.*

A. The neutron is an electrically neutral part of an atom.

Q. Define *molecule.*

A. The molecule is the smallest part of matter that can exist by itself and still show the characteristic properties of the original substance.

Q. Diagram the structure of matter.

A.
```
              Matter
                ↓
Simple --- Molecule --- Compound
                ↓
              Atom
           ↙   ↓   ↘
    Electron Neutron Proton
```

Q. When pressure has established a state of imbalance in an atom, how does the atom achieve a return to stability?

A. The atom has a natural tendency to return to a neutral state and it will immediately attract electrons from other sources to restore its neutrality.

Q. When an electron is removed from an atom, how is the atom charged?

A. Positively.

FORMULATING X-RAY TECHNIQUES

Q. When a free electron attaches to an atom, how does the atom become charged?

A. Negatively.

Q. What is electricity?

A. The flow of negatively charged particles, called electrons, along wire conductors.

Q. Define *ohm*.

A. An ohm is a unit of electrical resistance.

Q. Define *volt*.

A. A volt is a unit of electrical pressure. One volt is the amount of electrical pressure required to force one ampere of electrical current through one ohm of electrical resistance.

Q. Define *ampere*.

A. An ampere is a unit of electrical current. One ampere is the amount of electrical current forced through one ohm of resistance by the electrical pressure of one volt.

Q. Distinguish between a good conductor and a good insulator. Name one of each.

A. A good conductor is any material which permits a free flow of electrons, such as copper wire. A good insulator is any material that impedes the flow of electrons, such as glass.

Q. Define *milliampere*.

A. A milliampere is $1/1000$ of an ampere.

Q. Define *kilovolt*.

A. A kilovolt is equal to 1000 volts.

Q. Define *peak kilovolt*.

A. Peak kilovolt is the highest kilovoltage at any time in an electrical cycle.

Q. What is an ammeter?

A. A device used to measure amperes.

Q. What is a voltmeter?

A. A device used to measure volts.

Q. What is a galvanometer?

A. An instrument used to measure small amounts of current.

Q. What is a resistor?

A. A device which offers a great resistance to the flow of electrons. Some resistors offer resistance in varying degrees and can be manually controlled.

Q. What is an ohm?

A. The unit of resistance. An electromotive force of 1 volt will move an electric current of 1 ampere against the resistance of 1 ohm.

Q. What is a magnet?

Study Questions

A. A bar or horseshoe-shaped piece of iron which has the power to attract pieces of iron to its poles. This is called magnetism. A compass needle is said to be a bar magnet. The pole of the needle pointing to the north has a north-seeking or north pole. The earth is a big magnet with magnetic poles near its north and south geographical poles. In the space around the magnet there is a field of force.

Q. Do electric currents show magnetic effects?

A. Yes. A compass needle held close to a straight wire with direct current passing through it will turn its needle perpendicular to the wire and the current. This shows the presence of a magnetic field around the wire. There is no movement of electrons without this field of energy and this movement continues until the magnetic field disappears. It may be that each moving electron creates its own field of energy.

Q. What is electromagnetic induction?

A. This is the production of an electric current in a wire coil by placing it within a magnetic field which surrounds another wire coil. The current is produced even though there is no electrical connection between the coils.

Q. What is a magnetic field?

A. An area of magnetic force which surrounds an electric charge of current.

Q. Does a magnetic field exist at right angles to or parallel to an electric conductor?

A. At right angles.

Q. Distinguish between static and current electricity.

A. In static electricity the electric charge is at rest. In current electricity, the charged particles flow along a conductor.

Q. What is mutual inductance?

A. This is the establishment of a voltage in a wire coil either by moving a conductor across magnetic lines of force or by having the magnetic field change polarity, causing the magnetic lines to cut across a conductor.

Q. What is a transformer?

A. A device used to transfer electrical energy from one circuit to another and either raise or lower the voltage without the two circuits being electrically connected to one another.

Example: If the windings of wire in the primary circuit are 100 and those of the secondary circuit 100,000, the voltage in the secondary circuit will be 1000 times as great as that in the primary circuit.

Q. What is the structure of a step-up transformer?

A. The number of turns of wire is greater in the secondary coil than in the primary coil. This causes an increase in voltage.

Q. What is the structure of a step-down transformer?

A. The number of turns of copper wire in the primary coil is greater than those in the secondary coil. This results in a decrease in voltage.

Q. What is an autotransformer?

FORMULATING X-RAY TECHNIQUES

A. A device used to select the amount of voltage to introduce into the primary coil of the step-up transformer. It consists of a single winding of copper wire around an iron core. Leads are taken off from various turns of the coil, allowing a selection of the amount of voltage to let in. It is generally used as a step-down transformer.

Q. What is meant by the ratio of a transformer?

A. The ratio of a transformer is the relation of the number of turns on the primary to the number of turns on the secondary.

Q. What is meant by frequency of an alternating current? What frequencies are commonly used?

A. The frequency of an alternating current is the number of times the current changes from positive to negative to positive per second. The common frequencies are 25 cycles, 50 cycles, and 60 cycles.

Q. What are the properties of x-rays?

A.
1. The ability to penetrate solids and opaque media.
2. The ability to darken photographic film.
3. The ability to emit light (fluorescence) when they strike certain substances.

Q. Name the three necessary conditions for the production of x-rays.

A.
1. A concentration of electrons.
2. The movement of those electrons at a high speed.
3. Sudden stoppage of electrons by striking a target.

Q. How are x-rays produced?

A. The electrons, which are negatively charged particles traveling at a high speed through a metal conductor, are forced to cross a gap in the conductor and strike a metal target on the other side of the gap. The target is positively charged and thus attracts the negatively charged electrons. At the target the electrical energy is converted into light energy and we then have x-rays.

Q. What is the usual electric voltage used?

A. 110 or 220 volts.

Q. How may 110 or 220 volts be increased to say 50,000 volts?

A. By the use of a step-up transformer.

Q. How may 110 or 220 volts be decreased to say 5 volts?

A. By the use of a step-down transformer. This is used to heat the filament of the x-ray tube.

Q. Which is more penetrating, an x-ray with a short wave length or one with a long wave length?

A. The short wave length is more penetrating.

Q. What is the unit of measurement of wave lengths?

A. The angstrom unit (Å). One angstrom unit is equal to .00000001 centimeter ($1/100,000,000$ centimeter, or one one-hundred-millionth of a centimeter).

Study Questions

Q. What is the electromagnetic spectrum?

A. The grouping of electromagnetic waves or radiations according to their wave length.

Q. What are some of the rays of the electromagnetic spectrum?

A. Electric, microwaves, infrared, ultraviolet, television, radio, visible light, x-rays, gamma rays, cosmic rays.

Q. Upon what does the penetrability of x-rays produced depend?

A. The penetrability of x-rays depends on the kilovoltage at which they are produced or, more specifically, on their wave length.

Q. What is meant by *hard rays*? By *soft rays*?

A. Hard rays are rays produced at relatively high kilovoltage and are more penetrating than the soft rays, which are produced at relatively low kilovoltage. Hard rays are short-wave-length rays and soft rays are long-wave-length rays.

Q. What is the fundamental relation between kilovolts impressed on an x-ray tube and the quality of the emergent beam?

A. The quality of hardness of an x-ray beam increases as the voltage increases, decreases as the voltage decreases. The wave length of the beam becomes shorter as the kilovoltage increases and longer as the kilovoltage decreases.

Q. What meters are necessary in an x-ray machine? For what purpose is each used, and where is each located in the circuit?

A. The necessary meters in an x-ray machine are an ammeter, milliammeter, and a voltmeter. The ammeter measures the filament current and is in the primary circuit to the filament transformer. The Ma. meter measures the current flowing through the x-ray tube and is in the high-tension circuit. The voltmeter is in the primary circuit of the high-tension transformer and indicates the voltage applied to the primary of the high-tension transformer.

Q. How is electricity flowing through a conductor like water running through a pipe?

A. Water flowing through a pipe flows in one direction at a constant volume similar to direct current through a wire. It encounters resistance to its flow and therefore must have pressure behind it to cause the water to flow. In an electrical system the equivalent pressure is voltage and the resistance ohms. Flow of electricity may be likened to the flow of water in a pipe; the voltage corresponds to pressure — the higher the voltage, the more current or water flow. The current or amperage corresponds to gallons per minute. Resistance in the electrical flow corresponds to friction or resistance to the water flow,—the larger the wire or water pipe, the more current or water flow with the same voltage or water pressure.

Q. Can a direct current be used to operate a transformer? If only direct current is available, how could you operate an x-ray machine?

A. A direct current cannot be used to operate a transformer. If only direct current is available it must be converted to alternating current by a device called a rotary converter.

FORMULATING X-RAY TECHNIQUES

Q. Is the filament control in the low- or the high-voltage portion of the circuit?

A. In the low-voltage portion.

Q. What is self-rectification?

A. When high voltage is applied to an x-ray tube only those alternations above the base line are of value, and cause electrons to be cast off to the target of the tube. During the period of alternations below the base line no electrons are given off and thus no x-rays are produced. This is due to the fact that the anode of the tube (containing the target) is positive and negative alternatingly with relation to the cathode during each half cycle. When the anode is positive, the negative electrons at the cathode are attracted to the anode and x-rays are produced. When the anode is negative, electrons are not attracted. Self-rectification is used in portable and dental x-ray machines for light x-ray work.

Q. What is half-wave rectification?

A. If heavier work is demanded from an x-ray tube, it cannot act as a self-rectifier. A valve tube must be used in the circuit of high voltage which prevents the unused voltage (alternations below the base line) from being applied to the x-ray tube. This tube has a large cathode filament which produces an abundance of electrons which are bombarded against the entire face of the anode (target).

Q. What is valve-tube rectification (full-wave)?

A. This is the use of four valve tubes in the circuit so that the alternations above the base line fill in the gap ordinarily utilized by the alternations below the base line. The first two valve tubes carry electrons from the alternations above the base line to the x-ray tube. The next two valve tubes then complete the circuit. This gives maximum use of voltage and equipment.

Q. Why is alternating current better than direct current?

A. It can be sent over long distances with a minimum of loss in transit. It is also possible to cut it down from high voltage to the 110 or 220 voltage needed in homes and offices.

Check the statement below which is CORRECT:

The energy level of electrons in the inner orbits of atoms is:
- ☒ High
- ☐ Low

Check the statement below which is CORRECT:

In a normal atom, the following number of negative charges should be present to counteract the number of positive charges in the nucleus:
- ☐ Twice as many
- ☒ The same number
- ☐ Half as many
- ☐ Four times as many

Study Questions

Check the statement below which is CORRECT:

Electricity is a form of energy primarily because it:
- ☐ Occupies space
- ☒ Can do work
- ☐ Has weight
- ☐ Has inertia

Check the statement below which is CORRECT:

The voltage in the filament circuit of an x-ray tube usually is approximately:
- ☐ 220–240 volts
- ☒ 10–15 volts
- ☐ 110–115 volts
- ☐ 30–150 Kv.P.

Check the statement below which is CORRECT:

The purpose of the choke coil (variable resistor) in an x-ray circuit is to regulate the current delivered to the:
- ☐ Primary windings of the x-ray transformer
- ☐ Autotransformer
- ☐ Filament transformer of rectifier tube
- ☒ Filament of x-ray tube

Check the statement below which is CORRECT:

The following does not significantly affect the strength of an electromagnet:
- ☒ Voltage
- ☐ Amperage
- ☐ Turns in the coil
- ☐ The core

Check the statement below which is CORRECT:

The amount of electrical current flowing in a conductor is measured in
- ☐ Ma.
- ☐ Kilovolts
- ☒ Amperes
- ☐ Volts

Check the statement below which is CORRECT:

The current flowing between the transformer and the rectifier is:
- ☐ Direct current
- ☐ High frequency current
- ☐ Pulsating direct current
- ☐ Unidirectional current
- ☒ Alternating current

Check the statement below which is CORRECT:

Electrical pressure is measured in:
- ☐ Amperes
- ☒ Volts

FORMULATING X-RAY TECHNIQUES

☐ Ohms
☐ Watts
☐ Ergs

Check the statement below which is CORRECT:

A good insulator is:
☐ Copper
☐ Silver
☐ Salt water
☒ Oil
☐ Aluminum

Check the statement below which is CORRECT:

Since the voltage in the secondary of a step-up transformer is higher than in the primary:
☐ Electrical potential in the secondary is higher than in the primary
☐ The frequency of alternations is increased
☒ Milliamperage in the secondary is less than in the primary
☐ The milliamperage is increased in the secondary
☐ The frequency of alternations is decreased

Check the statement below which is CORRECT:

The ratio of a transformer is determined by:
☐ The relation of the size of the wires in the primary winding to those in the secondary
☐ The relation of the voltage impressed on the primary to the voltage produced in the secondary
☒ The relation of the number of turns in the primary to the number of turns in the secondary
☐ The relation of the current produced in the secondary to the resistance in the primary

Check the statement below which is CORRECT:

Of wires of identical material, the one that offers the least resistance to the flow of an electric current is:
☒ Short and thick
☐ Long and thin
☐ Short and thin
☐ Long and thick

Check the statement below which is CORRECT:

The wave lengths of x-radiation generally used in radiography are:
☐ Longer than visible light
☒ Longer than gamma rays
☐ Shorter than radium radiation
☐ Longer than ultraviolet rays
☐ Longer than infrared rays

Q. What is an impulse timer and what are its applications in radiography?

Study Questions

A. An impulse timer is a very accurate x-ray timer which times an x-ray exposure in exact multiples of one impulse; that is, it starts an exposure at a zero point of the alternating voltage supplied to the high voltage transformer and interrupts it at a zero point of some subsequent impulse. It permits the use of very accurately controlled high-energy exposures.

Check the statement below which is CORRECT:

The direction of electron flow through an x-ray tube is:
- ☐ From positive to negative terminal
- ☐ Determined by the heat of the filament
- ☐ From anode to cathode
- ☐ Determined by the shape of the focusing cup
- ☒ From negative to positive terminal

Check the statement below which is CORRECT:

In checking the timer of a full-wave rectified x-ray machine using a spinning top for $1/10$ of a second, the number of dots recorded should be:
- ☐ 6   ☒ 12   ☐ 18   ☐ 20   ☐ 60

Check the statement below which is CORRECT:

In half-wave rectified x-ray machines operating with a 60-cycle current the number of impulses per second passing through the x-ray tube is:
- ☐ 12   ☐ 6
- ☐ 18   ☒ 60
- ☐ 30   ☐ 120

Check the statement below which is CORRECT:

The flow of electrons through a conductor is termed:
- ☐ Static electricity
- ☐ Reticulation
- ☐ Rectification
- ☐ Chemical action
- ☒ Current electricity

Check the statement below which is CORRECT:

The term 'amperage' is used to describe:
- ☐ The direction of flow of electrons through a conductor
- ☐ The resistance offered to the flow of electricity
- ☒ The number of electrons passing a given point in a conductor in a given period of time
- ☐ The electromotive force impressed upon the conductor
- ☐ The amount of ionization produced in a given quantity of air in a given period of time

Check the statement below which is CORRECT:

A line voltage compensator is located:
- ☒ In the primary circuit
- ☐ In the secondary circuit
- ☐ Just before the rectifier
- ☐ Just after the rectifier
- ☐ In the filament circuit

FORMULATING X-RAY TECHNIQUES

Check the statement below which is CORRECT:
Ohm's Law is expressed by:
- ☒ Amperes equal $\dfrac{\text{Volts}}{\text{Ohms}}$
- ☐ Volts equal $\dfrac{\text{Watts}}{\text{Amperes}}$
- ☐ Horsepower is $\dfrac{\text{Watts}}{746}$
- ☐ Volts equal Amperes x Watts
- ☐ A equals ½ bh

Check the statement below which is CORRECT:
In checking the timer of a half-wave rectified machine using a spinning top for 1/10 of a second the following number of dots should be recorded:
☒ 6 ☐ 12 ☐ 24 ☐ 48 ☐ 60

Check the statement below which is CORRECT:
The pre-reading voltmeter is connected:
- ☐ In parallel with the x-ray tube
- ☐ Across the rectifier
- ☒ Across the primary of the step-up transformer
- ☐ In the filament circuit
- ☐ At the midpoint of the secondary of the high-voltage transformer

Check the statement below which is CORRECT:
With a self-rectified unit operating on a 60-cycle circuit the number of impulses of radiation striking the film in ½ second will be:
☐ 15 ☒ 30 ☐ 60 ☐ 120 ☐ 240

Opposite each term in Column 'A' place the number indicating its definition as given in Column 'B'.

A		B
3	Volt	1. Unit of electrical current
1	Ampere	2. Unit of electrical resistance
2	Ohm	3. Unit of electrical pressure
8	Watt	4. 1/1000 of an ampere
4	Milliampere	5. 1,000 amperes
7	Kilovolt	6. 1/1000 of a volt
		7. 1,000 volts
		8. Product of a volt and an ampere

Check the statement below which is CORRECT:
An instrument used to measure electromotive force is:
- ☐ An ammeter
- ☐ A microammeter
- ☐ A watt-meter
- ☐ An r-meter
- ☒ A voltmeter

Study Questions

Check the statement below which is CORRECT:

If a valve tube in a full-wave rectified machine burns out, the following will be noticed when an exposure is made:
- ☐ The milliammeter registers zero
- ☐ The voltmeter registers zero
- ☐ There are marked fluctuations in milliamperage
- ☐ The x-ray tube filament will fail to light up
- ☒ The milliamperage will be about half the normal amount

Q. Describe the principle and operation of the phototimer on the Morgan-Hodges principle.

A. The phototimer is a combination of a photoelectric cell and various electrical devices which, when incorporated in the primary circuit of an x-ray generator, will terminate the exposure when the desired radiographic density is reached.

Q. What apparatus is used to produce heat in the filament?

A. A filament transformer, sometimes called a Coolidge transformer, plus a filament control, is used to produce heat in the filament.

Q. What governs the milliamperage which passes through an x-ray tube? How is it varied?

A. The current passing through a tube filament will govern the milliamperage. This filament current is varied by means of a variable resistance called the filament regulator or control.

Q. For what purpose is an x-ray transformer used in an x-ray machine?

A. An x-ray transformer is used to generate the high voltage necessary for the passage of current through an x-ray tube.

Q. What is a milliampere-second meter? How is it used?

A. A milliampere-second meter is a milliammeter having a highly damped moving element. It is used to indicate the product of milliampere-seconds in short-time high-milliamperage procedures.

Q. What is the function of the fuse and circuit breaker? What is the difference between them?

A. Fuses and circuit breakers serve to disconnect the x-ray machine from the supply source whenever overloading or shortcircuiting occurs.

The essential difference between them is that a circuit breaker can be manually reset after each opening due to an excessive current, whereas fuses must be completely replaced each time overload causes their breakdown.

Q. If the controls are set for a certain exposure and then the milliamperage is increased—the other setting remaining the same—what is the result on the film produced? Why?

A. The radiographic density of the film will be increased by an amount proportional to the milliamperage increase. This occurs because the density is directly proportional to the milliamperage employed.

FORMULATING X-RAY TECHNIQUES

X-RAYS AND TUBES

Q. Explain the theory of the double-focus tube.

A. The double focus is designed to offer a small projected focal spot where low Ma. values can be used for a period of time long enough to obtain the quantity of radiation required. The large focal spot is used where involuntary motion is encountered in the subject requiring short exposure time. To obtain the required amount of exposure, higher Ma. values are necessary. As a limited amount of energy (Ma.) can be focused over a given area on the target for a certain period of time before the target will be damaged, double-focus tubes are necessary where the sharpest detail is desired.

Q. Explain the theory of operation and advantages of a "rotating-target" tube.

A. The amount of energy which can be focused over a given area on the target of the tube is limited by the size of the area and the melting point of the target material. The "rotating-target tube" has a beveled tungsten disk on the anode stem which is caused to rotate at a nonsynchronous speed. By this means relatively cool tungsten is brought under the electron stream, thus avoiding some of the limitations on the rating of the tube by the melting point of the target materials. With the "rotating-target" tube higher Ma. values are possible with smaller focal spots.

Q. From the standpoint of tube rating and factor of safety, which would be the more conservative method of increasing film density, increasing tube current (Ma.) or increasing Kv.P.?

A. From the standpoint of tube rating and factor of safety the more conservative method of increasing film density would call for increasing Kv.P. within the limits of the tube. Exposure time would be the second choice as a variable factor to increase density.

Q. What is meant by the term "gassy" tube, and to what condition or conditions is it attributed?

A. Usually a "gassy" tube is one which has had the vacuum affected by the liberation of gas molecules from the elements by excessive heating or where damage to the glass envelope has affected the vacuum. With a poor vacuum and gas molecules present, the high voltage will ionize the gas, permitting an unpredictable current to flow through the tube.

Q. What causes pitting of the target? Is this harmful to the tube?

A. Pitting of the target is usually due to overloading the focal area by the use of excessively high current values. If the pitting is severe the quantity of useful radiation will be diminished.

Q. Distinguish between actual and effective focal-spot size.

A. The effective focal spot is the projected focal-spot size of the tube as measured directly below the target area bombarded by electrons. The actual focal spot is the area bombarded by the electron stream and is approximately three times as long as it is wide.

Q. What are the advantages and disadvantages of a small focal spot?

Study Questions

A. The smaller focal spot produces radiographs with sharper detail. However, when the smaller focal spot is used, lower Ma. values must be employed.

Q. Describe how an x-ray tube functions.

A. The filament is electrically heated to the point where free electrons are liberated. High potential is placed across the tube focusing the electrons, accelerating the electrons to high velocity, and causing them to bombard a predetermined area on the target.

Q. What do you understand by the term "hot-cathode" tube?

A. The term describes the type of x-ray tube invented by Dr. Coolidge in which the operation depends upon the heated filament as an electron source.

Check the statement below which is CORRECT:

Each wave or quantum of x-ray energy travels at the speed of:
- ☐ 1180 feet per second
- ☐ 500 miles per hour
- ☒ 186,000 miles per second
- ☐ 53.7 feet per second
- ☐ 88 feet per second

Check the statement below which is CORRECT:

The quality of the x-ray beam is dependent on:
- ☐ The size of the focal spot
- ☒ The voltage impressed on the tube
- ☐ The heat of the filament
- ☐ The type and size of target
- ☐ The milliamperage

Check the statement below which is CORRECT:

The quantity of electrons in the cathode stream is dependent directly on:
- ☐ The size of the focal spot
- ☐ The voltage impressed on the tube
- ☒ The heat of the filament
- ☐ The type and size of target
- ☐ The kind of filter used

Check the statement below which is CORRECT:

The following is not a property of x-rays:
- ☐ Photographic effect
- ☐ Fluorescent effect
- ☒ Recoil effect
- ☐ Ionizing effect

Check the statement below which is CORRECT:

The heel effect is a variation in x-ray intensity output:
- ☐ At the tube window
- ☐ Along the cathode of the tube
- ☒ Along the longitudinal axis of the tube
- ☐ Along the transverse tube axis

FORMULATING X-RAY TECHNIQUES

Check the statement below which is CORRECT:

The heel effect is limited in its application when using:
- ☐ Short focal-film distance
- ☐ Long focal-film distance
- ☐ Long object-film distance
- ☒ A large film at short focal-film distance

Q. What are the fundamental properties of x-rays and how may they be detected?

A. Among the properties of x-rays the following are the most important.
- a. X-rays cause certain substances to fluoresce, thus producing visible light. Therefore, a fluoroscopic screen can be used to detect x-rays.
- b. X-rays produce a change in photographic film similar to the action of light. A film subjected to radiation will show blackening when developed. An unexposed film could be used to detect the presence of x-rays.
- c. X-rays increase the electrical conductivity of air through which they pass. This is called ionization and is used as a basis for measuring and detecting radiation.
- d. X-rays produce certain biological changes in cells that may stimulate or retard growth. In some cases the cell may be destroyed or the form of new cells may be altered.
- e. X-rays can be diffracted in much the same manner as light. This property makes x-rays a useful tool in the investigation of molecular structure of materials.

Q. How are x-rays produced?

A. A beam of rapidly moving electrons is caused to strike some form of matter. The bombardment of this "target" matter by the electrons results in the production of x-rays and heat.

Q. Can x-rays be controlled and how?

A. X-rays can be controlled by varying the voltage across the x-ray tube and by varying the current through the tube. The voltage across the tube determines the quality or penetrating power of the x-rays and also has considerable effect on the quantity. Variations of the current through the tube, which are dependent chiefly on the temperature of the filament, cause similar variations in quantity of x-rays produced but have very little effect on the quality.

Q. What portion of the total energy delivered to an x-ray tube at the target is given off as x-rays? What becomes of the remaining energy?

A. In most x-ray apparatus, less than 1 per cent of the total target energy is converted to x-rays. The remaining energy appears as heat and other forms of energy.

Q. If x-rays are invisible, how may their presence be detected?

A. The presence of the rays may be detected by their effects on photographic film and on fluorescent substances and by their ability to ionize the air through which they pass.

Study Questions

Q. If x-rays penetrate all materials, how then is it possible to apply them to radiography?

A. X-rays do not penetrate all matter to the same extent. The penetration of a given material will depend on its thickness and chemical composition. Because of the varying degrees of penetration for different materials, it is possible to differentiate between the various tissues in the body.

Q. What is primary radiation? secondary radiation?

A. Primary radiation is that radiation generated at the focal spot of the x-ray tube.

Secondary radiation is that radiation caused by the primary radiation striking some material. The quality of the secondary radiation is dependent on the atomic number of the material and is usually quite different from that of the primary radiation.

Q. Why is it necessary to have a filament in an x-ray tube? Explain fully.

A. The filament of the x-ray tube is the source of electrons. In order to produce x-rays, it is necessary to have a rapidly moving beam of electrons strike a target. The filament, when heated, emits electrons. These electrons are shaped into a beam by the cathode structure. The rapid motion of the electrons is caused by the potential difference between the anode and cathode.

Q. What is a line-focus tube?

A. A line-focus tube has a straight-line filament so arranged that the electron flow strikes the target, forming a narrow-strip focal spot. The angle at which the target tips is such that the projection of this strip on the film is a small rectangle called the effective focal spot.

Q. How do you determine the prime factors (Kv.P., time, Ma.) that may be safely employed with reference to a given tube and apparatus?

A. The prime factors that may be safely employed with a given tube and apparatus are determined from the equipment-rating charts supplied by the manufacturer.

Q. How would one check the timer of an x-ray machine for exposures of less than $2/10$ second?

A. To check the timer of an x-ray machine for exposures of less than $2/10$ second, a spinning top, consisting of a lead disc superimposed on a brass plate and revolving about a pivot point, is placed on a film beneath the x-ray tube. An exposure of $1/10$ or $2/10$ second is made, and the accuracy of the timer may be determined by counting the number of black dots which show on the processed film. At $1/10$ second, utilizing self or half-wave rectification, the dots should be six in number; for full-wave rectification, they should be twelve in number.

Q. When a spinning top is used for checking a timer, what effect does speed of rotation have?

A. Speed of rotation of a spinning top has no effect on results of checking a timer, providing the individual dots on the film can be distinguished.

FORMULATING X-RAY TECHNIQUES

Check the statement below which is CORRECT:

The advantage of the rotating-anode x-ray tube over the stationary-anode tube is:
- ☐ Its low cost
- ☐ It permits lower energies to be used
- ☐ It is small and easily manipulated
- ☒ It permits high energies with a small focal spot
- ☐ The focal spot gets hotter

Check the statement below which is CORRECT:

If an x-ray tube is gassy the following will usually be noted:
- ☐ No reading can be obtained on the primary voltmeter
- ☐ The tube filament does not light up
- ☐ The milliammeter does not register any current
- ☒ There are irregular fluctuations in milliamperage
- ☐ The valve tubes will not light up

Check the statement below which is CORRECT:

Like poles of a magnet:
- ☒ Repel each other
- ☐ Attract each other
- ☐ Neutralize each other
- ☐ Do not affect each other
- ☐ Must be made of different materials

Check the statement below which is CORRECT:

Milliamperage across the x-ray tube for any given exposure is correlated with:
- ☐ The heat of the anode
- ☒ The heat of the filament
- ☐ The size of the target
- ☐ The distance between anode and cathode
- ☐ The voltage applied to the tube

THERAPY AND PROTECTION

Q. What are the complications to the skin that may develop from x-ray therapy?

A. Redness, blistering, loss of hair, telangiectasia.

Name several different conditions treated with superficial x-ray therapy.

Skin Lesions
- a. Basal Cell
- b. Hyperkeratosis
- c. Acne
- d. Squamous cell
- e. Warts
- f. Keloid (scars)

Infections
- a. Otitis media
- b. Furunculosis (boils)
- c. Pneumonia
- d. Herpes simplex (fever blisters)
- e. Sty

Study Questions

Name several conditions treated with deep x-ray therapy.
    Hodgkin's disease
    Cancer
    Bursitis
    Brain tumors
    Leukemia
    Metastatic bone disease
    Herpes zoster (shingles)

Q. What is the difference between a cobalt beam and an x-ray beam?
A. The cobalt beam is made up of two wave lengths. An x-ray beam is a mixture (spectrum) of wave lengths.

Q. What are the signs and symptoms of radiation sickness?
A. Nausea, vomiting, headache.

Q. If you have a copper and aluminum filter, which filter is the exit filter (closest to the patient)? Why?
A. Aluminum: it filters out characteristic rays from copper.

Q. What is meant by the term "half-value layer"?
A. That thickness of material that will absorb 50 per cent of the radiation.

Q. What is the cone?
A. It is a mechanical device used to limit the field of radiation.

Q. What is its purpose?
A. The quantity of scattered radiation may be reduced by using a cone small enough to cover only the part to be radiographed or treated.

Q. What is the purpose of a lead shield?
A. To limit scatter and stray radiation as much as possible.

Q. What is meant by a "hot spot"?
A. An area of overlap from two or more areas of treatment.

Q. What do filters do to an x-ray beam?
A. The greater the filtration the greater the half-value layer; a filter affects the quality by decreasing the wave length of maximum intensity and by decreasing the effective wave length.

Q. Would you expect a skin lesion to require more or less filtration than a bone lesion? Why?
A. Less filtration, because it is not as hard to penetrate.

Check the statement below which is CORRECT:
    A thoreus filter is made of layers of:
        ☒ Aluminum, copper, tin
        ☐ Aluminum, copper, zinc
        ☐ Aluminum, copper, brass
        ☐ Aluminum, copper, lead

FORMULATING X-RAY TECHNIQUES

Check the statement below which is CORRECT:

The greatest radiation hazard to an embryo or fetus occurs during the:
- ☐ Period right after delivery
- ☒ First trimester
- ☐ Second trimester
- ☐ Third trimester

Check the statement below which is CORRECT:

The "r" unit is a measurement best suited to determine the:
- ☐ Quality of radiation
- ☐ Character of radiation
- ☒ Quantity of radiation
- ☐ Amount of gamma radiation

Check the statement below which is CORRECT:

The materials below which are commonly used for protective barriers against radiation are:
- ☒ Lead
- ☒ Poured concrete
- ☐ Polyethelene blocks
- ☒ Barium plaster

Check the statement below which is CORRECT:

Indicate which of the therapy field sizes given below will result in the greatest absorbed dose:
- ☐ A round area 10 cm. across
- ☐ A 10 cm. square area
- ☐ A rectangle 10 cm. x 15 cm.
- ☒ A 15 cm. x 15 cm. square area

Check the statement below which is CORRECT:

Beta rays consist of high-speed:
- ☒ Electrons
- ☐ Atoms
- ☐ Neutrons
- ☐ Protons

Check the statement below which is CORRECT:

The one type of radiation not commonly used in therapy is:
- ☒ Alpha particles
- ☐ Isotopes
- ☐ X-rays
- ☐ Gamma rays

Check the statement below which is CORRECT:

Check the item below which includes *both* instruments commonly used to measure gamma radiation:
- ☒ Ionization chamber and Geiger counter
- ☐ Geiger counter and ammeter
- ☐ Electrometer and voltmeter
- ☐ Galvanometer and Geiger counter

Study Questions

Check the statement below which is CORRECT:

The item below which will *increase* the radiation exposure to the patient's skin is the:
- ☐ Use of a cone
- ☐ Addition of aluminum filters
- ☐ Use of high Kv.P. and low Ma.S. technique
- ☒ Use of low Kv.P. and high Ma.S. technique

Check the statement below which is CORRECT:

The tissue listed below which is *most* sensitive to x-radiation is the:
- ☐ Brain
- ☐ Muscle
- ☒ Gonads
- ☐ Skin

Q. What are the chief dangers to the operator in a radiographic department where general radiographic work is done?

A. The chief dangers to the operator in a radiographic department are exposure to the radiation coming directly from the x-ray tube and exposure to the secondary and scattered radiation coming from the patient during an x-ray exposure.

Q. How do you protect yourself from stray radiation?

A. Stand behind a lead screen or, if a lead screen is not provided, stay at least 10 feet or more away from the patient during an exposure. If suitable lead screening is not provided, use radiographic cones of sizes just large enough to cover the part being radiographed. This will help to limit scattered and stray radiation from the patient.

Q. How much radiation can be given a patient with safety in radiographic work?

A. It is generally safe to expose a patient to about 2400 milliampere seconds, 85 Kv.P. at 30 inches, using only the inherent filtration of the tube. This figure must be lowered to about 1790 milliampere seconds for head work. If the patient receives the amounts of radiation mentioned, a period of 4 weeks should elapse before additional radiographs are taken.

Q. What are "scattered rays"? What measure can be taken to reduce their effect?

A. Scattered rays are the x-rays that are given off by anything in the path of the primary x-ray beam during an exposure. The main sources are the patient and the x-ray table. The quantity of scattered radiation may be reduced by using a cone small enough to cover only the part to be radiographed. The smaller the area of the primary beam, the less scattered radiation produced.

Q. What milliamperage is usually employed for fluoroscopic work?

A. Usually from one to five milliamperes are employed for fluoroscopic work.

FORMULATING X-RAY TECHNIQUES

Q. If you were operating the x-ray machine during radiation therapy, what would your duties be during the period of treatment?

A. During the treatment periodically check the positioning of the patient, making sure that no change in position has occurred. A constant check of the x-ray machine factors is also necessary so that proper dosage is given. Should the x-ray factors or patient-position change, corrections must be made immediately. CAUTION: do not attempt to reposition the patient without first turning off the x-ray unit.

Q. If an "r" meter is used to indicate the amount of x-ray being given, is a milliammeter necessary? Why?

A. Yes. Both meters are generally employed as a double check on the quantity of radiation being given to the patient. The Ma. meter is also used to set the machine for the desired exposure factors and used when calibrating the output of the generator.

Q. In handling filters what precautions should be taken before starting treatment?

A. Double check the filters in position for the treatment against the filters called for in the treatment being given to the patient. Request that the radiologist also carefully check the filters being used before treatment is started.

Q. What methods do you employ in checking the correct filter in therapy?

A. Visual inspection of the filters in the filter box, checking the filters by the indicating system on the control panel and/or by the "r" output as indicated by the dosage meter on the control panel against the treatment as described by the radiologist.

Q. What means are used for restricting the radiation to the desired areas?

A. Lead or leaded protective material, cones, or diaphragms, and the correct target-skin distance.

Q. What kind of dressing, ointments, solutions, etc., should be avoided on the skin in areas that are to be treated?

A. It is generally a good rule that all dressings, ointments, and solutions should be avoided unless specifically approved by the radiologist.

Q. What information (technical factors) is necessary to keep your therapy record?

A. The dose in "r" units, the Kv.P., Ma., length of treatment time, target-skin distance, filters and cones employed.

Q. How are the quantity and quality of radiation recorded?

A. Quantity—checked by ionization means. A Victoreen r-meter is generally used. Quality—checked by absorption in some metal, the metal generally being the same as the added filter material. The quality is thus checked by the amount of added filter required to reduce the given intensity by half or to the "half-value layer."

Q. Define: Depth dosage, erythema dose, radiation sickness, epithelioma, wave length.

Study Questions

A. Depth dose—amount of radiation absorbed at the desired depth in the body.

Erythema dose—amount of radiation necessary to produce a noticeable skin reaction.

Radiation sickness—general systemic disorder produced by the destruction of irradiated tissue.

Epithelioma—a malignant tumor consisting mainly of epithelial cells and primarily derived from the skin.

Wave length—since radiation is generally considered to be a wave disturbance it must have a wave length. The length of one wave is the linear distance, in the direction of propagation, between two points of the disturbance which are in the same phase; that is, the distance, for example between successive crests or troughs, so to speak, of the disturbance.

Check the statement below which is CORRECT:

The following devices are not used in measuring the adequacy of x-ray protection:
- ☐ Film badges
- ☐ Minometers
- ☒ Voltmeters
- ☐ Ionization chambers
- ☐ Dental films

Check the statement below which is CORRECT:

The safe tolerance amount of whole body radiation per week is about:
- ☐ 3.0 roentgens
- ☐ 10.0 roentgens
- ☐ 100.0 roentgens
- ☒ 0.3 roentgens (300 milliroentgens)
- ☐ 0.001 roentgens (1 milliroentgen)

Q. Why does the radiotherapist prefer two parallel opposed ports to one single port if the tumor is located in the midpelvis?

A. With two parallel ports more radiation is given to the tumor than to the skin.

Q. Which machine gives more backscatter on the skin, the cobalt-60 or the 250-Kv. machine?

A. The 250-Kv. machine.

Q. What will the treatment time be in minutes and seconds for 365 r if you have
Field size: 10 x 15 cm.
TSD: 85 cm.
Output on surface: 73 r/min.

A. 5 min.

Q. If the depth dose percentage at 6 cm. is 73.3 per cent and the patient received 785 r to the surface, how many r has the patient received at 6-cm. depth?

A. 575.4 r (rounded off).

Q. Which of the following ports would have to have the shorter treat-

343

FORMULATING X-RAY TECHNIQUES

ment time to deliver the same surface dose, a 6 x 10-cm. port or a 10 x 12-cm. port?

A. The 10 x 12-cm. port.

Q. How would you change your treatment time to give the same surface dose if you doubled the TSD?

A. Four times the treatment time (inverse square law).

Q. A patient is being treated on a cobalt-60 machine and has a bandage 5 mm. thick within the treated area. Where will the maximum dose be?

A. To the skin.

Q. What is the advantage of using a wedge?

A. The wedge helps prevent a "hot spot" in an area and gives uniform dosage throughout the treated area. For example, a wedge is used in treating the tonsil, which is not located in the center of the neck but to one side.

Q. Why is the surface dose always larger than the air dose?

A. The surface dose is the result of the air dose plus backscatter, whereas the air dose is only the dosage at a given point in the air.

Q. What does the filter on the superficial machine do to the beam?

A. The filter on the superficial machine screens out the soft rays, thus hardening the beam and giving more penetration.

FINAL EXAMINATION IN RADIOLOGIC TECHNOLOGY: TYPICAL QUESTIONS

Select the best answer from the following multiple-choice questions. Check the square for the answer which you believe to be correct.

1. Radiation doses to the occupational personnel are measured in units of
   - ☒ rem
   - ☐ rep
   - ☐ rad
   - ☐ roentgen

2. The accumulated occupational maximum permissible dose from x-, gamma, or beta radiation to the whole body is calculated by using the formula
   - ☒ MPD = 5(N − 18) rads
   - ☐ MPD = 5N − 18 rads
   - ☐ MPD = 5(18 − N) rads
   - ☐ MPD = 5(N) − 18 rads

3. One method that is useful to keep radiation exposure to a minimum is
   - ☒ the inverse square law
   - ☐ using the largest possible x-ray beam
   - ☐ standing as close as possible to the table during fluoroscopy
   - ☐ never wearing a lead protective apron

4. The allowable dose of radiation which will produce no detectable damage to the individual is known as the
   - ☒ maximum permissible dose
   - ☐ gonadal dose
   - ☐ whole-body dose
   - ☐ cancerocidal dose

5. The unit of absorbed dose is the
   - ☐ rem
   - ☒ rad
   - ☐ kilovolt
   - ☐ rep

6. The total filtration of the useful beam shall be equal to at least
   - ☐ 1 mm. lead
   - ☒ 2.5 mm. aluminum
   - ☐ 4.5 mm. aluminum
   - ☐ 3 mm. copper

FORMULATING X-RAY TECHNIQUES

7. If a lead apron is worn, the monitoring device should be worn
   - ☐ outside of the apron
   - ☒ under the apron
   - ☐ on the wrist
   - ☐ need not be worn at all

8. The area under bombardment by electrons is known as the
   - ☐ effective focal spot
   - ☒ actual focal spot
   - ☐ large focal spot
   - ☐ double focal spot

9. Heat units are a product of
   - ☐ Ma. × time
   - ☐ Kv.P. × time × 2
   - ☒ Kv.P. × Ma. × time
   - ☐ Ma. × time × distance

10. In x-ray production, kilovoltage and wave length are interdependent in the following way:
    - ☐ Wave length increases with increase of kilovoltage
    - ☒ Wave length decreases with increase of kilovoltage
    - ☐ Wave length is proportional to the square of kilovoltage
    - ☐ Wave length is proportional to the inverse square of kilovoltage

11. Beta particles are also called
    - ☐ protons
    - ☐ helium nuclei
    - ☒ electrons
    - ☐ neutrons

12. In electrification by induction the kind of charge conferred on a metallic object placed in the field of a charged object is
    - ☒ the opposite kind
    - ☐ the same kind
    - ☐ positive
    - ☐ negative

13. You get the electrons to move from the cathode to the anode of an x-ray tube
    - ☐ by heating the filament to a higher temperature
    - ☐ by having a vacuum inside the glass envelope
    - ☒ by putting a high voltage across the x-ray tube
    - ☐ by introducing a focusing cup

14. A type of radiation called secondary (scattered) would be that which
    - ☐ emerges from the tube and reaches the patient
    - ☐ emerges from the patient and reaches the film
    - ☒ scatters on contact with the patient
    - ☐ controls image distortion

15. The film emulsion is composed of
    - ☐ potassium bromide
    - ☐ silver plus gelatin
    - ☒ silver halide plus gelatin
    - ☐ gelatin

Final Examination Questions

16. Gamma rays are
    - ☐ high-speed electrons emitted by radioactive nuclei
    - ☒ electromagnetic radiations coming from atomic nuclei
    - ☐ produced when electrons jump between electron orbits in atoms
    - ☐ emitted by all radioisotopes

17. The pair of bones that form most of the lateral wall and part of the roof of the skull are
    - ☒ parietal bones
    - ☐ sphenoid bones
    - ☐ nasal bones
    - ☐ occipital bones

18. The immovable joint that separates the frontal from the parietal bones is
    - ☐ temporomandibular joint
    - ☐ lambdoidal suture
    - ☐ sagittal suture
    - ☒ coronal suture

19. The mastoid process is part of the bone called
    - ☐ occipital
    - ☒ temporal
    - ☐ sphenoid
    - ☐ zygoma

20. The process by which carbon dioxide and oxygen are exchanged in the body is known as
    - ☐ apnea
    - ☐ anoxia
    - ☐ expiration
    - ☒ respiration

21. In radial deviation the wrist is turned
    - ☐ inward
    - ☐ upward
    - ☒ outward
    - ☐ medially

Opposite each term in column I, place the letter representing the correct definition as listed in column II.

	I		II
22.	a oblique	a.	rotated from true AP
23.	e lateral decubitus	b.	straightening of the part
24.	b extension	c.	with part moved away from the midline
25.	c abducted	d.	toward the back
26.	d dorsal	e.	lying on the side
		f.	flexion

27. The malleoli are used as landmarks when making a radiograph of
    - ☒ AP ankle
    - ☐ PA knee

FORMULATING X-RAY TECHNIQUES

☐ AP shoulder
☐ AP elbow

28. With the patient in the supine position, the radiographic baseline is placed parallel to the film. This is called the
    ☐ posteroanterior position
    ☐ Towne position
    ☒ submentovertical position
    ☐ reverse Towne position

29. If the medial plane, radiographic baseline, and central ray beam are all perpendicular to the x-ray table, and the interorbital line and coronal plane are parallel to the table, the skull is positioned in a true
    ☒ posteroanterior view
    ☐ lateral view
    ☐ reverse Towne view
    ☐ base view

30. The size and shape of the spleen, liver, and kidneys are best visualized in the following view of the abdomen
    ☐ right anterior oblique
    ☒ anterior and posterior supine view
    ☐ lateral view
    ☐ anteroposterior view with x-ray beam horizontal

31. The following is (are) radiographed in the upright position to demonstrate fluid levels:
    ☐ parotid duct
    ☒ sinuses
    ☐ mandibular menti
    ☐ spinosum ovale

32. A line drawn between the pupils of the eye is called
    ☐ Reid's baseline
    ☐ the canthomeatal line
    ☐ the orbitomeatal line
    ☒ the interpupillary line

33. The view that best demonstrates the intercondyloid notch or space is (are) the
    ☐ anteroposterior view of the mandible
    ☒ tunnel view of the knee
    ☐ transthoracic view
    ☐ oblique views of the patella

34. The anteroposterior projection of the cervical spine through the open mouth will demonstrate the following:
    ☐ C-7
    ☐ upper and lower molars
    ☒ atlas, axis, and odontoid process
    ☐ foramen magnum

35. It is sometimes necessary to have the patient breathe during the exposure for a lateral thoracic spine
    ☐ to shorten the exposure

Final Examination Questions

☐ to blur out the vertebra
☒ to blur out the superimposed ribs
☐ to demonstrate the movement of the diaphragm

36. The shallow-breathing technique is used on the following examination:
    ☐ lateral view of the neck
    ☐ lateral view of the sternum
    ☐ lateral chest
    ☒ oblique view of the sternum

37. To visualize the ribs below the diaphragm to best advantage, the patient must be instructed to
    ☐ take in a deep breath and hold it
    ☒ exhale fully
    ☐ breathe normally
    ☐ hold his breath for 10 seconds

38. In adduction, the part is moved _____ the central axis of body.
    ☐ upward from
    ☐ downard from
    ☐ away from
    ☒ toward

39. In abduction, the part is moved _____ the central axis of the body.
    ☐ upward from
    ☐ downward from
    ☒ away from
    ☐ toward

40. The term extension refers to the _____ of a joint.
    ☐ bending
    ☐ turning inward
    ☒ straightening
    ☐ turning outward

41. Posterior, or dorsal, designates the _____ part of the body or organ.
    ☐ front
    ☒ back
    ☐ side
    ☐ top

42. Caudal refers to a part that is _____ the head of the body.
    ☒ away from
    ☐ toward
    ☐ in back of
    ☐ in front of

43. Distal refers to a part that is _____ the beginning or origin of a structure.
    ☐ adjacent to
    ☐ on top of
    ☒ away from
    ☐ near

FORMULATING X-RAY TECHNIQUES

44. Proximal refers to a part that is _____ the beginning or origin of a structure.
    - ☐ adjacent to
    - ☐ on top of
    - ☐ away from
    - ☒ near

45. The Trendelenburg position consists of the patient
    - ☒ supine with feet and legs elevated
    - ☐ supine with head elevated
    - ☐ in knee-chest position
    - ☐ lying on the side

46. When examining the lowest four pairs of ribs, it is best to project them
    - ☒ below the level of the diaphragm
    - ☐ above the level of the diaphragm
    - ☐ laterally
    - ☐ in flexion-extension

47. The largest tarsal bone, also known as the heel bone, is the
    - ☐ cuneiform
    - ☐ cuboid
    - ☐ talus
    - ☒ calcaneus

48. The ankle joint is formed by the articulation of the
    - ☐ talus with the calcaneus
    - ☐ calcaneus with the cuboid
    - ☒ talus with the tibia and fibula
    - ☐ talus with the navicular

49. The largest sesamoid bone in the body is the
    - ☐ femur
    - ☐ pelvis
    - ☐ calcaneus
    - ☒ patella

50. In radiography of the sacrum in the anteroposterior position, the central ray is directed
    - ☐ perpendicular to the film
    - ☒ cephalad
    - ☐ caudad
    - ☐ to a point 2 inches above the superior iliac spine

51. The three main components of the sternum are the body, xiphoid, and
    - ☐ acromion
    - ☐ glenoid
    - ☒ manubrium
    - ☐ pedicle

Final Examination Questions

52. The most satisfactory radiographic examination of a long bone suspected of being fractured should include
    - ☐ the joint proximal to the injury
    - ☐ a similar bone for comparison
    - ☐ the joint distal to the injury
    - ☒ joints both proximal and distal to the injury

53. The five metacarpal bones are located in the
    - ☐ wrist
    - ☐ ankle
    - ☒ hand
    - ☐ foot

54. Fractures of the facial bones are better demonstrated by
    - ☐ angiography
    - ☐ osseous venography
    - ☐ arthrography
    - ☒ laminography

55. The *primary* purpose of a pelvimetry examination is to determine the measurements of the
    - ☐ fetus and placenta
    - ☒ pelvis
    - ☐ fetal head
    - ☐ fetal age

56. An autotomogram during the erect filling phase of pneumoencephalography is taken to demonstrate the following structures
    - ☒ fourth ventricle
    - ☐ lateral ventricle
    - ☐ corpus callosum
    - ☐ anterior cerebral artery

57. A "blow out" fracture of the orbit will best be demonstrated on
    - ☐ a PA projection of the skull
    - ☒ a modified Waters projection
    - ☐ a lateral projection
    - ☐ none of the above

58. In a lateral projection of the knee, the C.R. is directed
    - ☐ perpendicular to the joint
    - ☒ at an angle of 5 degrees cephalic
    - ☐ at an angle of 5 degrees caudally
    - ☐ at an angle of 10 degrees caudally
    - ☐ at an an le of 10 degrees cephalic

59. In a radiograph of the cervical spine in the oblique projection, the structures demonstrated are
    - ☐ an oblique view of the cervical bodies
    - ☐ a profile view of the intervertebral foramina
    - ☐ the pedicles
    - ☒ all of the above
    - ☐ all of the above except the pedicles

FORMULATING X-RAY TECHNIQUES

60. Reid's baseline is also known as the
    - ☐ glabellomeatal line
    - ☒ infraorbitomeatal line
    - ☐ orbitomeatal line
    - ☐ acanthiomeatal line
    - ☐ interpupillary line

61. In examining the abdomen for a possible ruptured viscus, radiographs made in the upright and/or decubitus positions are primarily intended to demonstrate
    - ☐ gas and fluid levels
    - ☒ free gas in the peritoneal cavity
    - ☐ mobility of organs
    - ☐ presence or absence of psoas shadows

62. A fracture of the zygomatic arch may *best* be demonstrated in the
    - ☐ PA view of the skull
    - ☒ submentovertex view of the skull
    - ☐ anterioposterior view of the skull
    - ☐ parietoacanthial view of the sinuses

63. In making a radiograph of the coccyx in the AP position, the central ray is directed
    - ☐ perpendicular to the film
    - ☐ to a point 2 inches below the pubis
    - ☐ cephalad
    - ☒ caudad

Select the answer which would utilize the following position: patient prone; right side elevated away from the tabletop; left anterior portion of the body in contact with the tabletop.

64.
   - ☐ oblique stomach and duodenum
   - ☐ oblique of the right hip
   - ☐ oblique sternum
   - ☒ oblique gallbladder

65.
   - ☐ left anterior ribs—oblique
   - ☒ right anterior ribs—oblique
   - ☐ right scapula—lateral
   - ☐ right clavicle—oblique

Select the answer which would utilize the following position: patient prone, left side elevated away from the tabletop; right anterior portion of the body in contact with the tabletop.

66.
   - ☐ gallbladder—oblique
   - ☒ stomach and duodenum—oblique
   - ☐ left scapula—lateral
   - ☐ oblique of the left hip

Final Examination Questions

67. ☒ lateral right scapula
    ☐ lateral left scapula
    ☐ right anterior ribs—oblique
    ☐ gallbladder—oblique

68. The bones articulating at the knee joint are the
    ☒ femur and tibia
    ☐ femur and fibula
    ☐ fibula, tibia, and femur
    ☐ femur, patella, and fibula

The names of certain bony structures are listed below. For each, indicate the location of the structure by writing the proper letter beside the name of the process or foramen of the bone in which it is found in the list on the right.

69. b alveolar process   a. mandible
70. c olecranor process   b. maxilla
71. e obturator foramen   c. ulna
72. a mental foramen   d. occipital bone
                             e. innominate bone

73. In the group of anatomical words below, indicate the one which is not related to the others:
    ☐ psoas
    ☐ quadriceps
    ☒ sternoclavicular
    ☐ diaphragm

74. In the AP projection of the knee joint, the anatomical landmark centered to the film is the
    ☐ popliteal fossae
    ☒ lower border of the patella
    ☐ head of the fibula
    ☐ upper margin of the patella

75. In the group of anatomical words below, indicate the one which is *not related* to the others:
    ☐ symphysis
    ☐ coranoid
    ☒ coracoid
    ☐ angle

76. In the group of anatomical words below, indicate the one which is *not related* to the others:
    ☐ multangular
    ☐ navicular
    ☐ pisiform
    ☒ talus

Here are four sets of technical factors to be used in routine radiography of a particular anatomic region. In each question, select the set of factors which

FORMULATING X-RAY TECHNIQUES

would produce a radiograph with the *greatest density,* all factors not listed remaining the same:

	Ma.	Time in seconds	FFD	Kv.P.	Grid ratio	Screen speed
77.	☐ 50	1½	40	74	12:1	medium
	☐ 100	¾	40	76	12:1	medium
	☐ 150	½	40	74	8:1	medium
	☒ 200	⅜	40	76	6:1	medium
78.	☐ 50	1	36	78	12:1	slow
	☐ 100	½	40	76	12:1	medium
	☒ 150	½	36	74	12:1	medium
	☐ 200	¼	40	78	12:1	slow
79.	☐ 100	1	40	65	8:1	slow
	☐ 100	¾	40	65	8:1	slow
	☐ 200	½	36	65	8:1	medium
	☒ 150	1	36	65	8:1	medium
80.	☐ 150	1/10	36	72	12:1	medium
	☐ 200	3/20	36	76	12:1	medium
	☒ 300	½	72	76	12:1	medium
	☐ 100	3/10	40	72	12:1	medium
81.	☒ 200	⅛	40	76	12:1	high
	☐ 150	⅙	40	76	12:1	medium
	☐ 100	¼	40	68	12:1	medium
	☐ 50	½	40	68	12:1	slow

82. Radiographic contrast is chiefly influenced by the
 ☐ milliampere-seconds
 ☒ kilovoltage
 ☐ milliamperage
 ☐ time

83. Compared to primary radiation, secondary radiation has
 ☐ shorter average wave lengths
 ☒ longer average wave lengths
 ☐ greater average frequency
 ☐ similar average frequency

84. Exposure latitude is long or short according to the
 ☐ distance
 ☐ millamperes
 ☐ time
 ☒ kilovoltage

85. A patient's chest measures 23 cm. in the anteroposterior diameter. Body section radiographs are to be made in the anteroposterior position of a questionable lesion 3 cm. posterior to the anterior chest wall. The fulcrum should be set at

Final Examination Questions

- [ ] 3 cm.
- [ ] 2.0 cm. above the mid-plane of the chest
- [x] 20.0 cm.
- [ ] 23.0 cm.

If one is checking the timber of a full-wave rectified x-ray machine, the number of dots recorded on the film should be as follows:

86. At $1/10$ second:
    - [ ] 6
    - [x] 12
    - [ ] 3
    - [ ] 16

87. At $1/60$ second:
    - [x] 2
    - [ ] 4
    - [ ] 6
    - [ ] 8

88. At $1/30$ second:
    - [ ] 2
    - [x] 4
    - [ ] 6
    - [ ] 8

59. At $1/20$ second:
    - [ ] 2
    - [ ] 3
    - [x] 6
    - [ ] 4

90. At $1/120$ second:
    - [ ] 2
    - [x] 1
    - [ ] 3
    - [ ] 4

89. At $1/20$ second:

91. For calculating the heat units of an x-ray tube operating on full-rectified single-phase current, then changing the calculations to cover a three-phase machine, to accommodate the change to three-phase, the heat units formula must be multiplied by:
    - [ ] 0.7
    - [x] 1.3
    - [ ] 2.0
    - [ ] 3.0

92. In a grid which has lead strips 0.5 mm. apart and 4 mm. deep, the grid ratio is
    - [ ] 4:1
    - [ ] 6:1
    - [x] 8:1
    - [ ] 12:1

FORMULATING X-RAY TECHNIQUES

93. In stereoscopy, the amount of tube shift is *chiefly* determined by the
    - ☒ focus-film distance
    - ☐ object-film distance
    - ☐ thickness of the part
    - ☐ size of the focal spot

94. The function of contrast in a radiographic film is to
    - ☐ decrease latitude
    - ☐ increase the average density
    - ☐ provide background density
    - ☒ make detail visible

95. The higher the grid ratio, the greater the
    - ☐ radius of the grid
    - ☐ speed of exposure
    - ☒ "cleanup" of the grid
    - ☐ focus-film distance required

96. The geometric law of image formation is used in the following radiographic examination(s)
    - ☐ cardioangiography
    - ☒ cephalopelvimetry
    - ☐ discography
    - ☐ placentography

97. Three-phase generators are more efficient than are full-wave because
    - ☒ voltage never drops to zero
    - ☐ cables are larger
    - ☐ there is higher milliamperage at longer exposures
    - ☐ they are more expensive to purchase

98. The following is (are) not essential to the production of radiation:
    - ☐ source of electrons
    - ☒ oscilloscope
    - ☐ sudden stoppage of high-speed electrons
    - ☐ electrons in high-speed motion

99. Poor screen contact reduces
    - ☐ density
    - ☐ contrast
    - ☐ distortion
    - ☒ definition

100. The advantage of a rotating anode tube over a stationary tube is
     - ☐ a larger field coverage
     - ☒ a greater tube capacity
     - ☐ an increase in contrast
     - ☐ less expense in operating

101. A radiograph is made using an 8:1 grid. If a 16:1 grid replaces the original 8:1 grid, to maintain the same density we need to
     - ☐ decrease the amount of radiation
     - ☐ make no change

Final Examination Questions

☒ increase the amount of radiation
☐ use a large focal spot

102. A cone sufficient to cover a 14 × 17-inch film is used to produce a satisfactory radiograph. If a 4-inch cone is used to cone down on the gallbladder, with no other factor changes, the resulting radiograph will exhibit
☐ mottled density
☐ more density
☒ less density
☐ same density

103. The half-value layer (hvl) is
☒ the thickness of material that reduces the intensity of the x-ray beam by a factor of 2
☐ the kilovoltage used for measurement of intensity
☐ the milliamperage that reduces the intensity by a factor of 2
☐ the filter added on top of the x-ray tube

104. The following would produce radiographs with the best detail sharpness on a small part:
☐ detail screens
☐ ultra-detail screens
☐ high-speed screens
☒ direct-exposure technique

109. A film is made of the knee, using a cassette and tabletop exposure. Another x-ray is made with the film in the Bucky tray; all the exposure factors are the same for both exposures. The second film (Bucky) will exhibit
☐ more density
☐ no change in density
☐ greater detailed sharpness
☐ less detailed sharpness
☒ less density

106. Short-scale contrast is defined by
☒ high contrast
☐ low contrast
☐ product of high kilovoltage
☐ product of secondary radiation

Please read carefully.

A radiograph has been taken of a lateral skull. The film is entirely satisfactory. Having been properly processed, it is placed on a view box to be used as a standard for comparison with a series of films to be taken of the same skull. In each of the ensuing exposures only one factor or condition is changed from the original.

Each of the resulting radiographs is to be compared with the original in some respects. You are to determine from your own knowledge in what regard or regards each of the experimental films will differ. A 1.0-mm. focal spot. Intensifying screens. Develop 5 minutes at 68° F. Bucky diaphragm 8:1. Cone cover 10 times 12-inch film. 40-inch focus-film distance, 100 Ma., 0.5 second, 65 Kv.P.

FORMULATING X-RAY TECHNIQUES

The above information is to be used in answering questions 107–109 only.

107. Twenty-four-hour development would increase
     - ☐ detail
     - ☒ density
     - ☐ contrast
     - ☐ magnification and/or distortion

108. Increased object-film distance would primarily decrease
     - ☒ detail
     - ☐ density
     - ☐ contrast
     - ☐ magnification

109. A three-inch mastoid cone would increase
     - ☐ density
     - ☐ contrast
     - ☒ detail visibility
     - ☐ magnification and/or distortion

110. The type of radiation called primary is
     - ☒ that which emerges from the tube and reaches the patient
     - ☐ that which emerges from the patient and reaches the film
     - ☐ that which is controlled by Ma.S.
     - ☐ that which is controlled and cut off by cones

111. High-ratio grids, in the control of radiographic quality,
     - ☐ prevent distortion
     - ☐ filter out 100 percent of the remnant radiation
     - ☐ move back and forth under the x-ray table
     - ☒ filter out a high degree of scattered radiation
     - ☐ reduce expense or cost

112. Visual detail may be partially obliterated by
     - ☒ poor screen film contact
     - ☐ too great a tube-to-film distance, causing magnification
     - ☐ too great a distance between the cathode and the anode of the x-ray tube
     - ☐ decreasing Kv.P. and increasing Ma.S. in proper ratio
     - ☐ industrial film

113. A decrease in grid ratio would result in
     - ☐ no change in exposure
     - ☐ increase in exposure
     - ☒ decrease in exposure
     - ☐ out-of-focus exposure

114. Minor degrees of overloading of the tube will result in
     - ☐ a defective ohmmeter
     - ☒ pitting of the target
     - ☐ buildup of filtration on the tube window
     - ☐ filament burnout

115. A timer measuring impulses of alternating current starting at zero and terminating at zero is a

Final Examination Questions

- ☐ mechanical timer
- ☐ synchronous timer
- ☐ Geiger counter
- ☒ impulse timer

116. Three-phase equipment utilizes more of the peak Kv.P. than does conventional full-wave (four-valve tube) equipment. The percentage of efficiency of three-phase equipment is
   - ☒ 95
   - ☐ 70
   - ☐ 80
   - ☐ 100

117. An exposure is made at 40 inches focus-film distance, using 100 M.S. At 60 inches the exposure required would be
   - ☐ 50 Ma.S.
   - ☐ 150 Ma.S.
   - ☒ 225 Ma.S.
   - ☐ 300 Ma.S.

118. The sharpness of detail in a radiograph is decreased by the use of
   - ☒ a large focal spot
   - ☐ a grid
   - ☐ a decrease of 10 Kv.P.
   - ☐ increased filtration

119. In body-section radiography a thin section of the body may be obtained by
   - ☐ a short amplitude and a long target-film distance
   - ☒ a long amplitude and a short target-film distance
   - ☐ a short amplitude and a short target-film distance
   - ☐ a long amplitude and a long target-film distance

120. The following combination determines the thickness of the plane portrayed by body section radiography:
   - ☐ length of tube travel and part-film distance
   - ☒ target-film distance and length of tube travel
   - ☐ part-film distance and speed of tube travel
   - ☐ speed of tube travel and length of tube travel

121. The following instrument(s) would be used to demonstrate the effect of kilovoltage on contrast:
   - ☐ a spinning top
   - ☐ a ballistics meter
   - ☐ an oscilloscope
   - ☒ an aluminum step wedge

122. When proper radiographic detail cannot be obtained because of excessive part-film distance. The following change in technique may be used to improve the detail:
   - ☐ change the Kv.P.
   - ☐ increase the time
   - ☐ change the Ma.S.
   - ☒ increase the focus-film distance

FORMULATING X-RAY TECHNIQUES

123. When using a Bucky with a focused grid, if the lateral edges of the film lose density, it is an indication that the
    - ☐ grid travels too fast
    - ☒ focus-film distance is too great
    - ☐ tube is not perpendicular to the grid
    - ☐ part-film distance is too great

124. A radiograph is made using a 16:1 ratio Bucky. The resulting film shows longitudinal streaks of uneven densities. These are probably caused by the
    - ☒ central ray not being directed to the center of the table
    - ☐ Bucky moving unevenly during the exposure
    - ☐ Bucky stopping at some time during the exposure
    - ☐ film moving during the exposure

125. "The range between the minimum and maximum exposure that will produce a scale of translucent densities acceptable for diagnostic purposes": this is a definition of
    - ☐ contrast
    - ☐ wave amplitude
    - ☒ exposure latitude
    - ☐ absorption differential

126. The *chief* purpose of a filter of aluminum placed beneath the aperture of a radiographic tube is to
    - ☐ control the latitude of the radiographic image
    - ☐ eliminate the light given off by the filament
    - ☒ absorb some of the longer wave lengths
    - ☐ filter out undesirable stem radiation

127. The four possible sets of technical factors listed below are to be used in routine radiography of a particular anatomic region. Select the set of factors that would most likely produce a radiograph with the *most magnification,* with all factors listed remaining the same:
    - ☐ 25 Ma.S., 1-mm. focal spot, 40-inch focus-film distance, 4-inch part-film distance
    - ☐ 20 Ma.S., 2-mm. focal spot, 36-inch focus-film distance, 4-inch part-film distance
    - ☒ 25 Ma.S., 2-mm. focal spot, 36-inch focus-film distance, 6-inch part-film distance
    - ☐ 25 Ma.S., 1-mm. focal spot, 40-inch focus-film distance, 6-inch part-film distance

128. The single factor that does the *most* to control radiographic detail is the
    - ☐ kilovoltage
    - ☐ Potter-Bucky diaphragm
    - ☒ object-film distance
    - ☐ intensifying screen

129. To comply with Handbook No. 76, the total filtration in the useful beam should be
    - ☐ 1.0 mm. aluminum
    - ☐ 2.0 mm. aluminum

Final Examination Questions

- ☐ 3.0 mm. aluminum
- ☒ not less than 2.5 mm. aluminum
- ☐ 2.5 mm. aluminum

130. Currently used arteriography contrast agents all contain
    - ☐ sodium
    - ☐ meglamine (methyl glucamine)
    - ☒ iodine
    - ☐ benzene

131. A drip-infusion study is an examination of the
    - ☐ fallopian tubes
    - ☐ lymphatics
    - ☐ salivary ducts
    - ☒ renal pelves

132. Short exposure times are *most* helpful in
    - ☐ urography
    - ☐ pneumoencephalography
    - ☐ venography
    - ☒ angiocardiography

133. In this list of special examinations the following item does *not* belong in the series:
    - ☐ retrograde aortography
    - ☐ venacavography
    - ☒ hysterosalpingography
    - ☐ cerebral angiography

134. In the following list of special examination, the following item does *not* belong to the series:
    - ☐ peri-renal air insufflation
    - ☒ splenoportography
    - ☐ retrograde pyelography
    - ☐ nephrotomography

135. A pneumoencephalogram is an examination of the
    - ☒ ventricular system
    - ☐ retroperitoneal space
    - ☐ arteries of the brain
    - ☐ uterus and ovaries

136. The Sweet's localizer is likely to be used in an examination of the
    - ☐ sinuses
    - ☒ eye
    - ☐ GI tract
    - ☐ bladder

137. Three of the following items are used as contrast media in radiography. Select the one which is *not* so used.
    - ☐ Air
    - ☐ Carbon dioxide gas
    - ☒ Isotonic saline
    - ☐ Iodized poppy-seed oil

FORMULATING X-RAY TECHNIQUES

138. Compared with an x-ray tube used in radiography, a deep-therapy tube is operated at
- ☐ Higher Ma. and lower Kv.P.
- ☐ Higher Ma. and higher Kv.P.
- ☐ Lower Ma. and lower Kv.P.
- ☒ Lower Ma. and higher Kv.P.

139. In doing intravenous opaque studies, the following equipment should be provided for the *maximum* safety of the patient:
- ☐ Sphygmomanometer
- ☒ Emergency kit with oxygen
- ☐ Intravenous cutdown set
- ☐ 5% dextrose solution

Complete the following short answer questions:

What is the difference between the following?

140. Projection
141. Position
142. View
143. What views are taken of any anatomic part? Why?

BIBLIOGRAPHY

BOOKS

Cahoon, John B., Jr. 1948. *Formulating x-ray techniques.* Durham, N.C.: Carden Press, 1949, 2d ed.; 1952, 3d ed. 1953, 4th ed., Duke University Press; 1961, 5th ed.; 1965, 6th ed.; 1970, 7th ed.

Cullinan, John E. 1972. *Illustrated guide to x-ray technics.* Philadelphia: J. B. Lippincott.

Eastman Kodak Company. 1969. *Radiography in modern industry.*

Files, Glenn W., et al., 1943. *Medical roentgenographic technique.* Springfield, Ill.: Charles C Thomas.

Fuchs, Arthur W. 1955, 1958. *Principles of radiographic exposure and processing.* Springfield, Ill.: Charles C Thomas.

Hudson, Ralph G. 1939. *The Engineer's Manual.* New York: Wiley.

Jerman, E. C. 1928. *Modern x-ray technique.* St. Paul, Minn.: Bruce Publishing Company.

Mees, C. E. K. 1942. *The theory of the photographic process.* New York: Macmillan.

Merrill, Venita. 1967. *Atlas of roentgenographic positions.* St. Louis: Mosby.

Rhinehart, D. A. 1936. *Roentgenographic technique.* Philadelphia: Lea and Febiger.

Rollins, W. 1904. *Notes on x-light.* Cambridge, Mass.: Harvard Univ. Press.

Sante, L. R. 1947. *Manual of roentgenographic technique.* Ann Arbor, Mich.: Edwards Brothers.

ARTICLES

Andrews, J. F. 1936. Planigraphy—introduction and history. *American Journal of Roentgenology* 36: 575–87.

Ardran, G. M., and H. E. Crooks. 1951. The reduction of radiation dose in chest radiography. *British Journal of Radiology* 35: 22–26.

Bierman, A., and W. H. Boldingh. 1951. The relation between tension and exposure times in radiography. *Acta Radiologica* 35: 22–26.

Cahoon, John B., Jr. 1948. Barium plastic filters in roentgen diagnosis of placenta praevia. *X-Ray Technician* 19: 185–88.

_____. 1941. Lateral chest technique. *X-Ray Technician* 12: 2, 55, 56, 78.

_____. 1941. Radiography of the styloid process of the temporal bone. *X-Ray Technician* 12: 211–12.

_____. 1942. Radiography of the mandible. *Radiography and Clinical Photography* 18: 3, 71–73.

_____. 1942. Uses of opaque plastic filters in radiography of the lateral

FORMULATING X-RAY TECHNIQUES

lumbar-dorsal spine, lateral cervical-dorsal spine, and cases of suspected placenta praevia. *X-Ray Technician* 13: 242–43, 246.
———. 1946. Radiography of the foot. *Radiography and Photography* 22, no. 1: 2–9.
———. 1947. Radiography of the foot. *Yearbook of Radiology,* pp. 25–28.
———. 1948. Standardized technique in radiography of the labyrinth and petrous, employing a Lucite angle board. *X-Ray Technician,* 19 (Sept.): 80.
———. 1948. Recent advances in the use of opaque plastic filters in placenta roentgenography. *Radiography* (London).
———. 1948. The roentgen diagnosis of placenta praevia. *X-Ray Technician* 19: 185–188.
———. 1949. Lateral radiography of the mandible. *Medical Radiography and Photography,* 18, no. 3: 71–72.
——— and Reeves, Robert J. 1952. Lateral radiography of the pregnant uterus. *Medical Radiography and Photography* 28: 2–10.
———. 1970. New horizons in the technical and educational systems of radiologic technology. *Radiologic Technology* 42, no. 2: 83–90.
Carty, John R. 1936. Soft tissue roentgenography. *American Journal of Roentgenology* 35: 474–84.
Cornwell, William S. 1942. Lumbar vertebrae. *Radiography and Clinical Photography* 18: 2–11, 30–35, 54–61.
Crabtree, J. I., and R. W. Henn. 1947, 1948. Developer solutions for x-ray films. *Medical Radiography and Photography* 23: 2–12, 38–46; 24: 10–14.
Dotter, C. T., and I. Steinberg. 1952. Angiocardiography in congenital heart disease. *American Journal of Medicine* 12: 219–37.
———, I. Steinberg, and H. L. Temple. 1949. Automatic roentgen-ray roll-film magazine for angiocardiography and cerebral arteriography. *American Journal of Roentgenology* 62: 355–58.
Files, Glenn W. 1935. Maximum tissue differentiation. *X-Ray Technician* 7: 17–24.
———. 1926. The relation, radiographically, of kilovolt peak to time of exposure. *Radiology* 7: 255.
Friedman, J. S. 1951. The latent image in photography. *American Photographer* 45: 484–87.
Fuchs, Arthur W. 1947. Anode heel effect in radiography. *X-Ray Technician* 18: 158–63.
———. 1934. Radiology of the entire body. *Radiography and Clinical Photography* 10: 9–14.
———. 1938. Higher kilovoltage technique. *Radiography and Clinical Photography* 14: 2–8.
———. 1940. Balance and radiographic image. *X-Ray Technician* 12: 81–84, 118.
———. 1945. The optimum kilovoltage technique in military roentgenography. *American Journal of Roentgenology* 50: 358.
———. 1948. Relationship of tissue thickness to kilovoltage. *X-Ray Technician* 19: 287–93.
———. 1950. Control of radiographic density. *X-Ray Technician* 22: 62–68.

Bibliography

_____. 1950. Rationale of radiographic exposure. *X-Ray Technician* 22: 62–68.

_____. 1956. Evolution of roentgen film. *American Journal of Roentgenology* 75: 30–48.

Funke, T. 1955. Compensating filters in medical radiography. *X-Ray Technician* 27: 12–27.

Gianturco, C., and G. A. Miller. 1957. Low-exposure radiography. *Carle Memorial Hospital*, vol. 10.

Gifford, D., and D. E. Truscott. 1954. Use of additional filtration in medical radiography. *British Journal of Radiology* 27: 113–16.

Gould, D. R. 1940. Fundamentals of tissue differentiation. *Radiology* 6: 83–92.

Greening, J. R. 1949. Demonstration of the geometrical principles underlying radiography. *Radiography* 15: 268–69.

Henny, G. C. 1935. Artifacts in roentgen films. *Radiology* 24: 350–56.

Hodgson, M. B. 1919. A simple slide rule for computing x-ray exposures. *American Journal of Roentgenology*, March.

Holly, Elmer W. 1942. Some radiographic technics in which movement is utilized. *Radiography and Clinical Photography* 18: 78–83.

Huyler, W. C. 1938. Suggestions for simplifying technique in diagnostic roentgenology. *American Journal of Roentgenology* 39: 967–71.

Jaffke, Ruth C. 1942. Tissue thickness measurement technique. *X-Ray Technician* 13: 150–52, 180.

Jaundrell-Thompson, R. 1953. Radiography of air and fluids. *Radiography,* 19: 233–245.

Jerman, E. C. 1926. The analysis of the end result: the radiograph. *Radiology* 6: 59–62.

_____. 1926. Extremity technic. *Radiology* 6: 252.

_____. 1926. Potter-Bucky diaphragm technic. *Radiology* 6: 336–38.

Kieffner, J. 1938. The laminograph in its variations, implications, and applications of the planographic principles. *American Journal of Roentgenology* 39: 497–513.

Landfeldt, B. 1960. Tomography of the middle ear in columella operations. *Radiology* 53: 129–36.

Larson, E. T. 1951. Formation of the latent image by x-rays. *J.P.S.A.* 17B: 19–24.

Mahoney, G. J. 1959. A slide rule for Kv.P.-Ma.S. adjustments facilitating the use of high kilovoltage. *X-Ray Technician* 31: 35–38.

Mattisson, O. 1956. Reduction of static disturbances in dark rooms. *Acta Radiologica* 45: 383–88.

Mills, Walter R. 1917. The relation of body habitus to visceral form: position, tonus, motility. *American Journal of Roentgenology* 4: 155–69.

Morgan, R. H. 1950. An analysis of the physical factors controlling the diagnostic quality of the roentgen images. *American Journal of Roentgenology* 54: 128, 395.

_____. 1946. Analysis of physical factors controlling diagnostic quality of roentgen images; contrast and intensity distribution function of roentgen image. *American Journal of Roentgenology* 55: 67–89.

_____. 1946. Analysis of physical factors controlling diagnostic quality of roentgen images; contrast and film contrast factor. *American Journal of Roentgenology* 55: 627-33.

———— and W. W. Van Allen. 1949. Sensitometry of roentgenographic films and screens. *Radiology* 52: 832-45.

Newman, Gerbert. 1933. Relation of kilovolts to thickness of part in x-ray technique. *X-Ray Technician* 5: 21.

Rhinehart, D. A. 1933. Exposure technique chart. *X-Ray Technician* 4: 71.

————. 1949. This factor called voltage. *X-Ray Technician* 21: 21.

Roderick, J. F., and B. Southerland. 1952. Study of the static electricity problem in the x-ray darkroom. *X-Ray Technician* 23: 343-66.

Sanders, Aaron P., Kathryn Sharpe, John B. Cahoon, Jr., Robert J. Reeves, Joseph K. Isley, and George J. Baylin. 1960. Radiation dose to the skin in roentgen diagnostic procedures. *American Journal of Roentgenology* 84: 359-68.

Schoen, Cyrus, P. 1948. X-ray technique in pediatric cases. *X-Ray Technician* 19: 241-43.

Schwarz, G. S. 1960. Kilovoltage conversion in radiography. *X-Ray Technician* 31: 373-79, 436.

Seemann, H. E. 1940. The reduction of secondary radiation and of excessive radiographic contrast by filtration. *American Society for Testing Materials* 40: 1289-96.

————, and H. R. Splettstosser. 1955. The effect of kilovoltage and grid ratio on subject contrast in radiography. *Radiology* 64: 572-80.

————, and Splettstosser, H. R. 1954. Some physical characteristics of Potter-Bucky diaphragms. *Radiology* 62: 4:575-83.

Shearer, J. S. 1916. The physical aspect of roentgen ray measurement and dosage. *American Journal of Roentgenology* 6: 2-12.

————. 1917. X-ray physics, in *X-ray manual,* U.S. Army, chap. 2.

Shields, David G. 1937. General roentgenologic technic for infants and children. *X-Ray Technician* 5: 9, 42.

Spiegler, G. 1950. The story of contrast and definition. *Radiography,* 16: 177-82.

Teplick, J. G. 1946. Simplification of roentgenography by high kilovoltage technique. *American Journal of Roentgenology* 56: 660-67.

Trout, E. D., D. E. Graves, and D. B. Slauson. 1949. High-voltage radiography. *Radiology* 52: 669-83.

Tuddenham, W. J., G. H. McDonnel, T. A. Tristan, H. P. Pendergrass, and L. Stanton. 1957. Diagnostic megavoltage radiography. *Medical Radiography and Photography* 33: 58-65.

van Dijk, D. 1956. Some factors influencing the results in radiography. *Medica Mundi* 1: 27-32.

Watson, W. 1958. Gridless radiography at high kilovoltage with air gap technique. *X-Ray Focus* 2: 1: 12-13.

Webb, J. H. 1941. Formation of the photographic latent image. *J.P.S.A.* 7: 136-43.

Wilsey, R. B. 1921. Intensity of scattered x-ray in radiography. *American Journal of Roentgenology* 8: 328-38.

————. 1921. The effects of scattered x-rays in radiography. *American Journal of Roentgenology* 8: 589-98.

————. 1922. The efficiency of the Bucky-diaphragm principle. *American Journal of Roentgenology* 9: 58-66.

Bibliography

———. 1932. Stereoradiography and distortion. *Radiography and Clinical Photography* 8: 25.

———. 1933. The physical foundation of chest roentgenology. *American Journal of Roentgenology* 30: 235, 388.

Wolcott, Roy. 1937. Technics for unusual cases. *X-Ray Technician* 9: 38–42.

Wynroe, R. F. 1955. Some observations on kilovoltage variations. *Radiography* 21: 242–43.

PERSONAL COMMUNICATIONS

K. D. A. Allen, Denver, Colo.
C. J. Bodie, Winnipeg, Canada
Charles Bridgeman, Eastman Kodak Company
Tom Byrd, R. T., Danville, Va.
W. Edward Chamberlain, Temple University
William Conklin, Orangeburg, S.C.
John E. Cullinan, Albert Einstein Medical Center, Philadelphia, Pa.
Floyd Driver, R. T., Sumter, S.C.
Terry Eastman, E. I. du Pont Company
Charles T. Dotter, University of Oregon
James C. Fletcher, Baltimore, Md.
Don Fowler, R. T., Spartanburg, S.C.
Margaret Hoing, Chicago, Ill.
Jon Hough, R. T., Salisbury, N.C.
J. Kieffer, New London, Conn.
Larry G. Lambrecht, R. T., Milwaukee, Wis.
J. B. Langley, Eastman Kodak Company
Ted Lynch, Baltimore, Md.
Ben Martin, R. T., Charleston, S.C.
Venita Merrill, New York, N.Y.
Blanche Mowry, New London, Conn.
James Ohnysty, R. T., Greenville, S.C.
Richard A. Olden, Johns Hopkins Hospital
Ted Ott, R. T., California
Carl W. Reed, Minneapolis, Minn.
Ray Runge, Mayo Clinic Hospital, Minn.
Edward Rusin, Eastman Kodak Company
Aaron P. Sanders, Duke University Medical Center
L. R. Sante, St. Louis, Mo.
Harold Smythe, Machlett Laboratories, Conn.
Dick Stueve, R. T., Loma Linda, Calif.
E. V. Stober, Stamford, Conn.
Clark R. Warren, Royal Oak, Mich.
W. W. Wasson, Denver, Colo.

BROCHURES

E. I. du Pont Nemours Company. *Darkroom technique.*

———. *Split-second exposures* (using Du Pont Cronex XTRA Life intensifying screens).

FORMULATING X-RAY TECHNIQUES

Eastman Kodak Company. *A totally new approach to improved image quality.*
———. *ABC's of x-ray film processing.*
———. *Fundamentals of radiography.*
———. *Medical radiography and photography.*
———. *Radiographic duplicating film.*
———. *Subtraction film.*
———. *Time/temperature development chart.*
GAF X-ray Company. *Radiography—tool of medical science.*
General Electric Company. *How to prepare an x-ray technic chart.*
———. *A guide to radiological anatomy—a series of drawings of identified anatomical parts.*
———. *Phototiming.*
———. *Principles of x-ray generation.*
———. *Visual densities throughout the range of 40–130 Kv.P.*
Liebel-Flarsheim Company. *Characteristics and applications of x-ray grids.*
Picker X-Ray Company. *Outline of modern x-ray technique.*
———. *Production of x-rays—a matter of energy conversion.*

INDEX

Abdomen, children's, exposure guide, 221
  exposure guide for, 178, 215
  fistulae in, procedure, 147
  high Kv.P. guide, 235, 238
  pathology procedure, 147
  radiation dosage and, 258
Abscess, encapsulated, penetrability, 161
Absorption, air, 3
  of x-rays, bone and flesh, 139
  by grids, 47, 59
  by tissues, 135
Accidental motion, 158
Acetabulum, 307, 308
Acidity, of fixer, 31
Acromegaly, 161
Acromioclavicular joint, procedure, 144
Acromion process, procedure, 307
Actinomycosis, 161
Additive penetration, 161
Adjustment for equipment, 224
  for pathology, 224
Age, correction factors for children and infants, 105, 175
Air-contrast radiograph, 229, 231
Air-gap technique, 194, 198–99, 202, 239, 240
Air tubes, correcting, 40
Alignment of tube, and anode heel effect, 61
Alternating current, 326
Aluminum, in filters, 44–46, 155
Aluminum sulfate, in fixer, 31
Ampere, 324
Aneurysm, of aorta, 147, 161
Angiocardiogram, positions for, 241, 242
Angle of tube, 100–101
Ankle, exposure guide, 218, 221; high Kv.P., 237; with screen, 218
  procedure, 144, 176, 196
  thickness, 208
Anode heel effect, 59–61, 141
  chart, 60
Anthracosis, penetrability, 161
Aorta, aneurysm of, penetrability, 161; procedure, 147
Appendix, identified, 308
Arm, thickness, 207

Arterial system, of skull, procedure, 146
Arteriograms, screen for, 25
  cerebral, technique, 242
Arthritis, of sacroiliac, procedure, 146
  degenerative, penetrability, 161
Artifacts, in film, 12, 35–36
Asbestosis, penetrability, 161
Ascites, penetrability, 161
Ashes, in cassette, 29
Asthenic habitus, 155–56
Asymmetry, procedure, 155
Atelectasis, defined, 311
  penetrability, 161
Atlas, defined, 307
Atlas and axis, 307
  procedure, 144, 237, 317
Atrophy, allowance for, 211
  and measurement, 160
  penetrability, 161
  procedure, 224
Attenuation coefficient, 131–32
Auditory canal, identified, 308
Auditory ossicles, high-Kv.P. technique for, 198
Automatic processing, 30–35
  advantages, 34–35
  development, 29–30
  effect of temperature, 33
  film-feeding chart, 32
  and light-tightness, 26
  silver recovery, 29–30
  trouble chart, 38–41
Axis, identified, 307; see also Atlas and axis

Backscatter radiation, 18
  on skin, 343
Barium lead sulfate, phosphor, 23
Base, of film, 3
Beam restrictor, use, 83
Beam shape, of collimator, 42
Beck's sarcoid, penetrability, 161
Bierman and Boldingh, formula, 191
Biliary tract, procedure, 148
Bite-wing film, 5
Bladder, urinary, identified, 308, 309
  procedure, 148
Blank film, correcting, 37

369

Blastomycosis, penetrability, 161
Bleaching, by fixer, 32
Blotchiness, in film, 33
Blue fluorescence, 23
Blu-Ray duplication, 6-7
Bone, absorption of radiation, 134, 139
   density and, 143
   long, identified, 311
   petrous, radiographs, 101
   and secondary radiation, 115
Bone age, of ankle, 144
   of wrist, 143
Bone disease, allowance for, 210, 224
Bones, dried, 171-72
   facial, fracture, 147; exposure guide, 175
Bowel obstruction, penetrability, 161
Brachycephalic skull, 155
Breast, radiography of, 5, 148
   pendulous, penetrability, 161
Bronchial trees, procedure, 147
Bronchiectasis, defined, 311
   penetrability, 161
Bronchitis, defined, 311
Bronchogram, 228-29
   exposure guide, 241
Bucky, Gustav, 46
Bucky diaphragm (Potter-Bucky), 46-49, 82-83, 189-90
   adjustment, 263
   and cone, 77
   cutoff, 37
   effect on fog, 77
   with grid, 46, 48, 54, 57-58
   limitations, 52
   for radiation fog, 115
   rule for use, 57-58
   tables, 191
   technique, 155, 171
Bursa, subdeltoid, procedure, 144

Cahoon, John B., Jr., techniques of, 191, 197
Calcaneus, identified, 308
Calcification, penetrability, 161
   abdomen, procedure, 147
Calcinosis, penetrability, 161
Calcium tungstate, phosphor, 23
Caldwell projection, 51-52, 168
   radiation dosage, 253, 257
Calibration of radiographic unit, 21-22, 153
   importance, 94, 202
Calipers, in measuring, 160
Cancer, of lungs, 147
   and radiation dosage, 203
Canthus, identified, 308
Cardboard angles, use of, 155
Cardboard film holder, 4, 155, 290-91
   and exposure guide, 223
   exposure time with, 23

Cardboard film holder (*cont.*)
   and fogging, 28
   when impractical, 173-74
Carcinoma, penetrability, 161
Cardiac cycle, adjusting exposure to, 159
Carotid canals, procedure, 145
Carpal canal, procedure, 143
Cassette, 18-21
   dust in, 25
   faulty placement, 37
   phototimer, 18-19
   vacuum, 201
   warped, 19
Cassetteless radiography, 22
Cast, *see* Plaster cast
Cathode, hot, 335
Cecum, identified, 308
Cellulose, in film, 3-4
Centering the tube, 51
Central ray, intensity of, 60
Cerebral arteriogram, table, 242
Cervical spine, children, exposure guide, 221
   exposure guide, 176, 177, 214-15, 221; high Kv.P., 234, 237
   magnification, 243
   procedure, 144
   radiation dosage, 253, 257
   radiography with stationary grid, 52
Cervical vertebrae, thickness, 208
Charcot joint, penetrability, 161
Charts, exposure, making, 184-85
   formulating, 153-85
   value of, 202-3
Chassard projection, radiation dose, 255
Chest, adjustment of exposure, 224
   air-gap technique, 194, 198-99, 202, 239, 240
   child's, exposure, 162-64, 179, 219
   exposure guide, 176, 178, 179, 212-13
   with fluid, 163
   fogging of film and, 28
   graph of thickness, 209
   high-Kv.P. technique, 202, 233, 236, 240
   with Hodgkin's disease, 163
   infant's, 179, 219
   interlobar effusion, procedure, 147
   and Kardex, 227
   motion in, 159
   penetration, 162-64
   procedure, 146, 195
   radiation dosage, 252, 256
   radiation in exposure with grids, 47
   radiograph, 92-93; with grid, 252-53; high-Kv.P., 199
   rapid exposure for, 301
   thickness, 207, 209
Child(ren), chest exposure, 162-64, 179
   conversion factors for, 105, 175

Index

Child(ren) (cont.)
  exposure guide, 219
  fixed-Kv.P. technique, 197; examples, 231
  grids or Bucky with, 83
  skull, 168
Cholesterol stones, contrast for, 132
Circuit-breaker, fused, 333
  trouble with, 262
Circulatory system, penetrability, 161
Cirrhosis of the liver, penetrability, 161
Classification, for thickness, 205
Clavicle, fractured, procedure, 144
  high-Kv.P. guide, 237
  thickness, 207
Cleanliness, in darkroom, 28–29
Cleanup, grids and, 56
Clearing time, 32
Close subject, technique, 180
Coating, of film, 4
  for Polaroid prints, 11–12
Cobalt beam, 339
Cobalt treatment, 344
Coccidiomycosis, penetrability, 161
Coin, radiation fog example, 112–13
Collimators, 42–44, 155
  as beam restrictors, 83
Colon, 155
  air-contrast view, 229, 241
  exposure guide, 215, 238
  high-Kv.P. technique, 198, 235, 238
  and Kardex, 227
  lesion of, 146
  location of, 155
  radiation dosage, 254
  radiographs of, 130; with grids, 47
Color, of darkroom, 27
Color radiography, 8
Compensation, in converting from grid to non-grid technique, 83
  for density, experiment, 72
Compression, use of, 299
Compression bands, and measurement, 160
Computer, for special procedures, 201, 204
Condyles, femoral, procedure, 144
  identified, 307
Cone(s), 42–43, 155, 339
  allowance for, in exposure, 82
  and fog, 77, 113, 115, 133, 141
  and high Kv.P., 125
  size, 57–58, 223
  Videx, 191
Constant factors, in exposure, 82
Contrast, 115–20, 124–25, 134–35, 136–39, 152, 173
  with cone, 42
  diagnostic value, 135, 142, 202
  effect of lag, 25
  experimental study, 244–48

Contrast (cont.)
  in iodinated studies, 131–32
  and Kv.P., 81, 88, 128, 130, 141, 198, 231–33
  limitations, 129
  long-scale, 142
  scale, 117–19, 135, 142
  short-scale, 142
  with screen, test, 19–20
  sufficient and excessive, 115, 142
Contrast media, adjustment for, 210, 224
Conversion chart, General Electric, 189–90
Conversion curve, Ma.S. vs. Kv.P., 183–84
Conversion factors, for extension cylinder, 83
  Ma.S. vs. distance, 99–100
  Ma.S. vs. Kv.P., 87
Coolidge tube, 189, 335
Copper, in filters, 44–46
Coracoid process, procedure, 144
Correction, in Ma.S., 169
Cosmic rays, 203
Cranium, 311
Crinkle marks, in film 28–30, 294
Cronex printer, 8
Cross-hatched grid, 51, 54
Crown static, 14
Current, alternating, 328
  direct, 327
Curve, of sensitometry, 249–50
Cutoff, off-distance, 51–52
Cylinder, extension, as beam restrictor, conversion factors, 83
Cystic conditions, penetrability, 161

Dangers, to operator, 341
Darkroom, 26–29
Decimals, 62–63
  table of equivalent fractions, 94, 95
Definition, 120–21, 124–25, 135–37, 244
Densitometer, and stepwedge, 16
Density, 134–37, 153
  with cone, 42
  contrast and, 116, 333–34
  desirable, 106
  development time effect, experiment, 71
  and distance, 73, 85, 140
  experimental study, 68–69, 74, 244
  factors affecting, 110–15, 250
  how to increase, 301
  indicates exposure, 162
  and Kv.P., 73, 74, 75, 85, 139, 183–84
  and Ma.S., 68, 72, 75–76, 85, 140, 135
  30 per cent rule for, 94
  and time, 140
Detail, 106, 120–21, 135–38, 153
  with cone, 42

371

FORMULATING X-RAY TECHNIQUES

Detail (*cont.*)
   and contrast, 114
   experimental study, 244
Developer, contaminated, 38, 40
   and contrast, 118–20
   and density, 110
   dilution, 39
   exhausted, 34
   oxidized, 292
   replenishment of, 30
   smears from, 25
   and temperature, 33, 38, 71–72, 294
   troubles, 40–41
Development, 17, 292–93
   and density, experiment, 71–72
Diagnostic quality, 135, 205–6
Diaphragm excursion, procedure, 146
Digestive system, procedure, 147–48
Diplomat processor, 22
Direct exposure, Ma.S. for, 85–86
Dirt deposits on film, 35–36
Disc, vertebral, procedure, 145
Distal, definition, 309
Distance (focus-film), 152, 301
   with air-gap technique, 239–40
   with angled tube, 100–101
   close, 317
   conversion table, Ma.S., 104
   and density, 140; experiment, 67, 73, 74
   and detail, 121
   and distortion, 124
   as factor in exposure, 82, 223–24
   with focused grid, 52
   formula, for Ma.S. relation, 93
   and Kv.P., relation, 85
   and Ma.S., 91–93, 99–100, 104
   short, 180
   standardized, for guide, 222
   and x-ray intensity, 90–91
Distortion, 106, 121, 123–24, 134, 153, 299
Dolichocephalic skull, 155
Dorsal spine, guide, 176, 177, 179
   radiation dosage, 254
   technique, 237, 317
Dosage, radiation, 129, 203–4, 257, 258
   surface vs. air, 344
Dosimeter films, 6
Dryer, 31, 40
Drying of film, 33
Duke University Medical Center, research in radiation, 203
Duodenum, 308
Duplication of radiographs, 6–7

Echogram, procedures, 198
Edema, penetrability, 161
Elbow, exposure guide, 217, 221;
   with screen, 218
   high Kv.P. guide, 236

Elbow (*cont.*)
   procedures, 143
   radial head, 143
   thickness, 207
Electromagnetic spectrum, 327
Emaciation, penetrability, 160, 161
Emphysema, allowance for, 211, 224
   penetrability, 161
Emulsion, of film, 3–4
Epigastrium, 309
Epithelioma, 343
Equations, 63
Erythema dose, 343
Esophagus, 308
   exposure guide, 216; high Kv.P., 238
   procedure, 148
Estar base, 7
Evaluation, of radiograph quality, 153
Ewing's tumor, penetrability, 161
Excretory system, procedure, 148
Exophthalmos, procedure, 146
Exostosis, penetrability, 161
Experiment, fluid level, 151–52
Experiments, basic exposure, 66–80
Expiration date, for film, 12
Exposure, 81–82, 135–40
   with angled tube, 101
   charts, early, 186–90; making, 184–85; *see also* Exposure, guides
   compensative, 162
   correct, 136
   direct, 173–74, 223; tables, 86
   and distance, 98–100
   effect on detail, 121
   experiments in, 66–80
   factors in, 84
   fixed Kv.P. system, 195–97
   with grids, 59, 129–30
   guides, 175–79, 240–41; adjustment for equipment, 225; direct exposure, 223; extremities, 216–18, 221; fixed kilovoltage, 210–22; formulating, 210; high kilovoltage, 234–39; at 150 Kv.P., 237–39; how to use, 223
   Ma.S. values for, 222; with screen, 218
   intensity, 98
   and Kv.P., 84, 125–27; experiment, 80
   latitude, 160; and Kv.P., 128–29, 140; and Ma.S., 140; narrow, experiment, 78–79; wide, experiment, 77–78
   and Ma.S., 84, 98, 126, 140
   with screens, 23, 85–86, 218
   and sensitivity of film, 28
   special, guide, 179
   systems, 201; modern, 195–203
   technique, 104; modern, 195–203
   time of, 153–54; tables, 88, 89; vs. Kv.P. 87–88; and distance, 99–100; and Ma., 99–100
Extremities, children, exposure guide, 221

Index

Extremities (cont.)
  exposure guide, 176, 178, 216–18; high Kv.P., 236; with screen, 218
  and Kardex, 227
  magnification of, 243
  technique for, 171–72, 197–98

Face, bones of the, 308
  fracture, 146
  guide, 175
Factors, in exposure, 81–82
Fallopian tubes, procedure, 148
Fat, and Kv.P., 131–32
Female reproductive system, procedure, 148
Femur, 144, 308
  high-Kv.P guide, 237
Fibrosarcoma, penetrability, 161
Fibrosis, radiation, penetrability, 161
Fibula, guide, 217
  procedure, 144
  radiation dosage, 259
Field size, conversion factors for, 83
Fifteen per cent rule, 89–90
Filament, in tube, 337
Files, Glenn W., 190
Film, 3–17
  artifacts on, 35–36
  base, 3
  blank, correcting, 37
  color, 8
  contrast, 117, 120
  crinkle marks, 28–30
  dark, 37
  dental, 5
  density, correcting, 38
  dirty, 40
  dosimeter, 6
  not drying, 40
  duplicating, 6–7
  exposure tables, 86
  fine-grain, 4–5
  fogged, 40
  graininess, 244
  grayed-out, 34, 37
  handling, 14
  identification, 15
  industrial, 6
  light, 37
  loading and unloading, 14
  mammographic, 4
  marks on, 293–94
  Medichrome, 8
  non-screen, 86, 174, 291, 294
  outdated, 12
  packing, 12, 14
  Polaroid, 9–12
  regular (non-screen), table, 86; speed, 291
  and safelight, 28
  screen, exposure table, 86

Film (cont.)
  sensitivity of unexpired, 28
  sensitometry of, 249–51
  size, appropriate, 223
  speed, 250
  staining of, 293
  static affecting, 14–15
  sticking, 38–39
  storage, 12–15
  streaking, 39, 293
  subtraction, 7–8
  tests, 15–17; experiment, 69–70
  therapy-localizing, 5
  trouble charts, 37–41
  Xerox system, 22
  X-Omat, 5–8
  x-ray, 4–5
Film-feeding, 31–32
Filter(s), 44–46
  air, 40
  compensating, 46
  handling, 342
  for hardness, 344
  and radiation dosage, 203
  for safelight, 27–28
  thoreus, 339
  trough, 46
  wedge, 25, 46
Filtration, 155
  defective, 37
Fingers, thickness, 207
Fistulae, in abdomen, procedure, 147
Fixed Kv.P. technique, 195–97, 202–3, 205–43
  advantages, 199–200, 204
  constructing charts, 206–210
  examples, 230–31
  experiment for, 206–8
  Ma.S. conversion factors, for children, 105
Fixed vs. variable factors, 210
Fixer, contamination of, 38
  exhaustion of, 39
  pH of, 31
Fixing, effect of prolonged, 33
  washing after, 29
Fixing bath, effect of, 4
Flesh, absorption, and detail, 139
Fletcher, technique, 197
Fluid(s), body, 143
  in tissue, adjustment for, 224
Fluid level, in chest and sinuses, 146
  experiment, 151–52
Fluorescence, lag, 25
Fluorescent light, effect on exposure time, 93–94
Fluorescent screens, 22–23
Fluoroscopy, 341
  with grid, 52
Foam, in tanks, 39

373

FORMULATING X-RAY TECHNIQUES

Focal spot, damage and density, 110, 112
 and detail, 120–21
 size, 334–35
Focus, short, effect of, 60
Focus-film distance, see Distance
Fog, 18, 134, 292–93
 cones and grids, effect on, 42, 77
 control of, 140–41
 correcting, 37, 40
 in darkroom, 28
 effect of grid, experiment, 76–77
 and high Kv.P., 125
 postexposure, 26–27
 and Ma.S., experiment, 75–76
 secondary radiation, 42, 111–15, 133–34
Foot, exposure guide, 217
 high Kv.P. guide, 237
 procedure, 143, 171
 radiograph of, 196
 thickness, 207
Foramen magnum, 308
 procedure, 145
Foramen ovale, procedure, 146
Foramina, intervertebral, procedure, 145
Forearm, exposure guide, 216, 221; with screen, 218
 high Kv.P. guide, 236
 procedure, 143
 thickness, 207
Foreign body, in chest or trachea, procedure, 146
Formula, for time, Kv.P., Ma., and distance in exposure, 98
Fractions, and decimals, 94
 table of decimal equivalents, 94–95
Fractures, procedures for, 144–45, 147
Frames, cassette, 21
Fuchs, Arthur W., 90–91, 125, 191–92, 195–96, 205, 206
Fusion, thoracic, procedure, 145

Gallbladder, 155, 308
 contrast for radiography of, 132
 exposure guide, 175, 177, 215
 fogging of film for, 28
 high Kv.P. guide, 235, 238
 and Kardex, 227
 procedure, 148
 radiation dosage, 254
 radiography, 42
 stones, 132
Gamma rays, geometric laws for, 123
Gassy x-ray tube, 37
Gastrointestinal tract, radiography, 47, 148, 198, 200
 high Kv.P. guide, 235
 and Kardex, 227
Gelatin, in film, 4
Gelatin coat, on rollers, 34

Generators, effect on radiographic quality, 263
Genetic mutations, and radiation, 203–4
Geometry, of distortion, 122–24
 and image formation, 134
Giant cell sarcoma, procedure, 161
Gianturco, Miller, and Wenks, on dosage, 203; filter, 45
Glass plates, history, 186
Glenoid fossa, 307
Gout, procedure, 161
Gradient, intensification, 24–25
Graininess, of film, 244
Graph, in making exposure chart, 184–85
 in sensitometry, 249–50
Green fluorescence, 23
Grid(s), 155, 195
 absorption, 47, 59
 allowance in conversion, 83
 in Bucky, 46, 48, 58
 characteristics, chart, 55
 and contrast, 129
 conversion factors, 58–59
 crossed, 48, 51, 55
 cutoff, 20, 48–49, 55–57
 and equipment, 54–55
 faulty use, 56
 focused, 52, 54
 and high Kv.P. technique, 54–55, 125, 233
 high-ratio, 47, 54, 56–57, 200–201
 linear, 51, 55
 misalignment, 56–57
 non-grid, conversion to, 58, 82–83
 off-distance and off-level cutoff, 56
 parallel, 52, 54
 patterns, 51
 ratio, 46–50, 56–57, 200–1
 and secondary radiation fog, 54, 113, 115; experiment, 76–77
 selection of, 53–54
 stationary, 52; conversion to Bucky, 58–59
 and stereo shift, 51
 warped, 20–21
Gridlines, trouble with, 263, 298
Grounding, of film-loading bench, 15
Groves, 129
Guide, for fixed Kv.P. technique, 211–221
 for high Kv.P. technique, 234–39
 for variable Kv.P. technique, 174–77; rules of formulation, 179; special exposures, 179
Guide marks, scratches on film, 35–36
Gumma, penetrability, 161

Habitus, 155
Half-value layer, defined, 339

Index

Hand, exposure guide, 216, 223; high Kv.P., 236; with screen, 218
  fracture, 143
  with gout, 165
  procedures, 143
  radiation dosage, 258–59
  radiographs, 107–9, 116
  thickness, 207
Hand-processing, and darkroom, 27
Heart, action and motion, 158–59
  enlarged, penetrability, 161
  long focus-film distance for, 302
  motion of, 158–59, 193–94
  position for exposure, 241
  procedures, 146, 147
Heat in x-ray tube, and Kv.P., 140
Heel effect, 59–61, 141
  chart, 60
Hemangioma, penetrability, 161
Hepatic flexure, 308
Herpes zoster, therapy, 339
High Kv.P. technique, 198–200, 202–3, 231–40
  advantages, 204
  air-gap technique, 239–40
  examples, 233–34
  exposure guide, 234–39
  and motion, 158–59
  highlights, value of, 136
Hinges, cassette, 21
Hip, exposure guide, 215, 237
  and Kardex, 227
  magnification, 243
  procedure, 144
  radiation dosage, 254
  thickness, 208
History of radiographic technique, 186–204
Hodges, technique, 194
Hodgkin's disease, chest, 163
  penetrability, 161
  procedure, 147
Hospitals, adapting technique from one to another, 104–5
Hot spot, defined, 339
Humerus, exposure guide, 175
  high Kv.P. guide, 236
  procedure, 143
Humidity, effect on operator, 27
Hydrocephalus, radiograph, 165
Hydropneumothorax, penetrability, 161
Hypaque, 151
Hyperparathyroidism, 161
  skull with, 165
Hypersthenic habitus, 155–56
Hypo, effect of, 4
  removing, 32
  smears, 25
Hypochondrium, 309
Hypogastrium, 309
Hyposthenic habitus, 155–156

Ileum, 309
Iliac region, 309
Ilium, 307
Image, diagnostic, 3
  formation, 134–36
  intensifier, 17
  latent, 3, 17
  reversal of, 29, 31
Immobilization of patient, 158, 318; and detail, 121
Impulse-time-Ma.S. table, 102
Impulse timer, 330–31
Inductance, 325
Infant, chest, exposure, 179; radiograph, 227
  conversion factors for Ma.S., 105
  correction factors for exposure, 105, 175
  exposure guide, 219–22
  skull radiograph, 227
Inferior, defined, 311
Injury, procedures to show, 143–49
Intensity, and inverse square law, 91
Intercondyloid space, procedure, 144
Interleaving paper, effect, 12, 14–15
Interproximal film, 5
Intestines, 309
Inverse square law, 90–93, 300
  for distance and density, 72
  for Kv.P. conversion, 85
  for screen exposure, 85
  for secondary radiation, 112
Involuntary motion, control, 158
Iodinated contrast studies, 131, 200

Jejumum, 309
Jerman, early charts, 188–89

Kardex chart, 179, 226–27
Keleket chart, 188
Kelley, 129
Kidneys, 308, 309
Kilovolt, defined, 324
Kilovoltage, 153–54; see also Kv.P.
  adjusting, 209
  as factor in radiography, 224
  and fog, 124
  and generator, 263
  and image, 124
Knee, in cast, allowance for, 105
  conversion, non-grid to grid, 58
  exposure guide, 217–18, 221–22, 225, 237; children, 222
  phantom, 16
  procedure, 144, 170
  radiation dosage, 259
  thickness, 208
  views, 169
K.U.B., exposure guide, 176, 178
Kv.P. (peak kilovoltage), 132–33, 134–36
  constant, 133, 135

FORMULATING X-RAY TECHNIQUES

Kv.P. (*cont.*)
  and contrast, 116–17, 137, 139, 141
  conversion with Ma.S., tables, 84
  and density, 85, 139; experiment, 70–71, 74
  and distance, conversion, 85, 139, 140
  effective, 173
  as exposure factor, 79, 81–82; experiment, 79–80
  extending range, 47
  fixed, 133
  and fog, 139
  grid conversion factors, 58
  high, 47, 139–40
  increasing, 107–11; and density, experiment, 72
  insufficient, 126–27
  for iodinated contrast, 131–32
  and latitude, 139, 140
  limit to, 129
  and Ma., 85–88, 139; table, 87
  and penetration, 139
  and radiation dosage, 140
  and screen exposures, 85–86
  shift for compensation, 83
  and time, 87–89, 139; 15 per cent rule, 89–90
Kyphosis, procedure, 145
  penetrability, 161

Labyrinth, procedure, 146
Lag, test for, 25
Langfeldt, and high Kv.P. technique, 198
Lapine projection, radiation dosage, 255
Latent image, 3, 17
Lateral, defined, 311
Lateral dorsal spine, special exposure, 179
Lateral projection, stereo, 52
Latitude, and Kv.P., 128–29, 139, 140
Law position, 318
  guide, 211
  radiation dosage, 253, 256
Lead, in cassettes, 18
Lead foil strips, in grid, 48
Lead-lined bins, 12
Leaking, at mixing valve, 41
Leg, exposure guide, 218, 221
  thickness, 208
Leprosy, penetrability, 161
Leukemia, penetrability, 161
Light leak, 12, 18
Light source, and distortion, 123
Light-tightness, of darkroom, 26
Line voltage, low, 37
Linear attentuation coefficient, 131–32
Linear grid, 51
Line-focus tube, 337
Liver, 308
  functions, 311
  procedure, 148

LogEtronic equipment, 8
Long-scale contrast, 116–18, 128–29, 139, 142
Low Kv.P. technique, 196–98, 201–2
  obsolete, 204
Lumbar area, 309
Lumbar spine, children, exposure guide, 221
  exposure guide, 176, 177, 215, 221;
  high Kv.P., 234–35, 237
  high Kv.P. technique for, 198–200, 234–35, 237
  magnification, 243
  measuring, 160
  radiation dosage, 254, 257–58
  radiograph, 13
  technique, 145, 170
  thickness, 208
Lung abcess, penetrability, 161
Lung cancer, procedure, 147
Lungs, high Kv.P. guide, 236
  procedure, 146
Lynch, technique, 197

Ma., *see* Milliamperage
Magnetism, defined, 324–25
Magnification, 243, 317
Mahoney, slide rule, 194
Malar bone, 307
Malignancy, penetrability, 161
Malleolus, 307
  procedure, 144
Malnutrition, allowance for, 210, 224
Mammography, with Xerox, 22
Mammography film, 4–6
Mandible, 307
  child, exposure guide, 221
  exposure guide, 175, 177, 212, 221, 253
  high Kv.P. guide, 238
  magnification, 243
  procedure, 147
  radiation dosage, 253
  radiograph, 168
  thickness, 208
Manubrium, 307
Marble bone, penetrability, 161
Ma.S. (milliamperes per second), 134–36
  and contrast, 116
  corrections in, 169
  and density, 85, 94, 135, 140; experiments, 68–69, 70–71
  and distance, 91–93, 99–100; table, 104
  and fog, experiment, 75
  grid vs. non-grid conversion, 58–59, 83
  effect of increasing, 107–11
  high, 84
  with impulses, table, 102
  and Kv.P., 75–76, 85–88, 126, 183

Index

Ma.S. (*cont.*)
  and low Kv.P., 126
  meter, 333
  rule of thumb in fixed Kv.P., 75–76
  in screen exposures, 75–76
  and time, tables, 103, 140
  and time and distance, 99–100
  values, computing, 94; and fractions, 62; for exposure guide, 222
  as variable, 81
Markers, lead, for radiographs, 15
Mask, for subtraction film, 7–8
Mastoid, cells, 308
  children, exposure guide, 220
  exposure guide, 175, 177, 211, 220; high Kv.P., 238
  lateral, 167
  magnification, 243
  procedure, 146
  radiation dosage, 256, 257
Mathematics, 62–65
Maxillae, 307
Maxillary, exposure guide, 178
Maxillary view, radiation dosage, 253, 257
Measuring, of patient, 159–60
Medial, defined, 311
Mediastinal mass, procedure, 147
Medichrome film, 8
Mentovertex view, exposure guide, 177, 220
  radiation dosage, 253, 256
Mesocephalic skull, 155–56
Metacarpal, identified, 308
Metastasis, allowance for, 210
  penetrability, 161
Meter, Ma., troubles with, 261–62
  'r', 342
  in x-ray machine, 327
Miliary tuberculosis, penetrability, 161
Milliamperage, 153–54; *see also* Ma.S.
  and focus-film distance, experiment, 67–68
  and time, 84, 98; table, 103
Milliampere, defined, 324
Milliampere seconds, 154–55; *see also* Ma.S.
  as factor in technique, 224
Mitral stenosis, procedure, 147
Moisture, and static, 15
Morgan-Hodges phototimer, 333
Motion, 244
  in exposure, 82, 156, 158
  exposure technique for, 192–94
  kinds, 158
  radiograph showing, 159
Mottle, 12–13, 40
Mowry, W. W., 190
Muscle, absorption of x-rays, 135
  and Kv.P., 131–32
Myeloma, multiple and solitary, penetrability, 161

Nasal bones, procedure, 147
Nasal sinuses, *see* Sinuses
Neck, procedure, 147
Necrosis, aseptic, penetrability, 161
  radiation, penetrability, 161
Negative photography, 3
Neuroblastoma, penetrability, 161
New bone, penetrability, 161
Ninety-second film processing, 31–34; *see also* Automatic processing
Nomograms, exposure, 181–82
Non-grid technique, 83
Non-screen exposure tables, 86
Non-screen film, 4, 120
Nose, exposure guide, 212, 238
Nuclear medicine, technology, 198

Objective-film distance, detail and distortion with, 121, 124
Occipital view, exposure guide, 177
Occipital protuberance, defined, 309
Occlusal, defined, 309
Occlusal film, 5
  transport of, 31, 33
Odontoid, magnification, 243
Olecranon process, 143
Opacification, for heart, table, 242
Optic foramen, 168
  magnification, 243
  procedure, 146
  radiograph, 42
Optic position, guide, 175, 177, 211, 220
  radiation dosage, 253, 257
Orbital fissure, procedure, 146
Organs, locating, 155
Os calcis, exposure guide, 217
  procedure, 144
  radiation dosage, 255, 259
  radiographs, 132
Oscilloscope, 153
Osteitis, penetrability, 161
Osteoma, penetrability, 161
Osteomyelitis, penetrability, 161
Osteoporosis, senile, penetrability, 161
Overexposure, 37, 125, 136
Overpenetration, 302

Paget's disease, correction for, 164
  penetrability, 161
Parietal bone, 309
Parotid glands, procedure, 147
Parrafin block, and secondary radiation fog, 112–13
Patella, 308
  fracture, procedure, 144
  high Kv.P. exposure guide, 237
Pathology, adjustment for, 224
  and penetrability, 161–62
  positions to show, 143–49
Patient, immobilizing, 158
  intractable, 318–19
  judging the, 155–56

FORMULATING X-RAY TECHNIQUES

Patient (cont.)
  positioning and measuring, 158–59; for therapy, 342
Pediatric radiography, 83
Pelvimetry, 148
  exposure guide, 216
Pelvis, 309
  children, exposure guide, 221; radiographs, 228–31
  exposure guide, 176–78, 214, 215
  fracture, procedure, 144
  high Kv.P. guide, 235–37
  and Kardex, 227
  procedure, 144
  radiation dosage, 254, 258
  radiographs, 127
  thickness, 208
Penetration of x-rays, 106, 139, 327, 337
  and Kv.P., 81, 106–9
Penumbra, and detail, 121, 244
Percentages, 63–64
Periapical film, 5
Peristalsis, and motion, 159
Petrosae, procedure, 146
Petrous bone, 307
  exposure guide, 175, 177, 220
pH, of fixer, 31
Phalanges, radiograph, 132
Phantoms, for testing, 15–16, 47
Pharynx, procedure, 147
Phosphors, 22–23
Photofluorography, 23
Photograph, long- and short-scale contrast, 142
Photographic effect, experiment, 80
  formula, 98–99
Photography, 3
Phototimer, 201, 204, 333
Physique, judging, 155
Pi-lines, on film, 35–36, 40
Placenta, exposure guide, 179, 197–98; high Kv.P., 235
  and Kardex, 227
  radiation dosage, 255, 259
Plaster cast, correction for, 104
  of knee, 105
  with screen, 218
  technique for, 174
Pleural effusion, penetrability, 161
Pneumoconiosis, penetrability, 161
Pneumonia, penetrability, 161
Pneumoperitoneum, penetrability, 161
Pneumothorax, penetrability, 161
Polaroid process, 3, 9–12
  nomograms for exposure of TLX film, 180–82
Port of entry, and detail, 121
Portable x-ray machine, and grids, 55
Positioning the patient, 159–60
Positions, routine, to show pathology, 143–49

Positive photograph, 3, 11
Pregnancy, 47
  exposure guide, high Kv.P., 235, 239
  procedure, 148
Primary radiation, 111
Prime factors of radiography, 203
Procedure, routine, 143–49
  special, 228–31
Processing, 26–41
  manual necessary, 174
Projection, how to standardize, 223
Proportion, mathematical, problems, 65, 92–93
Prostate, procedure, 148
Protractors, 155
Punchcards, in exposure technique, 201
Pus, allowance for, 210, 224

'r' units, and meter, 342
Radiation, dosage, 230–4; from soft x-rays, 44–45; and Kv.P., 129, 133, 140
  dose to skin, table, 252–55, 256–59
  primary vs. remnant, 300, 337
  protection from, 341
  recording quantity and quality, 342
  remnant, 3, 111–15, 135
  safe, 341
  secondary, see Secondary radiation
Radiation fibrosis, penetrability, 161
Radiation necrosis, penetrability, 161
Radiation sickness, 339, 343
Radiograph, 153, 244–45
  checklist for quality, 304–5
  experiment with skull, 244–48
  history of technique, 186–204
  producing a, 81–105
  test, 195
  trouble chart, 262
Radiography, 3, 134–42
  cassetteless, 22
  historical charts, 188–89
Radiolucent material, 18
Rapido transport, 22
Ratio and division, problems, 64–65
Rays, hard and soft, 327
  scattered, 341
Reciprocity law, and exposure, 92–93
Recirculation, defective, 39
Rectification of current, 328
Reed, technique, 194
Reeves, technique, 198
Regular film, for radiographs, 4, 136, 138
Renal pelves, 148
Replenishment, 30–31, 34, 38, 39
Respiration, motion effects, 158–59, 319
Rinehart, D., 190–91
  diaphragms, 191
Rhombic grid, 51, 54
Ribs, 311
  exposure guide, 175; high Kv.P., 239

Index

Ribs (*cont.*)
   fracture, simulated by fog, 27
   procedure, 144
Roll film, loading, 31–32
Rollins, 186
Routine views, procedure, 143–49

Sacroiliac articulation, 308
Sacroiliac joint, arthritis, procedure, 145
Safelight, 27–28, 292
Sagittal plane, 309
Samuel, 199
Sante, L. R., and technology, 191
Scaphoid, procedure, 143
Scapula, procedure, 144; guide, 175
Scar-bone, penetrability, 161
Schönander, technology, 201
Schwarz, technology, 194
Sclerosis, allowance for, 210, 224
   penetrability, 161
Scoliosis, procedure, 145
Scotch tape, 31–32
Screen(s), 155, 244
   books, multisection, 24
   compensation for, 174
   contact, 19
   and detail, 23, 25, 121, 302
   exposure with, 82, 85–86, 92–93; tables, 86, 223
   film, contrast, 120
   grid, exposure, 223
   high-speed, 23–25
   intensifying, 22–25, 290–91
   medium-speed, 23–24
   radiograph with, 138
   reciprocity law with, 93–94
   slow-speed, 24
   speed, 23–25
Secondary radiation, 111–15, 200–201
   and cone, 42
   fog, 78, 133–34, 141; and Ma.S., experiment, 75
   grid effect on, 54, 59, 76, 129
   trapping, 48
Seemann, 47, 129
Sella, procedure, 146
Sensitivity, of unexposed film, 28
Sensitometry, 249–51
Shadow formation, geometry of, 122–23
Shearer's formula, 188–89, 191
Shift of tube, in stereoradiography, 50
Short-scale contrast, 116–17, 123–29, 139, 141–42
Shoulder, children, exposure guide, 222
   exposure guide, 175, 177, 178, 211–12, 217, 222; high Kv.P., 236
   magnification, 243
   procedure, 144
   radiation dosage, 255, 259
   radiograph, 126
   thickness, 207

Sickness, radiation, 339
Siderosis, penetrability, 161
Sigmoid flexure, 308
Silicosis, penetrability, 161
Silver, in latent image, 17
   in Polaroid process, 11
   recovery, 29–30
Silver bromide, in film, 3–4
Sinuses, 311
   children, exposure guide, 220
   exposure guide, 175, 178, 212; high Kv.P., 238
   and Kardex, 227
   magnification, 243
   procedure, 146
   radiation dosage, 253, 257
   in stereo, 51–52
   thickness, 208
Skin, and contrast scale, 118
   effects of x-rays on, 135, 338
Skin lesion, therapy, 339
Skull, 155–58
   arterial system of, 146
   child's, exposure guide, 220–21; view, 168
   experiments in projection, 244–48
   exposure guide, 175, 177, 178, 211–12, 221, 223, 225; high Kv.P., 238
   formulating technique for, 210
   fracture, procedure, 145
   habitus types, 155
   high Kv.P. technique, 198–99
   and Kardex, 227
   lateral, making chart for, 166–70; views, 84, 86, 165, 167
   low Kv.P. technique, 198–99
   phantom, 16
   radiation dosage, 252–53, 256
   radiographs, 88, 96–97, 110–11, 136–37
   thickness of, 208
   tumor, procedure, 145, 146
Slauson, 129
Slide rule, circular, 193
Smudge static, 14–15
Sodium carbonate, in developer, 119–20
Sodium hydroxide, in developer, 120
Spasm, 158–59
Sphenoid, exposure guide, 175, 177, 211, 220
   projection, stereo, 52
   radiation dosage, 253, 257
Spine, 311
   exposure guide, 176, 177, 214–15
   and Kardex, 227
   pathology shown, 228–29, 231
   procedure, 144
   radiograph, 228
   tumor, procedure, 145
Spinning top, and timer, 21, 152, 337–38
Spleen, 148, 308

FORMULATING X-RAY TECHNIQUES

Splettstosser, 47, 129
Spot exposures, 318
Stains, on screens, 25
Static marks, 14–15, 294
Stenvers position, 168, 318
    exposure guide, 175, 177, 211, 220
    radiation dosage, 253, 257
Step wedge, for tests, 15–17
    in Kv.P. experiment, 141–42
Sternoclavicular articulation, procedure, 144
Sternum, close subject-tube technique, 180
    low-voltage technique, 196
    exposure guide, 177
    procedure, 144
Stereoradiography, 15, 49–52, 298
    of thorax, 50–51
    shift, and grids, 51
Stereoscopic tube shifts, 53
Sthenic habitus, 155–56
Stomach, 155
    exposure guide, 179; high Kv.P., 238
    procedure, 148
    radiation dosage, 255, 259
    rapid exposure for, 301
Stone, gallbladder, contrast for, 132
Streaks, on film, 39–40
Styloid, temporal, procedure, 146
Submaxillary gland, procedure, 147
Superior, defined, 311
Symphysis, of mandible, procedure, 147
Symphysis pubis, 309
Syphilis (gumma), penetrability, 161

Tanks, 292
Target, rotating, pitting of, 334
Technique, defined, 152; limitations, 194–95
Technique charts, limitations of, 209–10
Technologist, defined, 204
Techron, machine, 190
Teeth, 308
Temperature, and density, 33–34, 71–72
Temperature chart, as example for sensitivity curve, 249–50
Temporal bone, 307
Temporomandibular articulation, procedure, 147
Test radiographs, 195
Therapy, x-ray, 338–39, 341–44
Thickness, average ranges, 207, 222
    classification, 205
    compensation in Kv.P. for, 81, 82
    exposure for, 162
    measurement, 160
    rule for uneven thickness, 141
    tissue, and secondary radiation fog, 113–15
Thigh, thickness, 208
Thiosulfate, *see* Hypo

Thomas position, exposure guide, 211
    radiation dosage, 252, 258
Thoracic spine, children, exposure guide, 221
    exposure guide, 177, 215, 221; high Kv.P., 234
    lateral, technique for, 170
    magnification, 243
    procedure, 145
    radiograph, and anode heel effect, 61
    thickness, 208
Thoracoplasty, penetrability, 161
Thorax, 309
    measurement, 160
    stereoradiography of, 50–51
Thoreus filter, 339
Three-phase unit, checking, 21
Thumb, thickness, 207
Tibia, 308
    exposure guide, 217
    procedure, 144
    radiation dosage, 255, 259
Tibiofibular articulation, procedure, 144
Time, clearing, 32
    and density, 140
    of development, and density, experiment, 71–72
    and distance and Ma., 99–100
    as exposure factor, 81–82
    and Kv.P., 87–88; 15 percent rule, 89–90; tables, 88, 89
    and Ma., table, 103
    of treatment, 343–44
Timer, checking, 21, 337
Timing, with cassette, 18
Tissue, absorption, 160
    classification, 160–62
    measurement, for radiation dose table, 256–58
    thickness, classes of, 172
Toes, procedure, 143
    radiographs of, 130, 132
Tone, defined, 135
    value, 136–38
Towne position, 318
    exposure guide, 211, 234
Trachea, procedure, 146
Transformer, 325–26
    Coolidge, 333
    and Kv.P. adjustment, 82
Transport of film, 30–32
Tree static, 14, 29
Tremor, and motion, 158–59
Trochanter, identified, 308
Trouble chart, for film, 37
    for x-ray unit, 260–63
Trough filter, 46
Trout, 44–47, 129
Tube, alignment, 59, 61
    angling, 101
Tube-rating chart, 154

Index

Tuberculosis, penetrability, 161
Tuberosities, 307
Tumor, procedure, 145, 147

Underexposure, 37, 125–27, 136
Underpenetration, 302
Unit system of exposure, 194
Ureters, 309
Urethra, 309
   procedure, 148
Urinary tract, 309

Valve tube failure, 37
Van Dijk, 191
Variable factors for radiography, 81–82
Variable Kv.P. method, 153–85, 201–2
   chart, 166–77, 197–98
   children, conversion factors, 105
   rule of chart formulation, 179
Veins, in tibia-fibula, procedure, 144
Venograms, 25, 242
Ventilation, of darkroom, 27
Vertebrae, 311
   procedure for, 144, 145
   thickness, 208
Vertex position, exposure guide, 173
   radiation dosage, 234
Videx cone, 191
Viscera, view, 149–50
Volt, 324
Voltage, see Kv.P.
   for x-rays, 326
Voluntary motion, 158

Warren, 192
Washing, in processing, 32
   improper, 34, 38, 39
Wasson, W. W., 192–94
Water, in processing, 40–41
Water spots on film, 294

Waters-Waldron position, 317–18
   exposure guide, 175, 177
   stereo, 52
Watson, air-gap technique, 239
Wave length, 326–27, 343
   and contrast, 117–18
   and density, 141
   and penetration, 106, 139
Wedge filter, 46–47, 344
Wilsey, 46–47, 129
Wratten filter, 27–28
Wrist, exposure guide, 216, 221; high
   Kv.P., 236; with screen, 218
   procedure, 143
   thickness, 207
Wynroe, formula, 191

Xerox radiography, 22
X-Omat, 5–8
X-ray film, 4–5, 32; see also Film
X-ray machine, 327–28
   portable, with grids, 55
X-ray therapy, 338–39
X-ray tube, double focus, 334
   hot cathode, 335; and Kv.P., 140
   rotating target, 334
X-ray unit, trouble chart, 260–63
X-rays, 134–35
   effect on exposed film, 28
   geometric principles of, 123
   intensity, and distance, 90–91;
      measuring, 59–60
   penetrating power, 106–9
   properties, 326, 336–37
   soft, effects, 44–45
Xyphoid process, 309

Zinc sulfide, phosphor, 23
Zygoma, 307
Zygomatic arch, procedure, 147

JOHN B. CAHOON

Occasionally a man walks into and up through a profession to its top rung, imbued with a sincerity and dedication that spread out to engulf all with whom he comes in contact. Such a man, determined to learn and teach the fundamental truths of his field, touches the lives of countless thousands and can kindle the spark that elevates the standards and stature of his whole profession. Such a man was John Cahoon.

He knew that to teach technology one must first be a technologist. He knew that to be a technologist one must have a sound understanding of the basic fundamentals of technology. To these ends he directed his life's effort—lecturing, teaching, writing—serving technology wherever his knowledge and talents could be helpful to an individual or a multitude.

John Cahoon was an educator—a teacher, a leader. He knew that the teacher must never cease to learn, and wherever his travels took him he sought knowledge—bits of information he might carry with him and share. To him his writing was a basis for study and understanding for students, and a repository of information and a reference work for experienced technologists.

It is the good fortune of teachers and students that this edition of his text was completed before his untimely death. It is an extension of his lifetime of service in the education of those who now follow him.

He stood and spoke out for what he believed was right for technology. No one can ever replace him—in his profession, in the regard and affection of the thousands for whom he did so much, or in the hearts of his friends.

Clark Warren